Dianna A. Redburn, Ph. D.
Department of Neurobiology and Anatomy
The University of Texas Medical School
P. O. Box 20708
Houston, Texas 77025

Synapses and Synaptosomes

Synapses and Synaptosomes

Morphological Aspects

D. G. JONES, B.Sc., M.B., B.S.
Senior Lecturer in Anatomy
University of Western Australia

CHAPMAN AND HALL
London
A HALSTED PRESS BOOK
JOHN WILEY & SONS
New York

First published 1975
by Chapman and Hall Ltd
11 New Fetter Lane, London EC4P 4EE
© *1975 D. G. Jones*
Printed in Great Britain by

Cox & Wyman Ltd, London, Fakenham and Reading

Library of Congress Cataloging in Publication Data
Jones, David Gareth.
    Synapses and synaptosomes.

    1. Synapses. 2. Synaptosomes. I. Title.
[DNLM: 1. Neural transmission. 2. Synapses.
3. Synaptosomes. WL102 J71s]
QL931. J58 1975 599′.01′88 74–26646
ISBN 0–470–44942–X

Contents

Preface

The late 1950s saw the adaptation of subcellular fractionation procedures to the study of the brain, and in particular to the study of neurons and their synaptic connections. This in turn provided neurochemistry with a revolutionary tool which has increasingly dominated synaptic investigations in the subsequent years. The pioneering laboratories of V. P. Whittaker and E. De Robertis, in which these advances were made, have now been supplemented by many others where these techniques are used daily on a wide variety of synaptic and related problems.

It would be unwise however, to view these developments as of relevance to biochemists alone. The significance of the fractions obtained by these techniques was realized initially in terms of their morphology, a procedure which has reasserted itself with each new technical development and which, ideally, should accompany each set of investigations. Furthermore, the conclusions emanating from fractionation studies require assimilation within the growing body of neurotransmitter concepts resulting from anatomical and physiological investigations.

Nowhere have fractionation techniques proved of greater value than in the study of the synapse. The synaptosome has proved a device of amazing versatility and its potentialities have been brilliantly exploited by neurochemists. This 'synapse in isolation' is proving of immense benefit to studies directed towards isolating and identifying neurotransmitters and synaptic populations, as well as providing a starting-point for the isolation of synaptic membranes and junctional complexes. The benefit of these studies lies not only in their neurochemical possibilities, but also in the fact that the subcellular components provided by them constitute highly segregated particles suitable for morphological analysis.

My aim in this book is to examine these developments in synaptosomal technology through the eyes of a morphologist. While this does not imply that only morphological considerations are dealt with, it does suggest that the burgeoning synaptosomal literature is viewed in a context grounded on a knowledge of synaptic ultrastructure. With this basis I have set out to examine ways in which synaptosomes and also subsynaptosomal particles can be regarded as structurally-intact entities. I have analysed the success of isolation procedures using primarily morphological criteria, although relevant biochemical data have been used where necessary. In order to bring together morphological and biochemical approaches to synaptic problems I have emphasized the role of autoradiographic, cytochemical and immunofluorescent techniques, while a discussion of current concepts of neurotransmitter release mechanisms has been introduced to highlight the difficulties as well as possibilities of present experimental procedures.

My purpose in these pages has been to provide a review of synaptic and synaptosomal literature, which is as up-to-date as possible and which it is hoped will prove a useful guide for those embarking on synaptosomal investigations. It is also my hope that it will prove a useful source of reference for those already engaged in some aspect of synaptic or synaptosomal work and wishing to become better acquainted with related investigations. Inevitably a review of this nature reflects the personal interests of the reviewer, although my principal aim has been to place in perspective the contributions of the many diverse groups of neurochemists and neurocytologists involved in synaptic and synaptosomal studies. It is for this reason that I have made liberal use of the published results of a wide range of investigators.

My initial interest in synaptosomes was nurtured by Dr V. P. Whittaker in whose laboratory I worked for a short time in the mid-1960s. The morphological emphasis I place on their study was due in no small part to Professor E. G. Gray who, in his early work with Whittaker, was responsible for recognizing and defining criteria by which synaptosomes may be characterized. The period of my emerging interest in synapses and synaptosomes was spent in University College London, where the ideas and questions generated by Professor J. Z. Young gave me a lasting enthusiasm for the central nervous system. More recently my collaboration with Dr H. F. Bradford on synaptosomal investigations has sustained my interest in this approach to synaptic problems and helped develop my concern that more sophisticated morphological approaches to these problems be found.

As is always the case with books, this one would not have been possible without the assistance of a large number of people. In particular I would like to mention Dr A. R. Lieberman who convinced me I should embark on the project, Dr A. M. Adinolfi and Dr H. F. Bradford each of whom has read various chapters, and all those who have so readily given me permission to use their published micrographs, diagrams and results. I am also indebted for the use of unpublished results and for help in many ways to members of my research group, especially Mrs S. E. Dyson, Mrs M-C Holst and Mr T. M. Nolan. I am extremely grateful to Mrs T. Johnson who has so willingly and efficiently undertaken the bulk of the typing, and Mrs Z. Gobby who has expertly carried out the artistic and photographic work. Finally, I would like to thank my wife not only for her practical help but also for her encouragement without which the book would never have seen the light of day.

Department of Anatomy,   D. G. J.
University of Western Australia
June, 1974

Acknowledgements

Thanks are due to the authors and publishers of the following journals and books for permission to use micrographs, figures and tables. The appropriate reference is given in each caption.

Albers, R. W., Siegel, G. J., Katzman, R. and Agranoff, B. W. (eds.) *Basic Neurochemistry* (Little, Brown and Company)

Anatomical Record (Wistar Institute Press)

Annals of the New York Academy of Sciences

Archives of Biochemistry and Biophysics (Academic Press)

Barondes, S. H. (ed.), *Cellular Dynamics of the Neuron, I.S.C.B. Symposium*, Vol. 8 (Academic Press)

Biochimica et Biophysica Acta (Elsevier)

Bourne, G. H. (ed.) *The Structure and Function of Nervous Tissue*, Vols. 3 and 6 (Academic Press)

Brain Research (Elsevier)

Clementi, F. and Ceccarelli, B. (eds.), *Advances in Cytopharmacology*, Vol. 1 (Raven Press)

Experimental Brain Research (Springer-Verlag)

Experimental Neurology (Academic Press)

Journal of Biological Chemistry (American Society of Biological Chemists)

Journal of Cell Biology (The Rockefeller University Press)

Journal of Cell Science (Company of Biologists)

Journal of Comparative Neurology (Wistar Institute Press)

Journal of Neurobiology (John Wiley)

Journal of Neurochemistry (Pergamon Press)

Journal of Neurocytology (Chapman and Hall)

Journal of Ultrastructure Research (Academic Press)

Marks, N. and Rodnight, R. (eds.) *Research Methods in Neurochemistry*, Vol. 1 (Plenum Press)

Nature (MacMillan)

Paoletti, R. and Davison, A. N. (eds.), *Chemistry and Brain Development* (Plenum Press)

Progress in Brain Research (Elsevier)

Science (American Association for the Advancement of Science)

Zambotti, V., Tettamanti, G. and Arrigoni, M. (eds.) *Glycolipids, Glycoproteins, and Mucopolysaccharides of the Nervous System* (Plenum Publishing Corporation)

Zeitschrift für Zellforschung und Mikroskopische Anatomie (Springer-Verlag)

Abbreviations and Glossary

ACh	acetylcholine	5-HT	5-hydroxytryptamine (serotonin)
AChE	acetylcholinesterase	LDH	lactate dehydrogenase
ATP	adenosine triphosphate	miniature	
BIUL	bismuth iodide-uranyl-lead	e.p.p.	miniature end-plate potential
ChAc	choline acetyltransferase	NANA	N-acetylneuraminic acid
ChE	cholinesterase	NE	norepinephrine (noradrenaline)
CNS	central nervous system	nm	nanometre (1 nm = 10Å =
con A	concanavalin A		10^{-9}m)
CsCl	caesium chloride	OsO_4	osmium tetroxide
cyclic AMP	cyclic adenosine monophosphate	P_1	nuclear fraction
DCV	dense-cored vesicle	P_2	mitochondrial fraction
DEAE	diethylaminoethyl	P_3	microsomal fraction
EGTA	ethylene glycol bis(2-aminoethyl ether) tetraacetic acid	PDE	cyclic 3′,5′-nucleotide phospho-diesterase
EM	electron microscope (-ical; -graph)	PTA	phosphotungstic acid
		SDH	succinate dehydrogenase
GABA	γ-aminobutyric acid	TPPase	thiamine pyrophosphatase
GAD	glutamic acid decarboxylase	μm	micron (1μm = 10^{-6}m)
HC-3	hemicholinium-3	ZIO	zinc iodide–osmium tetroxide

To
Beryl, Kathryn and Martyn

Chapter 1: Synapses

1.1 HISTORICAL CONCEPTS AND THE DEVELOPMENT OF MODERN IDEAS

1.1.1 The neuron

As soon as an understanding of the morphology of the nerve cell body and its processes had been gained another problem arose, that of the relationship between nerve cells. In answer to the question: 'How do nerve cells make contact with their neighbours?', neurohistologists gave two diametrically opposite solutions. On the one hand there were those, headed by His (1887), Forel (1887) and Ramón y Cajal (1888), who regarded the nerve cells and their processes as individual units. This developed into the *neuron theory* (Waldeyer, 1891). On the other side were the proponents of the nerve net or *reticular theory*, championed by Gerlach (1872) and Golgi (1883), and holding that the nerve cells and their fibres were not independent units but constituted instead an integral part of a continuous network.

Gerlach's ideas (1872) on a nerve net arose from his histological work employing carmine and gold stains and emphasized the role of the dendrites in this plexus. The advent of Golgi's silver staining method in 1873 placed neurohistology on a new footing by providing it with vastly superior preparations. For his part Golgi became an ardent supporter of the nerve net concept although he proposed an axonic as opposed to a dendritic network.

The reticular theory was first challenged in a serious way by His (1887) and Forel 1887), His demonstrating that nerve cells and their fibres grow as a unit and Forel that they also degenerate as a unit (Clarke and O'Malley, 1968). By far the most powerful exponent of the neuron theory however, was Cajal, working independently and producing a spate of papers over the period 1888 to 1933. It was he, above all others, who established that the functional connections between nerve cells are effected by close contacts and not by continuity in a syncytial network (Phillis, 1970).

In the 1930s and 1940s the neuron theory received strong support from degeneration studies. Amongst other things these showed that, following section of a presynaptic pathway, there was degeneration of the synaptic knobs but not of postsynaptic structures (see Bodian, 1942).

1.1.2 The synapse and neurochemical transmission

Mention of synaptic knobs presupposes the concept of the *synapse*, a term introduced by Sherrington in 1897 in an attempt to explain the characteristic features of the reflex arc. While Sherrington's use of the term had a firm grounding in morphology he used it in a functional sense, restricting it to those areas of close contact that were specialized for effective transmission from one neuron to another.

Having determined that neurons are separate entities, it remained to be decided how transmission occurs across synaptic junctions. In the 1870s Du Bois-Reymond suggested this may be either chemical or electrical in nature, but it was left to Elliott (1904) and later Dixon (1906) to suggest that a chemical transmitter might be released at the nerve endings, sympathetic nerve impulses liberating adrenaline and parasympathetic impulses a muscarine-like substance.

Dale in 1914, while working on ergot, discovered a substance which turned out to be acetylcholine (ACh). He speculated that it may have physiological significance because its effect resembled actions resulting from parasympathetic stimulation. At this stage there was no evidence for the liberation of either ACh or adrenaline at the nerve endings, a gap which was partially filled by Loewi (1921) when he demonstrated the release of ACh during stimulation of the vagus nerve with subsequent inhibition of the heart. The sympathetic side of the story was provided ten years later by Cannon and Bacq (1931).

Further work by Dale, Gaddum, Feldberg and others (Feldberg and Gaddum, 1934; Feldberg and Vartianen, 1934; Dale, Feldberg and Vogt, 1936; Brown, Dale and Feldberg, 1936) led to the extension of the chemical transmitter hypothesis to sympathetic ganglia and neuromuscular junctions with ACh as the transmitter. In 1935 Dale proposed that the chemical transmitter hypothesis also be applied to synapses of the central nervous system (CNS), an event of great moment for subsequent neurochemical and neuroanatomical studies.

In spite of this impressive evidence favouring chemical transmission, hypotheses advocating electrical synaptic transmission remained. There were two principal reasons for this: (a) the observed differences in latency periods in sympathetic ganglion and neuromuscular junctions on the one hand and in postganglionic junctions on the other, and (b) because it was envisaged that the primary transmitter in the CNS was ACh.

The controversy between the two forms of neurotransmission continued unabated until the early 1950's when the advent of intracellular recording techniques ousted electrical transmission as it had been generally envisaged. The anachronism is however, that just a few years after the conclusion of this debate Furshpan and Potter (1957, 1959) described a type of synapse in crustacea involving electrical transmission. Since then numerous examples of electrical transmission have come to light (e.g. Washizu 1960; Hagiwara and Morita, 1962; Bennett, Aljure, Nakajima and Pappas, 1963; Furukawa and Furshpan, 1963), although not in mammalian CNS. They are characterized morphologically by the close apposition of the adjacent membranes of the nerve terminals while they lack the distinctive features of chemically transmitting synapses, notably the synaptic vesicles (Robertson, Bodenheimer and Stage, 1963; Pappas, 1966; Pappas and Bennett, 1966; Bennett, Pappas, Giménez and Nakajima, 1967; Meszler, Pappas and Bennett, 1972). The apposed membranes at an *electrotonic synapse* (the term given to an electrical synapse) are separated by a 2–3 nm gap, which appears to comprise a network of channels continuous with the extracellular space (Pappas, Asada and Bennett, 1971).

1.1.3 The quantal nature of neurochemical transmission

In order to pursue further the development of ideas regarding the chemical nature of neurotransmission, reference must now be made to the early electron microscope (EM) studies on the morphology of the synaptic region. These, dating from 1953, provided the morphological basis for the concepts originating from the physiologists, and together opened the way for the subsequent development of neurochemical ideas and techniques.

The first descriptions of synaptic ultrastructure were made by Sjöstrand (1953), Palade (1954), Palay (1954), De Robertis and Bennett (1954, 1955) and Palay (1956). The essential features of the synaptic region to emerge from these studies were: (a) pre- and post-synaptic neuronal elements each invested by a membrane 7–10 nm thick, and separated from each other at the synaptic junction by a cleft, 10–20 nm across, (b) a granular or vesicular component, each 20–65 nm in diameter, within the cytoplasm of the presynaptic terminal and often closely related to the presynaptic membrane, (c) one or more mitochondria within the presynaptic terminal, and (d) localized regions of thickening and increased density of the apposed membranes.

Of these features the ones of most immediate interest were the presence of vesicles in the presynaptic terminal and the dimensions of the cleft separating the pre- and post-synaptic membranes at the junctional region. Sjöstrand (1953) described granules in the synaptic knobs of guinea-pig retina, Palade (1954) and Palay (1954, 1956) noted the presence of vesicles in the mammalian CNS, while Palade (1954) and Robertson (1956) described them in neuromuscular junctions. The term 'synaptic vesicle' however, was coined by De Robertis and Bennett (1955) studying frog sympathetic ganglia and earthworm nerve cord neuropil. The latter workers also concluded that the vesicles were located predominantly on one side of the synaptic junction, thereby polarizing the synapse.

The implication of synaptic vesicles in the transport of a chemical transmitter, such as ACh, to the presynaptic membrane was made by De Robertis and Bennett (1955), and also by Del Castillo and Katz (1955, 1956), Palay (1956) and Fernandez-Morán (1957). Working independently they were struck by the manner in which the newly-described synaptic vesicles possessed the appropriate size range and occupied the appropriate position expected of the *quantal units* of transmitter postulated a short time previously by Katz and co-workers (Fatt and Katz, 1952). This concept of the quantal release of transmitter stemmed from the recognition by Fatt and Katz (1950, 1952) at neuromuscular junctions of miniature end-plate potentials (miniature e.p.p.'s) that is, the existence of minute, transient fluctuations in voltage. Subsequently the same phenomenon was observed at central synapses in spinal motoneurons (Katz and Miledi, 1963).

Miniature e.p.p.'s exhibit a regular size and time course and from this it was concluded that they arise not from the leakage of single ACh molecules, but from a synchronous action of a quantum of ACh, the quantum containing thousands of molecules of the transmitter. Furthermore it was argued, the quantum must be highly concentrated and delivered at a very short distance from the postsynaptic receptors (Katz, 1966). These concepts form the basis of *quantal spontaneous release*, according to which concentrated multimolecular packets of ACh are secreted at random moments, in an all-or-none fashion, from discrete points of the terminal axon membrane (Katz, 1966).

Over the years 1952–1955 it was recognized that these quantal units were of a sub-cellular nature and probably corresponded therefore to a subcellular particle; hence the significance and timeliness of the descriptions of synaptic vesicles, and of the 20–40 nm wide synaptic cleft. For reviews on the quantal nature of synaptic transmission the ones by Martin (1966), Hubbard (1970), Katz (1971) and Kuno (1971) should be consulted. The present status of this concept as it relates to the vesicle hypothesis is considered in some detail in Chapter 5.

1.2 CHEMICAL SYNAPSES – AN OUTLINE

The following description of CNS synapses will be confined to cholinergic terminals, and will look principally at those found in areas such as the cerebral and cerebellar cortices. These limitations have been imposed because fractionation studies of brain have dealt largely with this particular type of synapse in these particular regions. Reference to other regions is only made when these throw light on our knowledge of synaptic ultrastructure in general terms. The emphasis in this description is also on *normal* synaptic appearances as opposed to degenerating ones, principally because degeneration studies have played little part as yet in synaptosomal investigations.

A number of reviews covering fields omitted from the present description as well as those considered here may be consulted. These include reviews concerning general synaptic organization in the CNS (De Robertis, 1964; Gray, 1964, 1966; Peters, Palay and Webster, 1970; Sotelo, 1971a), normal and degenerating synaptic morphology (Gray and Guillery, 1966), the morphological characteristics of excitatory and inhibitory synapses (Gray, 1969a), electrotonic junctions (Pappas, 1966; Bennett 1972), and synaptic vesicles in sympathetic neurons (Geffen and Livett, 1971), as well as a general assessment of the organization and connections of the cerebellum (Eccles, Ito and Szentagothai, 1967). In addition useful reviews on CNS white matter (Bunge, 1968) and peripheral nerve (Gray, 1970a; Morris, Hudson and Weddell, 1972 a–d) provide a background to some developing points in fractionation studies.

Early EM studies of the synaptic junction demonstrated the presence of three constituent elements, that is, pre- and postsynaptic terminals with an intervening gap or cleft region which is the extracellular space separating the two junctional membranes (Sjöstrand, 1953; Palade, 1954; Palay, 1954; De Robertis and Bennett, 1955). It remained for Gray (1959a, 1963) however, to define more precisely the nature of the densities along the junctional membranes, the *paramembranous densities* of current terminology (Jones and Revell, 1970b). According to Gray the synaptic region demonstrates a number of fundamental constituents in addition to the synaptic vesicles and mitochondria previously described. These are the regularly arranged *dense projections* projecting from the synaptic junctional membrane into the presynaptic cytoplasm (Gray, 1963), plus the thickenings found at the apposed pre- and post-synaptic membranes (Gray, 1959a; Fig. 1.1a). The synaptic junction with its paramembranous densities is co-extensive with the

4

active zone (Couteaux, 1961), that region where neurotransmission actually takes place from one neuron to another.

1.2.1 Two synaptic populations

In fact these thickenings of the synaptic membranes formed the basis of Gray's subdivision of cerebral cortical synaptic junctions into types 1 and 2 (Gray, 1959a), the principal distinction between the two types lying in the length and separation of the paramembranous thickenings, the depth of the postsynaptic thickening compared with the presynaptic and the clarity of the cleft material (Fig. 1.1a). Later, Gray (1961) extended this classification to the synapses of the cerebellar cortex. In these situations he concluded that type 1 synapses occur on dendritic trunks and spines* (axodendritic) and type 2 on neuronal perikarya (axosomatic) and a proportion of dendritic trunks. Useful as this distinction is, it does not have universal validity as Gray and Guillery (1966) later conceded. It appears to hold best in cortical situations as opposed to non-cortical, while intermediate forms are present in the brain stem and spinal cord.

It is also limited as a concept by the techniques on which it is based. Gray (1959a) employed osmium tetroxide (OsO_4) fixation and block staining in an ethanolic solution of phosphotungstic acid (PTA)† a technique rarely if ever used in synaptic investigations nowadays. More applicable today therefore is the classification of Colonnier (1968) who recognized two types of synaptic membrane differentiation in formalin-fixed cerebral cortex. These he termed *asymmetrical* and *symmetrical*, depending respectively upon the presence or absence of a thick cytoplasmic postsynaptic opacity bordering the postsynaptic membrane (Plate 1.1). While Colonnier regarded his synaptic types as corresponding to Gray's types 1 and 2 some of the distinguishing criteria used by Gray, notably the comparative width of the cleft, do not apply (Fig. 1.1). Furthermore there is not an exact parallel between the distribution of the synaptic types in the two classifications.

In order to determine whether the asymmetrical and symmetrical junctions represent distinct synaptic types or simply the two extremes of a single continuum Colonnier (1968) analysed a random series of 100 'normally' sectioned synapses. Study of these profiles revealed that the great majority of synaptic junctions can be classified as asymmetrical or symmetrical with very few junctions (three according to Colonnier's estimation) displaying a transitional appearance. With respect to the single criterion of the presence or absence of a postsynaptic opacity therefore, Colonnier concluded that synapses can be divided into two distinct populations.

The subdivision of synapses in this way has been criticized from a number of angles. The validity of Gray's classification has been questioned because of its non-reproducibility

---

* Dentritic spines are present on the distal sections of dendrites and are up to 3 μm in length (Ramón y Cajal, 1911; Sholl, 1956; Fox and Barnard, 1957). They are sites of synaptic contact, in that presynaptic processes with type 1 contacts occur at the distal ends of spines (Gray, 1959a, b).

† Throughout the synaptic literature phosphotungstic acid staining is taken to signify an ethanolic solution, with the result that it is sometimes referred to as E–PTA (Bloom and Aghajanian, 1968). The designation used in these pages however, is PTA, the ethanolic (E–) aspect being taken as read. Whenever it is used in an aqueous solution this is always stated (Pease, 1966; Meyer, 1969).

in other regions of the CNS (Karlsson, 1966), or simply because the profiles appear to represent the extremes of a continuum (Van der Loos, 1965). Colonnier's terminology is open to criticism on the grounds that the concept of the polarization of the synapse implies asymmetrical morphology in all cases (Sotelo, 1971a), and it must be admitted Colonnier's terms are far from ideal.

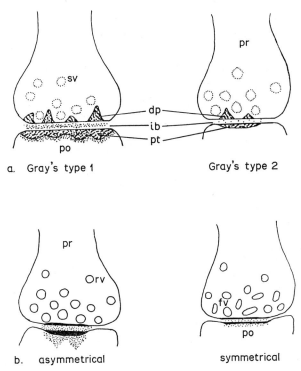

Figure 1.1   A schematic diagram to illustrate (a) Gray's types 1 and 2 synapses, prepared using the OsO$_4$–PTA method, and (b) Colonnier's asymmetrical and symmetrical synapses in aldehyde material postfixed in OsO$_4$ and stained with uranyl and lead salts. Dense projections (dp), an intermediate band (ib) within the cleft and a postsynaptic thickening (pt) are evident in (a), although the synaptic vesicles (sv) are not as clearly defined as in (b). Round vesicles (rv) occur almost exclusively in the asymmetrical synapse in (b), while flattened vesicles (fv) are also present in the symmetrical synapse. po, postsynaptic terminal; pr, presynaptic terminal.

While there are elements of truth in these statements Colonnier appears to have demonstrated fairly convincingly the reality of two populations.* It is unfortunate he chose to do this on qualitative rather than quantitative grounds, while his classification based as it is on a single criterion leaves a great deal to be desired. More recent preparative methods using non-osmicated tissue and block-staining with either PTA or a bismuth iodide complex (BIUL) have added significantly to our knowledge of the paramembranous densities and strengthen the case for distinct synaptic populations (Section 1.3.1).

* While this conclusion is clearly stated by Colonnier in his 1968 paper, he has been quoted by Peters *et al.* (1970) and Sotelo (1971a) as coming to the diametrically opposite conclusion, namely that the profiles represent a continuum. Perhaps this confusion results in part from the intensely subjective method of assessment used by Colonnier.

1.2.2 Synaptic vesicles

Of the organelles described in the presynaptic terminal, only the synaptic vesicles will be described here. The mitochondria, smooth-surfaced endoplasmic reticulum, neurofilaments (in certain situations), glycogen granules and synaptic ribbon (in the vertebrate retina, cochlea and pineal gland) will not be discussed.

Synaptic vesicles in vertebrates can be subdivided into *agranular* and *dense-cored varieties*, while the interesting *coated* (or complex) *vesicles* are best considered in conunction with the agranular vesicles.

By far the most commonly encountered type of vesicle is the agranular synaptic vesicle, referred to simply as synaptic vesicle in all succeeding discussion. In general these vesicles are spherical and are of the order of 40–50 nm in diameter, with a limiting unit membrane 6–10 nm across and a clear central zone. They are distributed throughout the presynaptic terminal (Plates 1.2 and 1.3). In some instances they line up along the presynaptic membrane and there may appear to be contact between some vesicles and the membrane itself. Little attention however, has been given to the detailed relationship between vesicles and the presynaptic membrane and much further work in this area is required before functional conclusions can be drawn (see Jones and Brearley, 1972a). Early reports purporting to demonstrate the passage of vesicles through the presynaptic membrane (De Robertis and Bennett, 1955) can be discounted as artefacts of sectioning. The exo- or endocytosis of vesicles from or into the presynaptic membrane (Andrès, 1964; Westrum, 1965) is occasionally observed, but cannot by itself be taken as conveying definite functional implications (Section 5.4.2).

The advent of aldehydes as primary fixatives heralded the appearance of a previously unrecognized variety of synaptic vesicle. This was the flattened or ellipsoidal-shaped vesicle which was initially described in a number of situations, including rat hypothalamus (Pellegrino de Iraldi, Duggan and De Robertis, 1963), cat cerebellum (Uchizono, 1965), cat spinal cord (Walberg, 1965), rat olfactory cortex and superior colliculus (Lund and Westrum, 1966) and goldfish brain (Robertson *et al.*, 1963). Further studies on the spinal cord of fishes (Gray, 1969b) and mammals (Bodian, 1966b; Ralston, 1968), and on mammalian cerebellum (Hirata, 1966; Larramendi and Victor, 1967; Larramendi, Fickenscher and Lemkey-Johnston, 1967; Uchizono, 1968) have confirmed the existence of the two varieties of vesicles, *round* and *flattened* (Plate 1.1; Fig. 1.1b). The distinction is not as clear-cut in invertebrates, although flattened vesicles have been noted in a number of situations including the crustacean stretch receptor (Uchizono, 1967) and *Octopus* supraoesophageal lobes (Jones, 1967; Gray,1970b).

The significance of the two vesicular types was first suggested by Uchizono (1965) who postulated that synapses containing rounded vesicles have an excitatory function whereas those with flattened vesicles* are inhibitory in nature. This conclusion, derived as it was from a correlation of morphological and neurophysiological findings in the molecular layer of the mammalian cerebellum, was a major advance in neuroanatomical

---

* Synapses containing flattened vesicles are sometimes referred to as *pleomorphic* because they contain a mixture of vesicle types and not the predominantly one type encountered in synapses with rounded vesicles.

investigations and has received increasing support as a general principle (see Gray 1969a, b).

A number of detailed points however, remain to be clarified. The use of the terms 'round' and 'flattened', or their equivalents, denotes a qualitative and hence partly subjective appraisal. This creates problems when endings containing vesicles of intermediate appearance are encountered, a relatively frequent occurrence in some situations. In an attempt to overcome this disadvantage Larramendi *et al.* (1967) carried out a statistical analysis of the synaptic vesicle populations in mouse cerebellum and concluded that the basic morphological difference between excitatory and inhibitory populations may be size rather than shape. They found that the synaptic vesicles within inhibitory terminals were significantly smaller and more elongated than those in excitatory terminals. Additionally, they noted a consistent decrease in size and increase in elongation of vesicles with ageing of animals. Lenn and Reese (1966) had previously noted a size difference between the vesicles in presumed excitatory and inhibitory endings in the ventral cochlear nucleus.

There is also a suggestion that vesicles may elongate during degeneration (Ralston, 1965; Walberg, 1966; Mugnaini and Walberg, 1967; Jones and Powell, 1970; Anderson and Westrum, 1972) because flattened vesicles may be observed apposed to asymmetrical contacts (as opposed to symmetrical—see Section 1.2.3) about 24 hours after the commencement of degeneration. Enlargement of vesicles is another phenomenon which may indicate early degeneration (Cuénod, Sandri and Akert, 1970; Akert, Cuénod and Moor, 1971; Mizuno and Nakamura, 1974) and although unreported by most workers is claimed to be independent of the method of fixation (Akert *et al.*, 1971).

These degenerative phenomena highlight the lability of synaptic vesicle morphology, a principle clearly demonstrated by the effect on morphology of changes in buffer osmolarity (Bodian, 1970; Valdivia, 1971). Bodian (1970) demonstrated the dramatic effect of the storage of aldehyde-perfused nervous tissue in cacodylate buffer containing sucrose prior to hardening in OsO_4. One type of vesicle was severely flattened by this procedure, a phenomenon which led Bodian to postulate the existence of a third type of vesicle in addition to the rounded and flattened varieties. This third type was characteristic of all cholinergic peripheral axon endings examined and also of large axosomatic synaptic bulbs of the spinal cord. When the buffer wash was omitted this type appeared as irregular, round vesicles. It is possible however, to interpret these findings as the result of exposing material to a buffer of low osmolarity as Valdivia (1971) has suggested. Valdivia (1971) himself, using rat cerebellum, again described three vesicle types – small round, large round and flattened (cf. entopeduncular nucleus; Adinolfi, 1969) – but observed that the proportion present in any axon depended upon the osmotic effect of the buffer (Plate 1.3). As the osmolarity of the buffer was increased the number of flattened vesicles increased.

It is clear therefore, that great care must be exercised in relating the structure of synaptic terminals to their presumed function solely in terms of the shapes of their constituent vesicles. Comparisons can only be made between different brain regions or cell types if *identical* fixation conditions have been employed, particular emphasis being placed on the osmolarity of the buffers and length of fixation, including exposure to buffer rinses. Even when these conditions have been observed however, and two or three vesicle types have been identified in a particular situation, the number of types may not have been exhausted. Synaptic vesicles of apparently similar morphology may display varying sedimentation properties (Jones, 1970c) and may therefore be structurally and perhaps functionally different.

The use of electron stereoscopy (Gray and Willis, 1968), although still in its infancy, has some bearing on vesicle classification as demonstrated by Dennison (1971). Working with aldehyde-perfused goldfish spinal cord and rat olfactory bulb, she distinguished two types of flattened vesicle in addition to a round or spherical type. The flattened vesicles may be 'cylindrical' or 'disc-shaped', the cylindrical variety being described only in the goldfish spinal cord. While direct correlations cannot be made at present between observations in different classes of vertebrate and brain regions, there is increasing evidence for the existence of more than one type of flattened vesicle (Bodian, 1970; Price and Powell, 1970; Dennison, 1971), and possibly therefore for a number of types of synaptic terminal (Bodian, 1970). This trend is in parallel with the recognition of an increasing number of transmitters at CNS synapses, and points to the possibility of recognizing a range of specific transmitters using morphological criteria. More information however, is required about the cytochemical characteristics of vesicles, the paramembranous densities at synaptic junctions (Sections 1.3.1, 4.4) and the sedimentation properties of synaptosomes and synaptic vesicles (Section 2.2).

In spite of the wealth of data accumulating about the appearance of aldehyde-fixed synaptic vesicles, the *rationale* for this effect remains somewhat elusive. Only rarely do vesicles flatten apart from initial fixation with aldehyde (Fukami, 1969). Valdivia's (1971) evidence concerning the osmotic effect of the buffer on a proportion of flattened or potentially flattenable vesicles strongly implicates the role of tonicity changes in altering the molecular architecture of the wall of these vesicles. As excitatory transmitters appear to be associated with rounded vesicles and inhibitory transmitters with flattened ones (Uchizono, 1965), the inhibitory transmitter or transmitters may be responsible for exposing the vesicular membrane to this tonicity effect. Alternatively, as Gray (1969a) has suggested, the aldehyde might be reacting with cytoplasmic factors which in turn influence the shape of the vesicle. Along similar lines is the suggestion that the presynaptic network (or grid), which is thought to have a close association with the dense projections, is rearranged and modifies the vesicles it encloses (Section 1.3.1). The role of cytoplasmic or network factors is an attractive one in view of the relative resistance of isolated synaptic vesicles to changes in osmotic pressure (Whittaker, Michaelson and Kirkland, 1964), and of the suggestion that they only become osmotically sensitive when removed from the protection of synaptosomes and hence of their enveloping cytoplasm (Marchbanks, 1968a; Jones, 1970c).

1.2.3 Correlating vesicular and synaptic types

Comparison of the results of electrophysiological and EM studies on the Purkinje cell (Gray, 1961; Andersen, Eccles and Voorhoeve, 1963b) and the pyramidal cell (Andersen,

Eccles and Loyning, 1963a; Blackstad and Flood, 1963; Hamlyn, 1963) of the cerebellum and hippocampus respectively, led to the suggestion that Gray type 1 synapses may be excitatory and Gray type 2 synapses inhibitory (Andersen *et al.*, 1963b; Eccles, 1964). If this generalization is accepted and if, as Colonnier (1968) has proposed, asymmetrical synapses in aldehyde-fixed tissues correspond to Gray type 1 synapses and symmetrical to Gray type 2, it follows that asymmetrical synapses are excitatory and symmetrical synapses inhibitory. This conclusion concurs with the complementary evidence also obtained from aldehyde-fixed material that round vesicles (excitatory) are associated with asymmetrical junctions and flattened vesicles (inhibitory) with symmetrical ones (Colonnier, 1968). This relationship worked out by Colonnier in the cerebral cortex had previously been demonstrated in equivalent terms by Uchizono (1965) in the cerebellar cortex and Lund and Westrum (1966) in the olfactory cortex and superior colliculus.

However, as Gray (1969a) has remarked, the analysis of this problem is still in its infancy. While the broad generalization outlined above is a useful guide for analysing synaptic contacts and viewing them in physiological terms there are a number of difficulties. Much of the work into this problem has centred on the cerebellum and in particular on the type of contacts made by the climbing fibres. This is not the place to go into detailed considerations of the relevant arguments, except to say that they revolve around the correct identification of climbing fibres (Gobel, 1968) and whether they make type 1 (Larramendi and Victor, 1967; Uchizono, 1967; Sotelo, 1969, 1971a) or type 2 (Palay, 1967) contacts.

A second difficulty stems from the intermediate appearance, or at best the lack of readily recognizable stereotyped features, of many junctions (Sotelo, 1971a). While a valid difficulty, this should not be used as an argument against attempts at relating morphological and functional patterns.

A third reason advanced for questioning the simple suggested relationship between morphology and physiology refers to axon terminals with synaptic junctions of both types (Palay, 1967; Mugnaini, 1970; Sotelo, 1971a). On the assumption that (a) different transmitters are related to the different synaptic junctions, and (b) different transmitters cannot be present in any one terminal at the same time, it may be concluded that the morphology of the junctions is not directly and intimately related to their function. It is as well to bear in mind however, that two assumptions have been made in reaching this conclusion, and that either or both may be incorrect. In particular, limitation of the number of transmitters per terminal to one has been challenged by a number of workers (Kerkut, Sedden and Walker, 1967; Martin, Barlow and Miralto, 1969).

As discussed in the previous section (1.2.2) the subdivision of vesicles into only two types is probably an oversimplification, as is the subdivision of synaptic junctions into only two categories. Until further progress is made in clarifying the additional classes of synapse in terms of vesicle and junctional criteria, little progress will be made in correlating the range of synaptic types on morphological and physiological grounds.

10

1.2.4 Dense-cored vesicles

As the emphasis in this chapter is on cholinergic systems rather than adrenergic, by far the greater part of the text is devoted to the agranular synaptic vesicles. These are the most commonly encountered vesicles in the nerve terminals studied in the CNS, although dense-cored vesicles (DCV; granular) are frequently seen in small numbers. For this reason reference is made to them at this juncture.

DCV are generally subdivided into *small* (40–60 nm in diameter) and *large* (80–100 nm across) vesicles of which the small vesicles are almost definitely the storage sites of norepinephrine (NE) in the peripheral nervous system (e.g. Wolfe, Potter, Richardson and Axelrod. 1962; Potter and Axelrod, 1963a, b; Iversen, 1967; Hökfelt, 1968; Tranzer, Thoenen, Snipes and Richards, 1969). There is also strong evidence implicating the small vesicles in monoamine storage in the brain (Hökfelt, 1967a, 1968). The large DCV may also contain NE although the evidence is not as clear-cut. Not only are they found in many NE nerve terminals, but those in adrenergic nerves may be relatively resistant to depletion by reserpine (Bloom and Barrnett, 1966; Bondareff and Gordon, 1966; Clementi, Mantegazza and Botturi, 1966a; Hökfelt, 1966). On the other hand presumed adrenergic nerves in some lower animals contain only large DCV (Burnstock, 1970). In certain regions of the CNS (e.g. striatum, hypothalamus) the dense core is visualized only with permanganate fixation.

The view that DCV contain NE and agranular vesicles ACh presents no major problem until consideration is given to those synapses containing both varieties. Most thought has been given to the *adrenergic* synapses in which this occurs. The problem can be overcome in one of two ways – either the agranular vesicles represent DCV which have discharged their contents (Pellegrino de Iraldi and De Robertis, 1963; Bloom and Barrnett, 1966; Bondareff and Gordon, 1966; Hökfelt, 1967b) or they actually contain ACh as suggested by Burn and Rand (1959, 1965). The experimental depletion of monoamine stores converts dense-cored into agranular vesicles (e.g. Pellegrino de Iraldi and De Robertis, 1963), while because the amount of osmiophilic material in vesicles depends on both the method of fixation and level of NE stores, mixed vesicle populations may represent varying levels of NE content (Tranzer and Thoenen, 1967). There is no experimental support for the Burn-Rand hypothesis (see Hubbard, 1970), while it has been strongly refuted by Tranzer *et al.* (1969) who concluded that all the vesicles of adrenergic nerve endings have the potential of taking up and storing NE. Indeed the presence of empty vesicles in these endings appears to be the result of poor preservation of the NE during fixation (Richardson, 1966; Tranzer and Thoenen, 1967; Tranzer *et al.*, 1969). With adequate fixation virtually all the vesicles of adrenergic nerve endings have an electron-dense core (Tranzer and Snipes, 1968).

The presence of occasional DCV alongside the agranular vesicles of cholinergic synaptic terminals is more difficult to explain. This is a widespread phenomenon in the CNS although practically no attention has been paid to its possible significance. One speculation, arising from the study of non-osmicated material (Section 1.3.1), is that the DCV may be involved in the transport and deposition of dense material at the presynaptic membrane (Pfenninger, Sandri, Akert and Eugster, 1969). This idea was prompted by the similar appearance of dense projections and the cores of DCV (Aghajanian and Bloom, 1967c), plus the frequent proximity of the projections and vesicles. Needless to say this is an indirect argument but one which, in view of the paucity of alternative ideas, warrants consideration.

The most commonly encountered DCV in CNS situations are generally of the order of 60–150 nm in diameter (e.g. Sotelo, 1971a). This is in marked contrast to *neurosecretory vesicles* which also possess dense-cores but are larger (up to 400 nm in diameter) and occur in, for example, the neurohypophysis (Green and van Breeman, 1955; Palay, 1957; Holmes, 1964). The relation between these neurosecretory vesicles and the smaller agranular vesicles in neurosecretory nerve terminals is unclear. They may be produced as a consequence of hormone release (Holmes and Knowles, 1960) or alternatively may be actively involved in stimulating this release (Gerschenfeld, Tramezzani and De Robertis, 1960). The distinction which some draw between the endocrine role characteristic of neurosecretory neurons and the secretory activity characteristic of neurons in general may have some bearing on a solution to this and other problems connected with neurosecretion (Knowles and Bern, 1966).

DCV similar in appearance to the neurosecretory vesicles of the vertebrate hypothalamo-hypophyseal system or of a smaller variety are observed in a wide range of neural situations in invertebrates (e.g. Scharrer and Brown, 1961; Hagadorn, Bern and Nishioka, 1963; Gray and Young, 1964; Barber, 1967; Martin, 1968; Rogers, 1968, Gray, 1970b). In *Octopus* for intance, up to 4% of the vesicles in the nerve terminals of the supraoesophageal brain lobes have dense cores (Dilly, Gray and Young, 1963; Jones, 1967, 1970c) with a size range of 30–150 nm in diameter (Gray and Young, 1964; Tonosaki, 1965; Jones, 1967). In a study of the relationship between vesicles associated with the Golgi apparatus and synaptic vesicles, Gray (1970c) demonstrated that 28% of the vesicles in one group of synaptic terminals in the vertical lobe were dense-cored. Two other groups by contrast contained exclusively agranular vesicles.

Another interesting point to emerge from *Octopus* and *Loligo* studies concerns the distinction between vesicles containing typical dense cores and those filled with diffuse dense contents (Martin *et al.*, 1969; Barlow and Martin, 1971). Neither type is stained by zinc iodide–OsO_4 (ZIO) impregnation (Section 1.3.4). The endings in which these vesicles are found constitute a majority of the endings in brain lobes having high levels of catecholamines (Juorio, 1970; Barlow and Martin, 1971), and it is tempting to speculate that the two vesicle types may be associated with different catecholamines.

1.2.5 Subsynaptic organelles

Of the regions making up the synaptic junction our knowledge of the *postsynaptic* terminal is by far the most rudimentary. Two features of this terminal will be discussed – the *subsynaptic apparatus* and *spine apparatus* (Fig. 1.2).

(i) *The subsynaptic apparatus.* While there have been a large number of reports of synapses displaying some form of subsynaptic apparatus it is difficult to correlate this information and postulate an underlying *rationale* of their functional connection with the junction. Profiles observed in the postsynaptic terminal may be closely related to the postsynaptic membrane and include the subsynaptic web (de Robertis, Pellegrino de Iraldi, Rodriguez de Lores Arnaiz and Salganicoff, 1961b; De Robertis, Rodriguez de Lores Arnaiz, Salganicoff, Pellegrino de Iraldi and Zieher, 1963) and subsynaptic organelle (Van der Loos, 1963). These are probably specializations of the membrane itself and can be incorporated within the more embracing concept of the postsynaptic

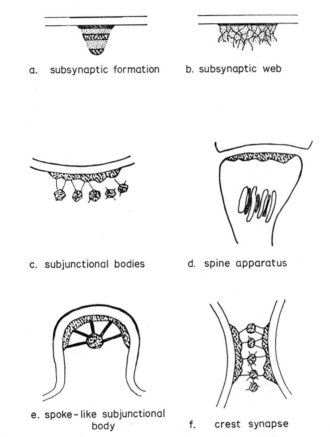

a. subsynaptic formation   b. subsynaptic web

c. subjunctional bodies   d. spine apparatus

e. spoke-like subjunctional body   f.   crest synapse

Figure 1.2 Diagram demonstrating various types of subsynaptic organelle. Details of the cleft regions and presynaptic terminals are omitted.

thickening or opacity of other workers (e.g. Gray, 1963; Colonnier, 1968). Although thickenings of this nature can be distinguished from the postsynaptic membrane in regions cut normal to the plane of section, they appear to be continuous with the membrane along their length (Colonnier, 1968; Jones, 1974).

There is in addition another group of profiles which, at low magnifications, appear as discrete entities subjacent to, and separated from, the junctional region. These profiles include variously-named structures – the subsynaptic formation (Taxi, 1961, 1967), subsynaptic sac (Gray and Guillery, 1966; Charlton and Gray, 1966), subsurface cistern (Rosenbluth, 1962; Plate 1.6). subsynaptic particles (Gray, 1963) and subjunctional bodies (Milhaud and Pappas, 1966a, b). In spite of the plethora of terms used to describe these postsynaptic structures they can be reduced to two principal categories on ultrastructural grounds, (a) those consisting of one or more dense bars (as in the subsynaptic formation) and (b) those consisting of one or more rows of dense circular bodies (as in the subjunctional bodies).* Although these structures are essentially separated from the postsynaptic thickening there may be connections between them and the thickening in the form of granules (subsynaptic formation; Taxi, 1961) or fine web-like extensions (subjunctional bodies; Akert, Pfenninger and Sandri, 1967).

The frequency with which some form of subsynaptic apparatus is encountered in postsynaptic terminals varies considerably. The subsynaptic formation (Plate 1.7) has only been described in autonomic ganglia (Taxi, 1961, 1967, 1969; Sotelo, 1968) while the subjunctional bodies (Plate 1.4) are remarkably frequent in one situation, that of the habenula and interpeduncular nuclei (Milhaud and Pappas, 1966a, b). They also commonly occur wedged between two junctions as in the crest synapses of the subfornical organ ('double-plug' synapses – Akert *et al.*, 1967; Akert, 1969; see also Milhaud and Pappas, 1966a; Lund, 1969; Plate 1.5). They are occasionally observed in other situations, and some form of subsynaptic apparatus, generally of the subjunctional body variety, has been described in spinal cord (Gray, 1962, 1963; Glees and Sheppard, 1964; Charlton and Gray, 1966; Nathaniel and Nathaniel, 1966; Malinsky, 1972, Jones, 1973a), cerebral cortex (Colonnier, 1964), optic tectum (Gray and Hamlyn, 1962), cerebellum (Szentagothai, 1962; Sotelo, 1971a; Jones, 1973a), hippocampus (Jones, 1973a), superior colliculus (Lund, 1969), lateral vestibular nucleus (Mugnaini, Walberg and Haugli-Hanssen, 1967b; Sotelo and Palay, 1970), interpeduncular nucleus (Mizuno and Nakamura, 1974) and olfactory tubercle (Anderson and Westrum, 1972). More recently they have been found in large numbers associated with junctions of the possum inferior olivary nucleus (Holst, 1974). Various postsynaptic membrane specializations, unlike CNS ones, have been described at certain neuromuscular junctions (e.g. Rosenbluth, 1973).

The subsynaptic apparatus has also played a part in aiding interpretation of degeneration studies. According to Taxi (1969) the subsynaptic formation may be considered an excellent criterion for recognizing synaptic junctions (or 'active zones') after section of preganglionic fibres and degeneration of presynaptic endings (Plate 1.7). This is because the subsynaptic apparatus persists after the disappearance of the presynaptic and cleft components of the junction (Mugnaini, Walberg and Brodal, 1967a; Koenig, 1967; Sotelo, 1968; Lund, 1969). From this it has been suggested that the apparatus, whatever its form or situation, is not dependent upon the functional integrity of the synapse (Sotelo, 1971a) and may not indeed be closely related to synaptic activity (Taxi, 1969). It would be interesting to know whether its appearance during development is in any way related to the appearance in a definitive form of synaptic components, particularly the postsynaptic thickening. Their persistence in degenerating terminals and their continued

---

* The term *subsynaptic apparatus* has been introduced into this discussion to include both categories, as it appears they are different entities for which different terms must be retained.

relationship to the postsynaptic thickening raises the question of the involvement of this thickening in synaptic events. Perhaps the subsynaptic apparatus and postsynaptic thickening have similar functions which are primarily concerned with adhesion and not neurotransmission.

Akert *et al.* (1967) contend that subjunctional bodies are obligatory in 'double-plug' crest synapses (Plate 1.5), but are encountered only rarely in 'single-plug' junctions. This may be true for some regions, although further evidence is required before making it a general principle. There appears no reason for even considering the concept in the case of the subsynaptic formation. Akert *et al.* (1967) postulate that in crest synapses the subjunctional bodies may separate the electrical and chemical processes occurring simultaneously in the two synaptic regions.

The presence of subjunctional bodies in all dendritic spines in the habenula and the interpeduncular nucleus is very striking (Milhaud and Pappas, 1966a, b), in view of their sparcity in most other areas. Whether their presence bears any relationship to biochemical parameters, such as the high concentration of monoamine oxidase in the habenula as suggested by Milhaud and Pappas, remains to be seen.

Subjunctional bodies with a spoke-like arrangement appear to characterize certain cerebellar junctions (Nolan, 1974). In these instances a central body is seen with spokes radiating from it to a highly concave postsynaptic thickening. The functional significance of these profiles is not clear, although their association with curved junctions and not straight ones suggests a mechanical role.

(ii) *The spine apparatus.* In 1959 Gray (1959a, b) described an organelle in the dendritic spines of rat occipital cortex to which he assigned the name *spine apparatus* (Plate 1.2; Fig. 1.2). According to Gray's original description this apparatus consists of at least two membrane-bound sacs, 30–50 nm apart, and separated from one another by 15–20 nm wide dense bands which are PTA positive (Adinolfi, 1971a). Although initially viewed as being confined to dendritic spines they have also been found in dendrites close to the base of spines (Westrum and Blackstad, 1962; Hamlyn, 1963) and in the basal portions of dendrites where spines are absent (Gray and Guillery, 1963). Similar profiles have been described in the initial segments of pyramidal cell axons (Palay, Sotelo, Peters and Orkand, 1968; Peters, Proskauer and Kaiserman-Abramof, 1968), observations which suggest that the apparatus or a related structure has an extra-dendritic localization in some instances.

Since its first description the spine apparatus has been recorded in numerous situations. The areas in which it is found include the neocortex of a range of mammals (e.g. Hamlyn, 1962; Westrum and Blackstad, 1962; Gray and Guillery, 1963; Gray, 1964), neostriatum (Adinolfi, 1971a), hippocampus (Hamlyn, 1962, 1963), ventral lateral geniculate nucleus (Colonnier and Guillery, 1964), and spinal cord (Gray and Guillery, 1963). A rudimentary form of the apparatus, excluding the dense bands, has been described in Purkinje cell dendritic spines in cerebellum (Gray and Guillery, 1963; Gray, 1964; Fox, Hillman, Siegesmund and Dutta, 1967).

In spite of the number of observations of the spine apparatus, little in the way of thorough investigations of its ultrastructure has been undertaken. The need for studies utilizing serial sections is paramount before the ultrastructure of the apparatus and its relationship to other organelles such as smooth-surfaced (Sotelo, 1971a) and rough endoplasmic reticulum can be elucidated. Comparative studies of the effects on it of different fixatives are also required in order to follow-up the work of Schultz and Karlsson (1966) relating its appearance to the mode of fixation. The possibility that it may be artefactual, as suggested by these workers, needs further consideration. Even if this does prove to be the case however, its consistency of appearance and location must be significant and may throw light on an underlying *in vivo* organelle, such as the smooth-surfaced endoplasmic reticulum, which may itself be significant for postsynaptic events (Sotelo, 1971a) and of which the spine apparatus may be a local specialization (Peters *et al.*, 1970).

With so many details still unresolved attempts to understand the apparatus in functional terms may be readily dismissed as premature. As it is not universally found in spines its presence cannot be critical to input–output spine function (Scheibel and Scheibel, 1968). During development the spine apparatus first becomes recognizable at approximately 16 days postnatal (rat occipital cortex – Gray, 1963, 1964), while the spines themselves appear at 4–10 days (cat superficial neocortex – Pappas and Purpura, 1961; Scheibel and Scheibel, 1964; see also Section 1.4.2). While care must be exercised in extrapolating from one species to another, there may be a period in mammalian cerebral cortex when the apparatus is not present in spines, its appearance being relatively late compared with most developmental parameters. The significance of this is not known, and even the possibility that it may be concerned in some aspect of learning (Gray, 1971) must await correlated behavioural and ultrastructural studies.

1.3 CHEMICAL SYNAPSES – ADDITIONAL FEATURES

In addition to the conventional preparative techniques considered in the previous section (1.2) a number of others have come into prominence in recent years and are contributing extensively to an understanding of synaptic ultrastructure. Chief amongst these is the use of a non-osmicated fixation procedure followed by block-staining in either PTA or BIUL. This procedure has already proved of considerable value in analysing the paramembranous densities. The other procedures to be discussed in this section are in a more preliminary stage of development but show signs of being useful ancillary techniques for synaptic studies. These are freeze-etching for the re-examination of synaptic ultrastructure, ZIO impregnation for the study of synaptic vesicles and the examination of unbuffered or incubated material as an aid to the investigation of coated vesicles.

1.3.1 Paramembranous densities

The stimulus to recent developments in our concept of the paramembranous densities* was provided by Bloom and Aghajanian (Aghajanian and Bloom, 1967c; Bloom and

---

* The term *paramembranous densities* covers the dense projections, cleft densities and postsynaptic-thickening (or postsynaptic focal densities).

Aghajanian 1966, 1968) with their demonstration that the paramembranous densities are highlighted when tissue fixed in glutaraldehyde alone is block-stained with PTA. Akert and co-workers (e.g. Akert and Pfenninger, 1969; Akert, Moor, Pfenninger and Sandri, 1969; Pfenninger *et al.*, 1969), using a parallel technique substituting a bismuth iodide complex for PTA and subsequently staining the sections with uranyl acetate and lead hydroxide (BIUL method), extended Bloom and Aghajanian's ideas and formulated the concept of a presynaptic vesicular grid (Fig. 1.3).

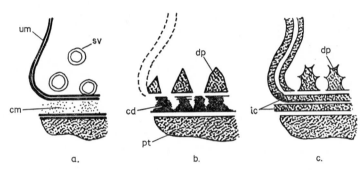

Figure 1.3   Comparison of synaptic junction appearances after three different preparative procedures: (a) aldehyde–OsO₄ fixation, double staining; (b) aldehyde fixation, PTA staining; (c) aldehyde fixation, BIUL staining. Details of the presynaptic network in (b) and of the presynaptic vesicular grid in (c) have been omitted. Dense projections are sometimes visible in (a). cd, cleft densities; cm, cleft material; dp, dense projections; ic, intracleft lines; pt, postsynaptic thickening; sv, synaptic vesicles; um, unit membrane.

These initial studies have been followed-up by a number of invesitgators either in developing ideas on synaptic ultrastructure or simply utilizing the techniques in conjunction with conventional ones. The glutaraldehyde–PTA method has been employed in studying brain tissue from a variety of angles and by a number of investigators as shown in Table 1.1. The BIUL technique by contrast has been employed almost exclusively by Akert's group. In addition to the 1969 papers referred to above, attempts have been made to correlate results arising from it with those derived from freeze-etching and ZIO studies (Akert and Sandri, 1970; see also Bloom, Iversen and Schmitt, 1970). Pfenninger (1971a, b, 1972) has carried out extensive cytochemical studies analysing the BIUL method and investigating the nature of the paramembranous densities and the binding mechanism between the synaptic membranes. His work taken in conjunction with other cytochemical studies on the synaptic region (e.g. Pease, 1966; Bondareff, 1967; Rambourg and Leblond, 1967; Bloom and Aghajanian, 1968; Bondareff and Sjöstrand, 1969; Meyer, 1969; Barrantes and Lunt, 1970) provides a basis for a more thorough appreciation of the chemical nature of the synapse (see Section 4.4).

While PTA and the BIUL complex are the stains routinely employed with non-osmicated material, a similar result is obtained with uranyl acetate and lead citrate. This is illustrated in Fig. 8 of Westrum and Lund's (1966) study on formalin fixation. While they realized that membranes occur as 'negative' images under these circumstances and that filamentous protein structures are accentuated, they failed to take their observations any further.

Regardless of the staining method, non-osmicated material is characterized by a number of features. These include: (a) a presynaptic network (Jones, 1969) or vesicular grid (Pfenninger *et al.*, 1969) within the presynaptic terminal, (b) dense projections (Gray, 1963; Bloom and Aghajanian, 1966) associated with the presynaptic membrane, (c) cleft material in the form of cleft densities (Jones, 1969) or a double intracleft line (Pfenninger *et al.*, 1969), and (d) a postsynaptic thickening (Jones, 1969) or band (Bloom and Aghajanian, 1966) subjacent to the postsynaptic membrane (Plates 1.8–1.10).

Table 1.1   Examples of CNS studies involving the use of the glutaraldehyde–PTA technique

Tissue	Investigators
INTACT TISSUE	
Rat cerebral cortex	Bloom and Aghajanian, 1966
	Aghajanian and Bloom, 1967c
	Meyer, 1969
	Jones and Brearley, 1972a, 1973
	West *et al.*, 1972
Rat cerebellar cortex	Woodward *et al.*, 1971
	Bloom, 1972b
	Hoffer *et al.*, 1972
	Nicholson and Altman, 1972c
Rat hypothalamus	Bloom and Aghajanian, 1968
Rat spinal cord	Jones, 1973a
	Nolan and Jones, 1973b, 1974
Rat thalamus, hippocampus	Jones, 1973a
Rat median eminence	Güldner and Wolff, 1973
Guinea-pig cerebral cortex	Jones, 1973c
	Jones *et al.*, 1974
Cat cerebral cortex (postnatal)	Adinolfi, 1972b
Cat putamen	Adinolfi, 1971a
Cat subfornical organ	Pfenninger *et al.*, 1969
Rabbit cerebral cortex	Vrensen and De Groot, 1973
Mouse cerebellar cortex	Hirano and Dembitzer, 1973
Monkey cerebral cortex	Sloper and Powell, 1973
Setonix lateral geniculate nucleus	Doran and Jones, 1971
	Jones *et al.*, 1972
FRACTIONATED TISSUE	
Rat cortical synaptosomes	Jones, 1969, 1972
	Jones and Brearley, 1972b
Rat cortical synaptosomes (postnatal)	Jones and Revell, 1970b
Octopus ganglia synaptosomes	Jones, 1970a, b
Isolated synaptic plasma membranes	McBride *et al.*, 1970
	Cotman *et al.*, 1971b
Isolated synaptic complexes	Cotman and Taylor, 1972
	Davis and Bloom, 1973
Isolated postsynaptic membranes	Garey *et al.*, 1972

In addition to these essential features others have also been noted. Electron-dense spheres (Bloom and Aghajanian, 1966) may be present within the presynaptic terminal and have been tentatively identified by Pfenninger *et al.* (1969) as the cores of DCV (Plate 1.11). In contrast to this mammalian situation, the profiles are far more numerous in *Octopus* terminals where they may represent a much wider range of synaptic vesicles including agranular ones (Jones, 1970b). Subjunctional bodies are sometimes visible in the postsynaptic terminal (Akert *et al.*, 1969; Pfenninger *et al.*, 1969; Jones, 1973a), although no attempt has been made either to study these in detail in this material or compare them with published reports of their appearance in conventional preparations (Section 1.2.5).

Underlying the essential features demonstrated by the synaptic junction in non-osmicated material is one basic principle, which is that *membranes are not stained* (Fig. 1.3). Instead what are stained are their internal and external coats which appear as prominent electron-opaque densities. Hence the internal coat of the presynaptic membrane gives rise to the dense projections and that of the postsynaptic membrane to the postsynaptic thickening. The external coats of both membranes contribute to the cleft material (either cleft densities or double intracleft lines) of the junctional region. The pre- and postsynaptic membranes are the electron-translucent bands intervening between the dense projections and cleft densities presynaptically and the postsynaptic thickening and cleft densities postsynaptically.

(i) *The presynaptic region.* A consequence of this staining phenomenon is that synaptic vesicles with their typical limiting membrane are not observed in the presynaptic terminal, which is occupied by a diffuse network (e.g. Jones, 1969, 1970b; Jones and Brearley, 1972a). In mammals, spaces are found between the strands of this network and it is assumed that many of these spaces contain the contours of synaptic vesicles (Jones, 1970b; compare Plates 1.12 and 1.14). The nature of the network itself is unclear but, in terms of the preceding discussion, it may well represent the coats of the vesicle membranes (Jones and Ellison, 1975). Alternatively, it may be a permanent structure, protein in composition, which is not rendered visible by uranyl-lead staining under 'normal' conditions (Barrantes and Lunt, 1970). A further possibility is that it is an artefact reflecting perhaps a breakdown of the vesicle membranes due to poor fixation. While this cannot be easily dismissed, the reproducibility of the network and the repeatedly observed orderliness of its appearance in the vicinity of the presynaptic membrane and lack of orderliness away from it (Jones and Brearley, 1972a) argues for its validity as a useful structural concept.

Akert and co-workers have concentrated their efforts mainly on the region of the presynaptic terminal close to the presynaptic membrane, emphasizing the orderly arrangement of the dense projections, their relationship to each other and their involvement in the presynaptic vesicular grid (Fig. 1.4). In addition to confirming the hexagonal arrangement of the dense projections (Gray, 1963, 1964), Akert's group has demonstrated their filamentous connections to each other to form a 'hexagonal peak-and-hole pattern' (Plate 1.13). This constitutes the presynaptic vesicular grid, with the dense projections as nodal points and each surrounded by a monolayer of synaptic vesicles (Akert *et al.*, 1969).

Detailed morphometric studies by Akert and co-workers (see Bloom *et al.*, 1970) have led them to recognize two populations on the basis of three indices: (a) the width of the synaptic cleft, (b) the spacing between the dense projections, and (c) the thickness of the postsynaptic element. Using a combination of the ZIO staining of synaptic vesicles and the BIUL impregnation of paramembranous densities (Akert and Sandri, 1970), dense projections and synaptic vesicles are visible in the same material (compare the PTA staining of unbuffered, incubated synaptosomes by Jones and Bradford, 1971b). While the EMs are not as clear-cut and easy to interpret as they might be, they allow a preliminary interpretation of the findings. From these it appears that round vesicles are associated with wider interprojection spacings, wider clefts and thicker postsynaptic bands than flattened visicles (see Bloom *et al.*, 1970; Akert, Pfenninger, Sandri and Moor, 1972). Freeze-etching has led to similar conclusions with the proviso that the vesicles are distinguishable in terms of size rather than shape (Akert *et al.*, 1972; Section 1.3.2).

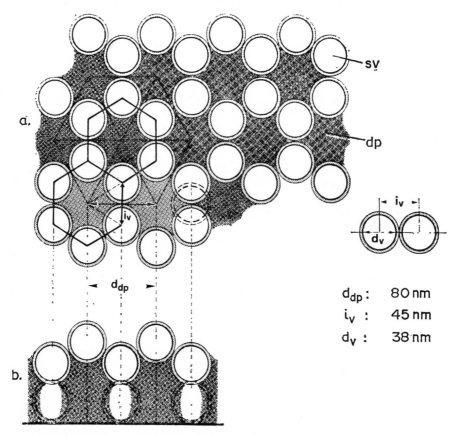

$$d_{dp}: \quad 80\,nm$$
$$i_v: \quad 45\,nm$$
$$d_v: \quad 38\,nm$$

Figure 1.4 Reconstruction of geometrical relationships between dense projections (dp) and synaptic vesicles (sv; v) as envisaged for the presynaptic vesicular grid in glutaraldehyde–BIUL material. Diagram (a) represents a tangential section of the grid, and diagram (b) a cross-section of it. d, diameter of dense projections or synaptic vesicles; i, interval between the central points of dense projections or synaptic vesicles. (From Akert *et al.*, 1969.)

At a more general level these results indicate that the presynaptic grid (and one also imagines the presynaptic network) is not an exclusive feature of excitatory junctions, but is also present in slightly modified form at inhibitory junctions (Akert and Sandri, 1970). They also introduce a postsynaptic criterion into the discussion of morphological differences between the two synaptic types.

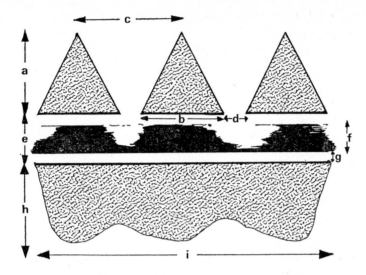

Figure 1.5 Diagram to illustrate the principal indices measured in glutaraldehyde–PTA studies of adult rat synaptic junctions. a, height of dense projection; b, width of dense projection at its base along the presynaptic membrane; c, distance between central points of adjacent dense projections; d, gap between nearest points of adjacent dense projections at their bases; e, distance between internal electronopaque coats of pre- and postsynaptic membranes; f, width of intracleft electronopacity; g, width of intermediate, electrontranslucent coat of postsynaptic membrane; h, height of postsynaptic thickening; i, length of postsynaptic thickening. (From Jones and Brearley, 1972a.)

Table 1.2 Dimensions of the indices outlined in Fig. 1.5 (from Jones and Brearley, 1972a)

Indices	Number measured	Mean value in nm (except i)	Standard deviation (S.D.) in nm (except i)
a	108	35·3	10·8
b	85	33·9	12·5
c	93	49·7	15·0
d	53	10·3	4·7
e	37	22·1	2·1
f	45	12·2	3·9
g	36	3·8	0·8
h	38	32·1	8·4
i	39	0·29 μm	0·087 μm

Another attempt at analysing the synaptic junction quantitatively is that of Jones and Brearley (1972a) on non-osmicated, PTA-stained rat cerebral cortex. Fig. 1.5 shows the indices, *a–i*, used in this study, and Table 1.2 the mean values and standard deviations of the indices. There is a considerable range of variation in the dimensions of the para-membranous densities, and this may be due in part to the sectioning.* This factor how-ever, is a limited one, especially for the intracleft structures.

With the exception of *f* and *g*, histograms of the indices have two peaks, thereby

* In a study of the effects of sectioning on the apparent distribution of dense projections along the presynaptic membrane, Jones and Brearley (1973) confirmed their regular and orderly arrangement. Unexpectedly large interprojection distances result from a failure to section some of the dense projections, and not from an absence of projections.

lending support to the concept of two synaptic populations (Jones and Brearley, 1972a). Unfortunately it was not found possible to relate the morphology of many individual synaptic junctions to the two types of junction depicted by the quantitative results.

Two further points remain to be considered at this juncture. First, concepts of both the grid and network require an intimate connection between dense projections and strands of the grid or network (e.g. Pfenninger et al., 1969; Jones, 1970b). Second, the arrangement of the dense projections at the presynaptic membrane is such as to allow only one synaptic vesicle between adjacent dense projections at any one time (e.g. Akert and Pfenninger, 1969). This is the basis of the orderliness observed at the presynaptic membrane, the morphological counterpart of quantal theories of neurotransmission (e.g. Fatt and Katz, 1950, 1952; Hubbard, 1970; Section 5.1). It has therefore generally been concluded that, in the light of this, synaptic vesicles pass between adjacent dense projections to contact the membrane and hence release their transmitter substance into the cleft (Akert et al., 1969). The distance between the bases of adjacent dense projections in transverse sections is of the order of 10 nm (Jones and Brearley 1972a), quite inadequate for such a phenomenon. Assuming this calculation to be valid it has consequences, not for the orderliness of the presynaptic region, but for the manner in which the transmitter is released in the vicinity of the membrane. The significance of this observation and of possible interpretations stemming from it will become clearer in the light of the discussion on synaptopores (Section 1.3.2) and on the vesicle hypothesis itself (Section 5.4).

Dense projections were first described in the presynaptic terminals of mammalian spinal cord by Gray (1963), although he had seen them earlier in other regions of the CNS including the cerebral cortex (Gray, 1959a). He described them as 'a series of regularly arranged dense structures projecting from the synaptic membrane into the presynaptic cytoplasm' (1963). When sectioned transversely they often appeared as triangular profiles with an irregular spikey appearance, whereas in tangential sections their hexagonal arrangement was pronounced (Gray, 1963, 1966; compare Plates 1.9 and 1.13).

The material examined by Gray was OsO_4–fixed and PTA–stained, an effective combination for demonstrating the *relationship* of dense projections to one another, although surprisingly disappointing in demonstrating the relationship of synaptic vesicles to dense projections. Akert and co-workers, using their non-osmicated technique, took up this theme of the relationship between presynaptic organelles, resulting in the formulation of their concept of the presynaptic vesicular grid.

Our knowledge of the ultrastructure of dense projections is rudimentary. Although they are often depicted as triangular profiles in cross-section and hence pyramidal in shape (e.g. Gray, 1963; Jones, 1969), this is variable (Plate 1.9). They are probably better described as truncated pyramids or polyhedric bodies (Akert and Pfenninger, 1969), although such terms should not conceal their irregular outline due to the protrusion of spikes or filaments (Plate 1.10).

Although initially conceived as solid bodies there is evidence to suggest a subunit structure (Jones and Bradford, 1971b) and possibly a central electron–translucent core

(Jones and Brearley, 1972a, b). While the latter feature has, to date, been noted only occasionally in rat cerebral cortex, it may be a commoner occurrence in other groups of animals. For instance, some dense projections studied in the lateral geniculate nucleus of the Australian marsupial *Setonix brachyurus* appear to consist of an outer 'skin' of spikes around a central electron-translucent area (Jones, Brearley and Doran, 1972; Plate 1.10). What one would like to know is whether minor differences in the preparation of the tissue, for example the amount of water and the nature and level of impurities in the PTA, affect the appearance of the dense projections in a similar way to its effect on the appearance of the presynaptic network and cleft material (Jones, 1973a).

The equidensitometric analysis of EMs of PTA–stained synaptic junctions emphasizes the lack of homogeneity of dense projections, which have a central dense core with dense protrusions into a less dense peripheral region in the screen equidensities technique (Nolan and Jones, 1973a, b, 1974; Plate 1.15). The exact configuration of this densely-staining framework may well vary with the functional state of the terminal, while its appearance may also depend upon the plane of sectioning. Nevertheless, the results of equidensitometric techniques leave little room for a homogeneous concept of dense projection ultrastructure. Kadota and Kadota (1973b, c) for their part suggest that dense projections may contain two classes of material, shell fragments and flocculent material, the shell fragments corresponding to the hexagonal and pentagonal units described in dense projections by Jones and Bradford (1971b) and the flocculent material consisting of the tetrasome units described by themselves.

The functional connection between dense projections and other presynaptic organelles, such as coated vesicles, synaptic vesicles and the presynaptic membrane, is a matter for speculation. Gray and Willis (1970) have suggested that dense projections may be derived from fragments of the shell or basket of coated vesicles, a suggestion supported by Jones and Bradford (1971b) using unbuffered, incubated, PTA–stained synaptosomes. This issue is taken up again in Section 1.3.3.

(ii) *Cleft material.* Material within the cleft separating the pre- and postsynaptic terminals represents the external coats of the pre- and postsynaptic membranes. Its appearance differs in non-osmicated tissue depending on whether PTA or BIUL staining is employed (Fig. 1.3). With the latter it takes the form of two lines running parallel to the synaptic membranes (Plate 1.11). These constitute the 'double intracleft line' of Akert's group (Pfenninger *et al.* 1969). These lines are continuous with nonsynaptic external membrane or outer 'fuzz' coats (Pfenninger, 1971a) which are thickened at the synaptic junction (Akert *et al.*, 1969). The intracleft lines are separated from the presynaptic dense projections and postsynaptic thickening by the unstained pre- and postsynaptic membranes respectively.

In PTA-stained, non-osmicated tissue the cleft material takes the form of interconnected *cleft densities* (Jones, 1969), which are electron-opacities within the cleft sometimes subjacent to the profiles of the dense projections (Plate 1.9). The term cleft density was originated to describe the appearance of the cleft material in synaptosomes, and it is true that cleft densities are more discrete in fractionated than intact tissue (Jones and

Brearley, 1972b). However, the cleft material in intact tissue, while it may appear more-or-less continuous along the length of the junction in low power micrographs, is clearly discontinuous when viewed at higher magnifications (Jones and Brearley, 1972a). Moreover there may be a correspondence between the positions of the opacities and the overlying dense projections.

The confusion over the appearance of the cleft material in PTA–stained synaptic junctions has arisen because of the way it has been depicted in the diagrams of certain authors (Aghajanian and Bloom, 1967c; Bloom et al., 1970; Pfenninger, 1971a, 1972). In these instances it has been shown as a continuous thickened line with no variation in opacity along its length. This however, does not correspond to its appearance in micrographs published either by these workers (Bloom and Aghajanian, 1966, 1968; Pfenninger et al., 1969) or others (Adinolfi, 1972b; Doran and Jones, 1971; Garey, Harper, Best and Goodman, 1972; Jones and Brearley, 1972a; Jones et al., 1972; Nolan and Jones, 1973a, b, 1774). It is recommended therefore that the term cleft densities be applied to the electron-opacities found within the cleft of PTA–stained, intact synaptic junctions.

While cleft densities are found within a majority of junctions there are exceptions. In some junctions the external coats of the synaptic membranes are visible as two distinct lines with transverse bars between them (Jones, 1969; Jones and Brearley, 1972a). This type of junctional profile is reminiscent of the appearance of cleft material in BIUL–stained junctions, and is present in both intact and fractionated cerebral cortex. These different appearances of the cleft material in PTA–stained junctions parallel differences of the internal coats, and so may point to functionally divergent types of synapse (Sections 1.2.2 and 1.2.3). Cytochemical analysis of the two types is required, along the lines of Pfenninger (1971a, b) on BIUL–stained material (Section 4.4.2).

(iii) *Postsynaptic thickening.* Only minor differences have been noted between the postsynaptic thickening in non-osmicated and osmicated tissue (compare Plates 1.2 and 1.8; Fig. 1.3). It extends the length of the synaptic junction, is continuous along its cleft aspect and uneven on its cytoplasmic side (e.g. Akert and Pfenninger, 1969; Jones and Brearley, 1972a). Its thickness varies, the regions of increased thickness corresponding approximately to the positions of the dense projections and cleft densities (Adinolfi, 1972b). Such areas have been referred to as postsynaptic focal densities (Jones and Revell, 1970b) which occur in intact junctions but are most pronounced in synaptosomes (Jones, 1969; Jones and Brearley, 1972b).

In most synaptic junctions so far examined the postsynaptic thickening is homogeneously electron–opaque (except Cotman and Taylor, 1972; Section 2.5.2). To date however, one exception has been noted – this encompasses certain junctions in the spinal cord, in which the postsynaptic thickening is of a fragmented nature giving the appearance of being separated from the postsynaptic membrane at a number of points (Jones, 1973a). Further investigation of this phenomenon is required, in order to decide whether it is an isolated one or whether it calls for a reappraisal of currently accepted views of the postsynaptic thickening.

The recent application of equidensitometric techniques for analysing the EMs of synaptic junctions (Nolan and Jones, 1973a, b, 1974), has cast doubt even on the homogeneity of the postsynaptic thickening. In all junctions so far examined its heterogeneity is demonstrated with screen equidensities which reveal a central dense framework enclosing and bordered by regions of lesser density (Plate 1.15). Furthermore, these less dense areas also vary from one another by small differences of density represented by one or two optical density symbols (Nolan and Jones, 1974).

The relationship of the postsynaptic thickening to subsynaptic organelles has been discussed above (Section 1.2.5 (i)). While non-osmicated preparatory techniques may have much to contribute to this debate, their contribution has not been exploited to date.

1.3.2 Freeze-etching

The advent of freeze-etching in recent years (Steere, 1957; Moor and Mühlethaler, 1963; Moor, 1966) has been welcomed, its significance arising from the fact that it involves neither dehydrating agents nor chemical fixatives. In practice however, the latter ideal has not generally been attained, at least not in synaptic studies, in which according to Pfenninger, Akert, Moor and Sandri (1972) unfixed material shows conspicuous damage from dissection and glycerination. A comparison of fixed and unfixed material by Akert *et al.* (1972) demonstrated that material fixed in glutaraldehyde contained no less important information than the unfixed replicas.

Interpretations of membrane ultrastructure based on freeze-etching have been controversial due to conflicting ideas regarding the site of fracturing (Plattner, 1970). According to some workers it occurs along surfaces (Moor and Mühlethaler, 1963), whereas others assert it reveals inner membrane faces (Branton, 1966). The interpretation of synaptic sites by Akert and co-workers, while unclear in their earlier papers, was later modified as discussed below to accord with Branton's view that freeze-fracturing separates the two leaflets of the unit membrane (Akert *et al.*, 1972; Sandri, Akert, Livingston and Moor, 1972).

Following the successful application of the freeze-etching technique to the study of myelin (Bischoff and Moor, 1967; Branton, 1967), it was adapted for the study of synaptic terminals. In particular, attention has been directed towards the appearance of synaptic vesicles (Moor, Pfenninger and Akert, 1969; Akert and Sandri, 1970; Nickel and Potter, 1970; Sotelo, 1971a), and the presynaptic (Akert *et al.*, 1969; Pfenninger, Akert, Moor and Sandri, 1971; Pfenninger *et al.*, 1972; Streit, Akert, Sandri, Livingston and Moor, 1972) and postsynaptic membranes (Sandri *et al.*, 1972).

(i) *Synaptic vesicles.* The most significant finding in relation to synaptic vesicles concerns their shape (Plates 1.18 and 1.19). In general only round vesicles have been reported (Akert *et al.*, 1969, 1972; Moor *et al.*, 1969) even in aldehyde-fixed spinal cord (Sotelo, 1971a), indicating that the flattening of vesicles in routinely fixed, dehydrated and embedded material occurs during tissue preparation. This is not to say that all vesicles in aldehyde-fixed, freeze-etched material are of the same size. There appear to be at least two vesicle populations based on their diameters. For example, careful measurements by Akert *et al.* (1972) in the spinal cord of cat and monkey, where round and flattened vesicles are found in conventionally prepared material, revealed a clear-cut difference in size – 48 nm diameter as opposed to 39 nm (compare Plates 1.18 and 1.19).

Furthermore the vesicles are disconnected, an observation in support of the existence of vesicular structures as opposed to tubules. This accords with their appearance in freeze-substituted tissues (Van Harreveld, Crowell and Malhotra, 1965). Vesicle diameter in freeze-etched material also corresponds closely to that in conventionally prepared material, regardless of whether the freeze-etched material is fixed or unfixed (Moor *et al.*, 1969).

The vesicles themselves appear either as concave, saucer-like profiles or convex protrusions into the terminal. According to Nickel and Potter (1970) the number of vesicles seen in cross-fractured terminals is highly variable, and although these workers demonstrated that vesicles may accumulate in the vicinity of the synaptic cleft (in the electric tissue of *Torpedo*) vesicular profiles in the majority of published micrographs appear fairly evenly distributed throughout the presynaptic terminal (e.g. Akert *et al.*, 1969). The apparent fusion of some synaptic vesicles with the presynaptic membrane (Nickel and Potter, 1970) is reminiscent of similar occurrences in conventionally prepared tissue (Westrum, 1965). Whether or not such appearances point to an exocytotic process of functional significance for neurotransmission is a matter which cannot be resolved by morphological studies alone (Sections 5.4 and 5.5.1).

(ii) *Pre- and postsynaptic membranes.* Attempts at understanding the structure of pre- and postsynaptic membranes in freeze-etched material cannot be considered in isolation from the interpretative principles of the authors. In this regard it is significant that papers published by Akert's group prior to 1972 appear to use the 'surface' concept of Moor and Mühlethaler (1963), whereas more recent publications (Sandri *et al.*, 1972) adopt the 'unit membrane-splitting' concept of Branton (1966). The difference between the concepts is reflected at a superficial level in the terminology adopted. Whereas the earlier papers of this group would have referred to the internal and external surfaces of a membrane, later ones speak about the external and internal surfaces respectively of the inner and outer leaflets of a membrane (cf. Akert *et al.*, 1969 with Sandri *et al.*, 1972 and Akert *et al.*, 1972). In spite of this, no discernible change in the interpretation of profiles is evident, a reflection perhaps of the dependence of the authors upon ideas derived from conventionally prepared material rather than the interpretative principles of freeze-etching.

Intramembranous fracturing of synaptic membranes very often produces an appearance comparable to that depicted in Fig. 1.6. The presynaptic membrane is viewed only as an internal surface, either as the outer face of its inner leaflet (pr-of) as seen from the postsynaptic side, or as the inner face of its outer leaflet (pr-if) from its presynaptic aspect. Adjacent to these two views of the presynaptic membrane are equivalent views of that part of the postsynaptic membrane lying alongside the synaptic region. Except at synaptic junctional areas, the inner face of outer leaflets is smoother and contains fewer and smaller granules than the outer face of inner leaflets. These granules or particles are 8–13 nm in diameter, and their common occurrence gives to the inner leaflets a rough appearance (Akert *et al.*, 1969; Plate 1.21).

Both leaflets of the postsynaptic membrane are characterized by these particles (Sandri *et al.*, 1972). They are however, more common on the outer leaflets, where they are especially abundant in the vicinity of postsynaptic sites. This is a reversal of the general distribution of particles on inner and outer leaflets away from immediate postsynaptic sites. These specialized aggregations of particles on the internal surfaces of both postsynaptic leaflets are localized to correspond with specific synaptic sites and may represent the hydrophobic portions of the unit membranes (Sandri *et al.*, 1972).

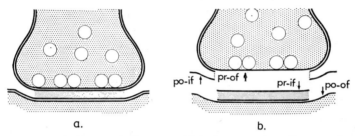

a. b.

Figure 1.6   Fracture plane in freeze-etched synapses. If the interpretation of intramembranous fracturing is correct, (b) represents the fragments obtained after fracturing of synapse (a). pr-if, inner face of the outer leaflet of the presynaptic membrane; pr-of, outer face of the inner leaflet of the presynaptic membrane; po-if, inner face of the outer leaflet of the postsynaptic membrane; po-of, outer face of the inner leaflet of the postsynaptic membrane. (Modified from Pfenninger *et al.*, 1972.)

In terms of this limited data it would be premature to link the particles to entities postulated to exist at conventionally prepared synaptic junctions, for example, Van der Loos's (1963) interlemmal elements or Gray's (1966) intracleft filaments (Sandri *et al.*, 1972). They may be artefactual, although as suggested above it is more likely they represent molecules integral to the architecture of the membrane (e.g. Branton, 1969). In some replicas there is a suggestion of their continuation through the outer postsynaptic leaflet and into the cleft, while particle-free spaces often occur within densely studded areas of postsynaptic active sites (Nolan, 1974). The significance of such observations remains to be determined, although the unique localization of these postsynaptic particles may provide an additional criterion for the identification of active synaptic sites.

(iii) *Presynaptic area.* The presynaptic area can be distinguished using three structural criteria: (a) a slight bulge or lifting of the membrane of the active zone towards the presynaptic cytoplasm, (b) the accumulation of intramembranous particles (9–11 nm) over the lifted area and near or attached to the pits or craters, and (c) the aggregation of 20 nm pits or protuberances (Pfenninger *et al.*, 1971, 1972; Streit *et al.*, 1972; Akert, 1973). It is possible that presynaptic areas may be identified using only two of these criteria, usually the former two (Nolan, 1974; Plate 1.20). If this is valid, the absence of the pits or craters may reflect decreased synaptic activity under the effects of barbiturate anaesthesia (Weakly, 1969; Barker and Gainer, 1973),* or alternatively, variability of morphology in response to a range of functional requirements.

Perhaps of greatest interest for synaptic investigations are the protuberances or pits which are confined to synaptic areas. Protuberances are seen on examination of the inner face of the outer leaflet of the presynaptic membrane (Plate 1.20) and pits on the corresponding outer face of the inner leaflet (Plate 1.21). In other words, protuberances are seen when a junction is viewed from the presynaptic cytoplasmic side, and pits when the junction is examined from the extracellular space. These characteristic deformations of the presynaptic plasmalemma are sometimes referred to as *synaptopores* (Akert et al., 1972), or as *presynaptic membrane modulations* (Streit et al., 1972), the two terms embracing both views. On other occasions they are termed respectively protuberances and micropits (e.g. Pfenninger et al., 1972). They are often arranged in small groups of 10 or 20, having a hexagonal distribution. The protuberances measure 20 nm across at their bases and are approximately 50 nm apart. Their summits sometimes have a crater-like opening. While they are reminiscent of pinocytotic or plasmalemmal vesicles (e.g. in capillary endothelia, Nickel and Grieshaber, 1969 or at extrasynaptic sites of nerve terminals, Akert et al., 1967, 1972), they are much smaller (20 nm compared with 35 nm) and have a hexagonal pattern in contrast to the triagonal one of pinocytotic stomata (Pfenninger et al., 1972).

The significance of the synaptopores is a matter for conjecture. Akert et al. (1972) put forward the idea that they are vesicular attachment sites, although conceding their inability to demonstrate synaptic vesicles actually attached to synaptopores. (Streit et al. (1972) claim to have detected very infrequently a presumed vesicular attachment rising intact from the presynaptic membrane and being continuous with an intact globule.) The principle data in favour of this concept are the intervals between synaptopores (47–58 nm), these being less than those between dense projections (60–80 nm) as measured in BIUL material. This led Akert and co-workers to postulate that synaptopores correspond to the positions of the holes in the presynaptic grid, and so to the synaptic vesicles, rather than to the positions of the dense projections. Taking this line of argument further, Pfenninger et al. (1972) regard synaptopores either as the fusion or fission sites of vesicles with the plasmalemmal membrane, or temporary attachments between them. In line with these alternatives they may represent native diffusion channels arising from gap or tight junctions (Bloom et al., 1970). The possible relevance of synaptopores to the vesicle hypothesis is considered in Section 5.5.1.

Little definitive information has been gained from freeze-etched studies concerning the paramembranous densities. Finely granular material in the region of the cleft and on its pre- and postsynaptic sides is occasionally seen (e.g. Akert et al., 1969; Akert and Sandri, 1970). This technique has not so far contributed any new data to existing knowledge based on thin-sectioned studies.

The freeze-etched studies from which the above results were obtained employed, one must assume, material from animals anaesthetized with barbiturates, although the

---

* Barbiturates decrease the turnover of brain ACh (Schuberth, Sparf and Sundwall, 1969), increase free and labile-bound ACh (Beani, Bianchi, Megazzini, Ballotti and Bernard, 1969) and decrease the mean quantum content in spinal monosynaptic pathways (Weakly, 1969).

studies as a whole do not make this clear. The significance of this particular experimental procedure has been demonstrated by another study from Akert's laboratory, that by Streit *et al.* (1972), who compared the ultrastructural characteristics of synaptic sites from anaesthetized and unanaesthetized animals, using both freeze-etching and thin-sectioning techniques. The three characteristic features of synaptic sites in freeze-etched tissues are more pronounced in unanaesthetized than in anaesthetized material, while Streit and co-workers noted two main differences. The synaptic sites are more convex and hence more conspicuous in the unanaesthetized state, while the presynaptic membrane modulations (synaptopores) have open, crater-like appearances. Examination of thin-sectioned material confirmed these differences, the unanaesthetized junctions having an uneven, wrinkled, convex presynaptic membrane with occasionally omega-shaped indentations. A glutaraldehyde–PTA study by Cooke, Nolan, Dyson and Jones (1974) has demonstrated quantitatively the increasing convexity of the presynaptic membrane towards the postsynaptic terminal with increasing doses of barbiturate. The contribution of these studies to our knowledge of the dynamic properties of the synapse is discussed in Section 5.5.1.

1.3.3 Coated vesicles

Complex (Gray, 1961; Gray and Willis, 1970) or coated (Roth and Porter, 1962; Friend and Farquhar, 1967; Kanaseki and Kadota, 1969) vesicles have been recognized for some time in a variety of tissues. Roth and Porter (1962) were the first to suggest that the 'coating' of the coated vesicle may play a role in the mechanism of the infolding and fissioning of the cell membrane. Bowers (1964) looked upon the coating as the binding site for protein, while other workers have viewed the vesicles in their entirety as being active in the cellular uptake and transport of either protein (Roth and Porter, 1963, 1964; Rosenbluth and Wissig, 1964; Friend and Farquhar, 1967) or enzymes (Bruni and Porter, 1965; Holtzman, Novikoff and Villaverde, 1967).

In the nervous system they were first recognized and commented upon by Gray (1961, 1962, 1963), and were alluded to in negatively-stained vesicle fractions by De Robertis *et al.* (1963). Andrès (1964), while describing structures akin to coated vesicles in rat synapses, postulated a continuum between the synaptic membranes, Golgi apparatus, the pinocytotic spiky vesicles and synaptic vesicles. They have been studied in some detail in fractions of guinea-pig brain (Kanaseki and Kadota, 1969), rat cerebral cortex (Gray and Willis, 1970; Gray, 1972), rat cortical synaptosomes (Jones and Bradford, 1971a, b), frog and fish spinal cord (Gray and Willis, 1970), neurosecretory terminals of rat posterior pituitary gland (Douglas, Nagasawa and Schultz, 1971a; Nagasawa, Douglas and Schultz, 1971), cat medial superior olive (Schwartz, 1972), rat and mouse neuromuscular junctions (Nickel, Vogel and Waser, 1967; Hubbard and Kwanbun-bumpen, 1968; Miledi and Slater, 1970; Korneliussen, 1972; Heuser and Reese, 1973), vertebrate retinal rod- and cone-bipolar synapses (Evans, 1966; Gray and Pease, 1971), developing rat cerebellar cortex (Altman, 1971), degenerating inferior colliculus (Jones and Rockel, 1973), crustacean neurosecretory terminals (Bunt, 1969) and *Helix* visceral ganglia (Chalazonitis, 1969). Attempts are in progress to isolate and characterize bio-chemically the vesicles themselves and their various constituents (Kadota and Kadota, 1973b, c; Section 2.4.4). For instance the coated vesicle fractions are preferentially associated with a nucleoside diphosphate phosphohydrolase, suggesting perhaps that they exert some control over energy metabolism and subsequent ACh synthesis in nerve endings (Kadota and Kadota, 1973a).

Different terms have been used to describe them in addition to complex or coated vesicles. These include annular vesicles (De Robertis *et al.*, 1963), alveolate vesicles (Palay, 1963), micropinosomes (Andrès, 1964), micropinocytotic vesicles (Fawcett, 1965), and acanthosomes (Fawcett, 1965; Bunt, 1969). In spite of this variety of terms my principal concern in this section is to consider the vesicles in general rather than attempt to distinguish between what may or may not be different vesicle types.

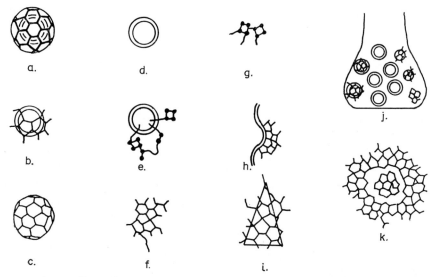

Figure 1.7 Diagram illustrating some of the profiles present in presynaptic terminals under a variety of experimental conditions. These observations constitute the basis for the various theories regarding coated vesicles in synapses. (a) complete coated vesicle; (b) coated vesicle with incomplete shell; (c) empty shell or reticulosome; (d) plain or agranular synaptic vesicle; (e) synaptic vesicle with attached tetrasomes; (f) presynaptic network (cytonet) consisting in some instances of recognizable pentagonal and hexagonal units; (g) isolated tetrasomes; (h) infolding of the limiting membrane of the terminal with attached spikes; (i) dense projection demonstrating a subunit substructure; (j) a presynaptic terminal with coated vesicles and reticulosomes occupying its marginal regions; (k) a reticulosome surrounded by a clear zone. Not to scale. Based on the observations and theories of Kanaseki and Kadota (1969), Gray and Willis (1970), Jones and Bradford (1971a), Gray (1972) and Kadota and Kadota (1973b, c).

In essence coated vesicles consist of a central vesicle surrounded by a network of baskets or a dense spiny arrangement (Plate 1.16; Fig. 1.7). According to Kanaseki and Kadota (1969), who employed an unbuffered fixation technique to demonstrate them, the baskets are composed of regular pentagons and hexagons with sides of equal length. Apart from the profiles composed of a central vesicle plus complete basket, there are others presenting a range of appearances from a vesicle with an incomplete basket to a complete basket lacking a vesicle (Plates 1.16 and 1.17). The latter appearance, that is, the empty basket (Kanaseki and Kadota, 1969) or shell of the coated vesicle (Gray and Willis, 1970; the 'reticulosome' of Gray, 1972) has been interpreted as the end result of the process whereby the central vesicle escapes from the basket of the coated vesicle. Kanaseki and Kadota (1969) repeated Roth and Porter's (1962) hypothesis that the basket of the coated vesicle plays a role in the mechanism of the infolding and fissioning of the membrane. In addition they proposed that these events result from the transformation of the regular hexagons of the basket into regular pentagons. A predominantly quantitative study of coated vesicles in cat medial superior olive by Schwartz (1972) demonstrated their preferential distribution next to or in contact with membrane abutting onto intercellular substance. This may suggest their implication in the production or recycling of some substance associated with intercellular substance, although it is not known whether this is a general phenomenon or even what is the fate of these coated vesicles.

The majority of studies on coated vesicles highlight *inter alia* their micropinocytotic origin. Invagination of the cell membrane results in the formation of micropits which, when covered by a filamentous or spiny coat, pinch-off to form coated vesicles (e.g. Kanaseki and Kadota, 1969; Gray and Willis, 1970). In this way substances from the extracellular space may be transported into the cell interior. Such substances could include proteins and, in the case of neurons, substances more directly involved in neurotransmission such as choline (Korneliussen, 1972). Such micropinocytosis is a general cytological phenomenon and its role in providing the cell with its nutritional requirements is generally accepted. Furthermore there can be little doubt that coated vesicles of one type or another are intimately involved in this process (see for example the tracer studies of Bunt, 1969; Nagasawa et al., 1971; and Nagasawa and Douglas, 1972). A situation which lends itself to the study of exocytosis is the posterior pituitary gland, where neurohypophysial hormones are extruded by this mechanism (refer to Fig. 5.2). The membrane of the neurosecretory granules is incorporated into the cell surface during this process, subsequently to be removed by a phenomenon of vesiculation in which caveolae form within the exocytotic pits. These then pinch off forming microvesicles which are, at first coated, and later smooth (Nagasawa et al., 1971; Douglas et al., 1971a; Douglas, Nagasawa and Schultz, 1971b). A similar phenomenon has been observed in adrenal medullary cells (Douglas and Nagasawa, 1971; Nagasawa and Douglas, 1972).

What is not so clear is the relationship of these processes to neurotransmission, and in particular the part played by coated vesicles in the formation of agranular synaptic vesicles and the paramembranous densities of the neuron. Andrès (1964) for instance suggested that, having resorbed transmitter substances, coated vesicles move from the limiting membrane of the presynaptic terminal towards the Golgi apparatus with which they fuse. Synaptic vesicles in turn bud-off from this system. Altman (1971) by contrast, working on developing cerebellar cortex, postulated that it is the coated vesicles which are pinched-off from the Golgi apparatus and agranular endoplasmic reticulum. Once formed they migrate to the surface of cells where they provide future synapses with transient adhesion membranes or lasting synaptic dense membranes.

Whatever may be the merit of these particular contributions they both overlook a point of fundamental importance, the direct relationship between coated vesicles and uncoated, agranular synaptic vesicles. As demonstrated by Kanaseki and Kadota (1969) and confirmed by other workers (Gray and Willis, 1970; Jones and Bradford, 1971b; Douglas et al., 1971a) there appears to be a continuum between the complete coated vesicle at one extreme and the uncoated agranular vesicle at the other. An interesting, if unusual, finding tending to support the reality of this continuum is that of Jones and Rockel (1973) who, in a degeneration study, noted that the synaptic vesicles of a few terminals disappeared during the early stages of degeneration only to be 'replaced' by a mass of empty shells of coated vesicles. More recently, however, Kanaseki (1973) has questioned this continuum because the 'elementary particles' observed by him attached to synaptic vesicle membranes are not visible in association with coated vesicles.

Using micropinocytosis as an important source of coated vesicles and accepting that they in turn give rise to synaptic vesicles, Gray and Willis (1970) postulated that in the nerve terminal the shell or basket of the coated vesicle helps form the presynaptic dense projections (Fig. 1.7). In an attempt to test this experimentally Jones and Bradford (1971b) studied unbuffered, PTA–stained synaptosomes. In a previous investigation (Jones and Bradford, 1971a) it had been found that coated vesicles decrease in number following the incubation and electrical stimulation of synaptosomes. With coated vesicles and dense projections visualized together in the same material, the dense projections had an irregular outline and were continuous with an enveloping network of spikelike processes (Jones and Bradford, 1971b). It was concluded that these spikes may be derived from the shells of coated vesicles, as this appearance was commonly encountered in stimulated synapto-somes but not in unstimulated ones.

In dynamic terms therefore, the shell of the coated vesicle may be transported either with or independent of a central vesicle towards a dense projection to become incorporated into it (Jones and Bradford, 1971b; Jones, 1972). This is basic to some of the profiles illustrated diagrammatically in Fig. 1.7. It has further been suggested that the basket or shell of coated vesicles corresponds to the presynaptic network (Jones, 1972), both in turn being intimately associated with synaptic vesicles and dense projections.

In terms of these concepts the fate of coated vesicles can be envisaged without invoking an exocytotic mechanism, although the fate of the central vesicle remains unresolved. While exocytosis may account for the disappearance of this latter vesicle, a recycling process may well occur within the terminal (Section 5.5.3). Another outstanding issue is the proportion of coated vesicles which originate by micropinocytosis from the limiting membrane of the nerve terminal, and hence the percentage of synaptic vesicles formed locally from sources within the terminal itself.

The apparent assurance of the preceding discussion should not be taken to imply that coated vesicles are well-defined or universally accepted entities. Their definition in micro-graphs is largely dependent upon the method of preparation of the material. For instance they are well-defined and occur in relatively large numbers in unbuffered material (Kan-aseki and Kadota, 1969), while in fractionated preparations they are more readily seen in incubated tissue than in unincubated (Jones and Bradford, 1971a, b). Even before these findings it had been suggested that they are a common occurrence in poorly fixed material (Ceccarelli and Pensa, 1968). Any attempt at integrating them into a broad view of synaptic function therefore must pay close attention to the procedures employed in demonstrating them.

Scepticism concerning their reality led Gray (1972, 1973) to make a further detailed investigation of their appearance using a variety of preparative procedures. Unlike his earlier paper (Gray and Willis, 1970) in which he had concentrated solely on the coated vesicle profiles, on this occasion he examined them in terms of *background* cytoplasmic appearances. Contending that the coats of coated vesicles as well as the empty shells are artefacts, Gray (1972, 1973) put forward an alternative theory which according to him accounts more satisfactorily than Kanaseki and Kadota's (1969) explanations for a number of observations, including the pale zone around coated vesicles and the occur-rence of complete but empty coats. The essence of Gray's theory is that synaptic vesicles lie in a fine protein skeleton in the cytoplasm, the *cytonet*, which may appear as a *stranded cytonet* or *polygonal cytonet*, depending upon preparative conditions (Fig. 1.7). These may also be responsible for causing the cytonet to condense into balls, the *reticulosomes* (corresponding to empty shells), or onto the surface of a vesicle to form a coated vesicle.

Gray's ideas deserve a sympathetic hearing as they fill in a number of explanatory gaps left by Kanaseki and Kadota. They also help to account for the preferential demon-stration of coated vesicles under a variety of preparative procedures. Furthermore his ideas fit in well with the concept of a presynaptic network and its relationship to dense projections, a concept formulated on PTA–stained material (Jones, 1969, 1970b). However, the evidence presented so far is not sufficiently convincing in terms of the raw data to abolish altogether the idea of coated vesicles. Certainly they must be viewed in cytoplasmic and not simply vesicular terms, but justification may now reasonably be demanded in support of the reality of the cytonet. Its relationship to the cytoplasmic flocculent material of Kadota and Kadota (1973b, c), with its 'tetrasome' units rather than the polygonal structured shell of coated vesicles, also requires clarification (Section 2.4.4; Fig. 1.7). Furthermore, it is necessary to ask how it accounts for the large degree of separation of synaptic and coated vesicles achieved by Kadota and Kadota (1973b, c) in their fractionation studies, in which synaptic and coated vesicles appear as distinct morphological entities although prepared and viewed under identical conditions.

1.3.4 Zinc iodide – osmium tetroxide impregnation

Considerable interest was aroused by Akert and Sandri's demonstration in 1968 that synaptic vesicles are selectively stained by the ZIO stain, which had originally been developed for light microscopy by Maillet (1962) and then adapted for EM by Jabonero (1964) and Taxi (1965). Of even greater significance was their suggestion that there may be a correlation between this stain and the presence of ACh within nerve endings.

Vesicles which stain positively on ZIO impregnation are filled with a black precipitate, only the vesicular membrane appearing as a discrete unstained entity around the precipitate (Plate 1.22). In deciding whether this staining is specific for cholinergic mechanisms it is important to be able to distinguish between ZIO positive agranular vesicles and ZIO positive DCV, as the latter appearance would point to the involvement of adrenergic organelles. As the dense cores or granules of DCV are obliterated by the precipitate, the distinction must be in terms of size.

Akert and Sandri (1968) originally postulated a relationship between ZIO positivity and cholinergic mechanisms because the agranular vesicles of the subfornical organ were positive, whereas DCV and spinal cord agranular vesicles were negative. It was soon discovered however, that the synaptic vesicles of non-cholinergic systems also responded to ZIO treatment (for review see Akert, Kawana and Sandri, 1971). In particular, Pellegrino de Iraldi and Gueudet (1968, 1969) investigating pineal nerves and retinal synapses, Kawana, Akert and Sandri (1969) spinal cord nerve terminals, and Matus (1970) the superior cervical ganglion, demonstrated that presumptive catecholaminergic endings contained ZIO positive vesicles, both agranular and dense-cored. Adopting a physiological approach to the problem, Párducz, Halász and Joó (1971b) pretreated the preganglionic terminals in sympathetic ganglia with hemicholinium (HC–3). They found that such treatment had no effect on ZIO positivity, whether or not there had been preganglionic stimulation. This, together with the other investigations cited, constitute strong evidence against a direct link between ZIO positivity in axon terminals and cholinergic transmission.

An important advance in the ZIO staining technique was made by Martin et al. (1969) who introduced aldehyde fixation into the procedure, a step omitted in the original study of Akert and Sandri (1968). Working with cephalopod nervous tissue Martin and co-workers obtained better preservation of ultrastructure than previously reported, and consequently were able to distinguish several types of synaptic vesicles and nerve terminals (Plate 1.22). Follow-up studies by the same workers (Barlow and Martin, 1971; Froesch and Martin, 1972) have further developed the potentialities of the ZIO reaction as a cytological stain, which is proving valuable in mapping synaptic vesicles in squid brain. This role of the ZIO technique is not dependent on its relationship to various transmitters and has since been used to differentiate between ZIO positive and negative components of the mammalian neuron (Akert et al., 1971) and to study the origin of synaptic vesicles during postnatal development (Stelzner, 1971).

The mode of action of the ZIO staining is still far from clear. As already indicated it is unlikely that the material being stained in the synaptic vesicles is the neurotransmitter since flattened as well as spherical vesicles may be stained (Kawana et al., 1969; Martin et al., 1969: Akert and Sandri, 1970), while DCV may also react in a positive manner (Pellegrino de Iraldi and Gueudet, 1968, 1969).

The ZIO reactive material disappears after reserpine (Pellegrino de Iraldi and Gueudet, 1968) and tyramine (Pellegrino de Iraldi and Suburo, 1972) treatment of the DCV in pineal nerve endings. By varying the iodide employed in the staining mixture Pellegrino de Iraldi and Suburo (1970) were able to demonstrate that the DCV, namely the matrix and the dense core, react in different ways depending on the iodide used and the final pH of the mixture. Niebauer, Krawczyk, Kidd and Wilgram (1969) noted that the ZIO material is lost after lipid extraction procedures, indicating that it may be either lipid or lipid-related.

In spite of the refutation of the idea that a specific transmitter is stained by the technique, it is possible that it may be involved in the synthesis, transport (Stelzner, 1971) or binding of the neurotransmitter, whether this be cholinergic or catecholaminergic in nature. The ZIO technique stains organelles other than synaptic vesicles, including the Golgi complex (in some situations) and the smooth endoplasmic reticulum, and this fact may be used as an argument either for or against its association with a neurotransmitter-producing process. If used in favour of this association, the diverse staining of axonal elements may throw light on the origin of ZIO positive synaptic vesicles (Stelzner, 1971).

An interesting and perhaps disturbing sidelight of the neurotransmitter discussion is the consistent failure of coated vesicles to react with the ZIO technique (Akert *et al.*, 1971; Stelzner, 1971). As they appear to give rise to agranular synaptic vesicles, the difference between the two vesicular types with regard to their ZIO reactivity suggests they are functionally dissimilar or that during the formation of the synaptic vesicle the matrix undergoes some structural transformation. Gray's (1972) artefact hypothesis (Section 1.3.3) is even more difficult to reconcile with this observation, unless it is argued that the build-up of the cytoplasmic matrix or cytonet around vesicles prevents adequate penetration of the stain.

1.4 SYNAPTOGENESIS

As the details of adult morphology clarify, increasing interest is being shown in the processes leading up to the adult configuration. An additional stimulus derives from the growing awareness that insults to the developing brain may result in major consequences for the adult.

The latter factor is resulting in a multi-pronged research emphasis ranging from the consequences of malnutrition on the developing brain (e.g. Dobbing, 1968, 1972; Dobbing and Sands, 1970; Bass, Netsky and Young, 1970; Cragg, 1972a; Gambetti, Autilio-Gambetti, Gonatas, Shafer and Stieber, 1972), to more specific synaptic problems such as the effect of hypo- and hyperthyroidism on the timing of synaptogenesis, the increase in number of synaptic profiles and the development of dendritic spines (Cragg, 1970; Nicholson and Altman, 1972a, b, c; Shapiro, Vukovich and Globus, 1973) and the effects of dark- and light-exposure on developing synapses in the retina and lateral geniculate nucleus (Cragg, 1969a, b).

Closely associated with these synaptogenic studies are parallel ones on adult synaptic junctions, investigating for instance the consequences of visual deprivation on the number of synapses in the retinal inner plexiform layer (Sosula and Glow, 1971; Fifkova, 1972), the effect on synaptic ultrastructure produced by various metabolic conditions including glucose deprivation, anoxia and high oxygen pressure (Webster and Ames, 1965; Van

Harreveld and Khattab, 1967; Dolivo and Rouiller, 1969; Williams and Grossman, 1970) and the influence of enriched or impoverished environments on the size and number of synaptic junctions (Møllgaard Diamond, Bennett, Rosenzweig and Lindner, 1971). The overall relevance of such studies, and the reason for their importance to an understanding of synaptogenesis, is that they raise the question of brain and neuronal plasticity (Bennett, Diamond, Krech and Rosenzweig, 1964; Bernstein and Bernstein, 1973) and more specifically of synaptic plasticity (Cragg, 1968; 1971).

Underlying present concepts of synaptogenesis at the ultrastructural level is a firm light microscope base which has contributed much useful information on the major changes occurring during the cytoarchitectural differentiation of various brain regions (e.g. Ramón y Cajal, 1911; Eayrs and Goodhead, 1959; Schadé and Baxter, 1960; Noback and Purpura, 1961). Also of relevance are the EM investigations directed towards identifying neuronal and neuroglial cell types, as a background to synaptic morphogenesis. In addition to morphological studies of synaptic development therefore, others have concentrated on an understanding of the maturation of neurons (Caley and Maxwell, 1968a; Meller, Breipohl and Glees, 1968, 1969; Schwartz, Pappas and Purpura, 1968), neuroglia (Caley and Maxwell, 1968b), blood vessels (Pappas and Purpura, 1964; Caley and Maxwell, 1970), extracellular space (Karlsson, 1967; Pysh, 1969; Caley and Maxwell, 1970) and neuronal mitochondria (Pysh, 1970).

Synaptic studies are diverse and numerous, although the majority have concentrated on cerebral cortex, with an increasing number investigating cerebellar cortex and spinal cord. Table 1.3 summarizes some of the principal studies to date.

Table 1.3   Representative ultrastructural studies of vertebrate synaptogenesis

Species and brain region	Investigators
Rat cerebral cortex	Aghajanian and Bloom, 1967c
	Armstrong-James and Johnson, 1970
	Johnson and Armstrong-James, 1970
	Gelzer, 1970
	Caley and Maxwell, 1971
Rat cerebellar cortex	Altman, 1971
	Bloom, 1972b
Rat dentate gyrus	Cotman et al., 1973
	Crain et al., 1973
Rat superior colliculus; inferior colliculus	Lund and Lund, 1972; Pysh, 1969
Rat spinal cord cultures	Bunge et al., 1967
Cat cerebral cortex	Voeller et al., 1963
	Adinolfi, 1971b, 1972a, b
	Cragg, 1972b
Mouse cerebellum	Larramendi, 1969
Mouse hypothalamus cultures	Masurovsky et al., 1971
Chick cerebellar cortex	Mugnaini and Forstrønen, 1967
	Mugnaini, 1970
Chick spinal cord	Glees and Sheppard, 1964
	Oppenheim and Foelix, 1972
	Stelzner et al., 1973
Chick ciliary ganglion	Hamori and Dyachkova, 1964
Monkey spinal cord	Bodian, 1966a, 1968
Dog cerebral cortex	Molliver and Van der Loos, 1970
Human spinal cord	Malinský, 1972
	Purpura, 1973

1.4.1 Quantitative studies

Quantitative data on synaptogenesis are sparse and uncoordinated. Employing the glutaraldehyde–PTA method Aghajanian and Bloom (1967c) reported a rapid increase in the number of synaptic junctions in the molecular layer of rat parietal cortex between the 14th and 26th postnatal days, whereas Armstrong-James and Johnson (1970) using osmicated material noted a sharp rise between 4 and 14 days postnatal in superficial motor cortex of the rat. The disparity between these estimates may reflect any one of a number of factors. Aghajanian and Bloom (1967c) did not examine material younger than 12 days postnatal, thereby excluding the critical period of postnatal development. The different methods of tissue preparation may have introduced a difference factor (see Jones, Dittmer and Reading,1974), although discriminating use of both methods should yield reliable results. It is not clear whether the same layers of cortex were examined; if not, the differential rate of synaptic development in different layers may account for some discrepancy (Molliver and Van der Loos, 1970; Cragg, 1972b), although it is unlikely that this alone would account for such a large one.

In the molecular layer of rat cerebellar cortex Bloom (1972b) noted that the rate of synapse formation accelerated after 9 days postnatal and even more so between 14 and 20 days. Analysis of his figures however, reveals that the most dramatic increase is between 12 and 14 days, with a gradual overall increase throughout the postnatal period up to 20 days. Karlsson (1967), working on rat lateral geniculate nucleus, observed a sharp rise in synaptic numbers 7 to 13 days after birth.

Turning to cat visual cortex Cragg (1972b) noted a steep increase in synapses from 7 days after birth to a peak at 36 days, while the number of synapses per neuron followed a similar curve. One of the surprising features commented on by Cragg was that at 8 days after birth the average number of synapses per cell is 112, 1·5% of the adult number, although the specificity of some cortical units for orientation and direction of stimulus movement has developed by this age (Cragg, 1972b). In line with this, Crain, Cotman, Taylor and Lynch (1973), examining the molecular layer of rat dentate gyrus, noted that less than 1% of the adult number of synapses are present 4 days after birth and less than 5% at 11 days. They also noted that the total number of synapses doubles each day between 4 and 11 days, while it increases 100-fold between 4 days and the adult condition.

The above studies suffer from two major drawbacks: not only are they confined to one parameter, they are also based on the assumption that the synapses within the brain area under investigation develop at a uniform rate. In order to overcome these limiting factors, it is necessary to distinguish between regions within any one brain area and investigate synaptic development within each of these. A start has been made in this direction by Molliver and Van der Loos (1970) by investigating the spatial distribution of synapses in somesthetic cortex of newborn dog. They were able to demonstrate that synaptic contacts develop at different rates depending on their depth within the cortex. Strata of high synaptic density alternate with strata of low synaptic density, and these in turn bear a definite relationship to cytoarchitectonic layers. Furthermore they postulated that the earliest synapses are established deep in the cortex. Cragg (1972b) found equivalent strata in foetal cat visual cortex and demonstrated that, by contrast, the density of synapses is remarkably even in the adult. Cragg also observed that a large increase in synaptic density occurs in the deeper layers of cat visual cortex between postnatal days 1 to 8, and in the superficial layers between days 8 to 27.

1.4.2 Sequences of synaptic development

One of the remarkable features of synaptic development is the general nature of the processes involved. As the developmental sequences are followed in a wide range of species and CNS regions similar principles emerge with almost monotonous regularity (e.g. Purpura, Shofer, Housepian and Noback, 1964; Larramendi, 1969; Adinolfi, 1972a; Lund and Lund, 1972). Consequently it is not difficult to sketch an overall scheme of synaptogenesis in vertebrates as depicted in Table 1.4, with the proviso that the seq-

Table 1.4   Principal stages in synaptogenesis

Stage 1*	Synapses recognizable as short contacts plus few vesicles presynaptically
	Vesicles variable in shape; mainly round
	Only axodendritic synapses†
	Membranes undifferentiated or symmetrically thickened
	Ribosomes presynaptically†
Stage 2	Increasing number of synaptic vesicles
	Flattened vesicles in addition to round ones
	Axosomatic synapses present
	Membranes thickening, leading to asymmetry of axodendritic junctions
	Dendritic spines appear
Stage 3	Further increases in vesicle numbers
	Considerable increase in number of junctions
	Further increase in membrane thickening
	Greater percentage of junctions demonstrate adult features
	Spine apparatus appears

* The distinction between the stages is arbitrary, individual junctions varying greatly in their maturity
† There is no universal agreement over these points

quence of events follows a different time course in the different situations, while the relationship between synaptic and behavioural development may be variable in different species (Stelzner, Martin and Scott, 1973). For accounts of synaptic development in a number of specific loci consult Voeller, Pappas and Purpura, (1963), Schwartz *et al.* (1968), Johnson and Armstrong-James (1970), Masurovsky, Benitez and Murray (1971), Oppenheim and Foelix (1972), Adinolfi (1972a), Bloom (1972b), Malinsky (1972), Alley (1973), Cotman, Taylor and Lynch (1973) and Stelzner *et al.* (1973). The observations of Jones and Revell (1970a) on synaptosomal development are also relevant (see Section 3.5.3).

Synaptic junctions first appear as short contacts with a minimal number of synaptic vesicles alongside the presynaptic membrane, and lacking any clear ultrastructural distinction between pre- and postsynaptic membranes (Plate 1.23 inset). This latter feature may be so marked as to suggest a desmosome-like appearance and function for these early synapses. Poorly-defined electron–opaque material is usually present at the cleft region, constituting part of the extracellular space which is relatively extensive in early development (Pysh, 1969; Johnson and Armstrong-James, 1970).

Not only are the synaptic vesicles small in number in the initial stages of synaptic development, they are variable in size and possibly also in shape (Jones and Revell, 1970a). They are however, spherical rather than flattened in aldehyde-fixed material (Oppenheimer and Foelix, 1972), as befits the axodendritic character of the endings (compare Plates 1.23 and 1.24). It is usually acknowledged that the appearance of axodendritic endings precedes that of axosomatic ones (Voeller *et al.*, 1963), although it is possible to find reports to the contrary, for example, Cragg (1972b) in cat visual cortex and Alley (1973) in the trigeminal mesencephalic nucleus. In accordance with this general theory it has been suggested by Mugnaini (1970) that the asymmetrical axodendritic contacts are formed at an earlier stage of maturation of the postsynaptic element than the symmetrical axosomatic ones.

The presence of synaptic vesicles in the initial stages of synaptic development may appear to prejudge an important issue in synaptogenesis, namely whether vesicles or membrane thickenings constitute the first step in the development of a synapse. Discussion on this point is better delayed until consideration of paramembranous densities in the next section (1.4.3). It is pertinent to point out however, that synaptic vesicles constitute the only reliable criterion of a primitive synaptic junction, as symmetrical membrane thickenings are just as likely to be nonsynaptic in origin in the absence of specific synaptic characteristics. This does not preclude the possibility that, due to the plane of section, asymmetrical synaptic junctions may be seen in the absence of vesicles (Molliver and Van der Loos, 1970).

With further development synaptic vesicles increase in number in the presynaptic terminal and are more frequently accompanied by at least one mitochondrion (Plate 1.24). The ribosomes, which some workers claim occur presynaptically in early development (Bunge, Bunge and Peterson, 1967; Caley and Maxwell, 1968a), become confined to their adult postsynaptic and dendritic situation. As the area of contact between pre- and postsynaptic terminals increases the electron–density of the membranes is transformed into conspicuous thickenings. This applies particularly to the postsynaptic membrane which adopts its characteristic thickened aspect, giving to the junctions their typical asymmetrical appearance in axodendritic junctions. Axosomatic synapses increase in number, as do flattened vesicles in certain terminals (Plate 1.24). Dendritic spines make their appearance by the tenth postnatal day (cat neocortex – Adinolfi, 1971b; Cragg, 1972b), although a readily identifiable spine apparatus is not present until the third postnatal week (Adinolfi, 1971b). Shapiro *et al.* (1973) observed spines as early as 4 days in rat visual cortex, although it was not until 12 to 14 days after birth that their density had increased to approximately 50% of that at maturity, their most rapid growth occurring at 8 to 14 days. An interesting observation was made by Cotman *et al.* (1973) in dentate gyrus where at 25 days complex spine formation was still incomplete, in contrast to synaptogenesis itself.

While it is possible to categorize synaptic development in a systematic fashion, it is unwise to adopt too rigid a scheme. The synaptic junctions observed at any one day during early development vary considerably in appearance and stage of maturation. Furthermore junctional components may be at different stages of development, so that for instance the membrane thickenings at a junction may appear more mature than the synaptic vesicles (e.g. Johnson and Armstrong-James, 1970, Fig. 8).

Although we are not directly concerned here with correlating ultrastructural and electrical changes during development (e.g. Crain and Bornstein, 1964 in cultures of mouse cerebral cortex; Nilsson and Crescitelli, 1969, 1970 in frog retina), an interesting study deserves mention. Model, Bornstein, Crain and Pappas (1971), after exposing explants of foetal mouse cerebral cortex to xylocaine, examined their synaptic junctions at various intervals following explanation. They found that, in spite of the absence of electrical impulse activity, synaptic development continued normally. From these observations they concluded that the potential for complex bioelectrical activity can develop in the absence of its expression, and that organized neuronal assemblies are formed in forward reference to their ultimate function. Further studies are required to relate these findings to those in which failure of synaptic transmission is produced by other factors, such as ischaemia and glucose deprivation (Webster and Ames, 1965; Dolivo and Rouiller, 1969).

1.4.3 Paramembranous densities

The essential features of the paramembranous densities at adult synaptic junctions have already been considered (Section 1.3.1). They are principally delineated by fixation in glutaraldehyde and block-staining with PTA (or BIUL), techniques of outstanding importance for study of the dense projections, cleft densities and postsynaptic thickening and focal densities. The use of this technique for analysing the maturation of the paramembranous densities is in its infancy, but is already provoking searching questions and suggesting intriguing concepts.

Aghajanian and Bloom (1967c) first made use of this stain to examine the formation of synaptic junctions in rat cerebral cortex. Their chief concern was to sample areas of brain at relatively low magnifications. A similar study by Bloom (1972b) repeated and extended these initial observations in rat cerebellar cortex. Jones and Revell (1970b) working with synaptosomes, outlined the essential changes in paramembranous densities during postnatal development of rat cerebral cortex (Section 3.5.3), work repeated by Adinolfi (1972b) on intact cat cerebral cortex. Further investigations by Jones and co-workers (Jones, 1973c; Jones et al., 1974; Nolan, 1974) have concentrated on the developmental sequences in guinea-pig cerebral and cerebellar cortices.

In the brain regions of rat and cat so far examined, there is strong evidence that the paramembranous densities first appear as continuous plaques (Aghajanian and Bloom, 1967c; Jones and Revell, 1970b; Adinolfi, 1972b). As development proceeds these undergo gradual differentiation giving rise presynaptically to interconnected dense triangular profiles (Jones and Revell, 1970b) which enlarge and separate to form discrete dense projections. The solid plate-like form of the cleft material focalizes to form the cleft densities of the adult, while the continuous postsynaptic thickening undergoes a limited degree of aggregation to produce the postsynaptic focal densities of the mature junction. In general terms early synaptic junctions are roughly symmetrical in outline, and become asymmetrical with maturation (refer to Fig. 3.7 for synaptosomal development).

While this evidence strongly suggests that the dense projections pre-exist in the form of a solid plaque or membrane thickening, it provides no information concerning the factor or factors responsible for their emergence. Akert and Pfenninger (1969) postulated that it is the presence of synaptic vesicles in the presynaptic terminal which provides the required stimulus. In an attempt to test this theory Jones and Revell (1970b) obtained data from both conventional and non-osmicated material, and compared the increase in height of dense projections and the increase in numbers of synaptic vesicles during post-natal development. They found a close correlation between the two, pointing to the possibility of a functional connection between the presence in the presynaptic ending of synaptic vesicles and the maturation of dense projections.

The question of the primacy of synaptic vesicles or dense projections remains. Vesicles are present however, when pre- and postsynaptic membranes are plaque-like in conventional and non-osmicated material (Jones and Revell, 1970a, b), from which it may be concluded that synaptic vesicles appear prior to dense projections but not necessarily prior to the thickening of the membranes at future synaptic sites. The evidence required to answer this latter point is disputable, in view of the inevitable difficulty encountered in identifying future synaptic sites in the absence of vesicles. However, once the process by which dense projections originate has been inaugurated, further enlargement and the establishment of adult connections are closely associated with the presence of a requisite number of synaptic vesicles (Jones and Revell, 1970b).

A number of investigators have stated that membrane thickenings are formed before synaptic vesicles (e.g. Glees and Sheppard, 1964, Hámori and Dyachkova, 1964; Larramendi, 1969; Tennyson, 1970; Alley, 1973; Stelzner et al., 1973), although the evidence presented by different workers varies regarding its reliability and the significance of its findings. In addition these studies were performed on osmicated material. Others have viewed the appearance of the vesicles and membranes as simultaneous events (Ochi, 1967; Bodian, 1968).

As it is hazardous to draw firm conclusions on the exact sequence of events, alternative approaches merit consideration. One of these revolves around the role of coated vesicles (Section 1.3.3). These are frequently observed in developing neurons, either as formed vesicles or invaginations of a limiting membrane (e.g. Johnson and Armstrong-James, 1970; Altman, 1971; Masurovsky et al., 1971; Stelzner, 1971; Stelzner et al., 1973), and they assume the major role in synaptogenesis according to the theory propounded by Altman (1971). This states that the coated vesicles provide future synapses with transient adhesion membranes or lasting synaptic dense membranes. Underlying it is the assumption that the formation of adhesion sites is the first step in synaptogenesis (Weiss, 1947), while the most direct evidence presented in favour of the theory is the presence of coated vesicles in the vicinity of cell processes characterized by synaptic relationships in older animals (Altman, 1971). Attractive as this theory is, it does not answer the question of the primacy of thickened membranes or synaptic vesicles in synaptogenesis, although it does highlight the possible role of coated vesicles in certain aspects of this process.

41

It is also pertinent to point out that coated vesicle fusions were observed recipro-
cally on apposed membranes, even though these membranes were not related synaptically
in a reciprocal way (Stelzner *et al.*, 1973). An adaptation of this theory is that of Stelzner
and co-workers who postulate that coated vesicles may be involved, not in the formation
of synaptic junctions, but in their subsequent growth or maintenance.

Leaving aside these questions, the study of the development of the paramembranous
densities is important in providing criteria for judging the extent of synaptic maturation.
Bloom (1972b), for instance, in a study of postnatal (3 to 20 days) rat cerebellar cortex,
reported an increase in the number of dense projections per junction with development.
This, coupled with a failure to detect any changes in the dimensions of dense projections
or of the cleft, led him to conclude that the principal morphological change during
maturation is a gradual increase in the number and density of dense projections.

From a complementary study by Jones and co-workers (Jones, 1973c; Jones *et al.*, 1974)
on pre- and postnatal guinea-pig cerebral cortex three indices emerged as important
indicators of synaptic maturity, namely, the height and base width of the dense projections which increase during development and the cleft width which decreases (Fig. 1.8).

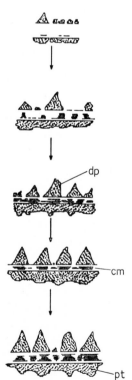

Figure 1.8   Diagram to illustrate the principal stages in the development of synaptic junctions in PTA-stained guinea-pig cerebral cortex.
There is a narrowing of the cleft with maturation, an increase in the
size and orderliness of the dense projections (dp), plus building-up
of the cleft material (cm) and focalization of the postsynaptic thickening (pt). (Modified from Jones *et al.*, 1974.)

Other indices examined, such as the number of dense projections per junction and the
length of the junction could not be correlated with developmental stages. The discrepancy
between these results and those of Bloom may be due in part to a real difference in

paramembranous maturational processes in guinea-pig and rat, and in part to a differential staining reaction on the part of the PTA (Jones *et al.*, 1974). Both possibilities need be borne in mind on account of the unusual initial appearances of guinea-pig synaptic junctions which are characterized by a dense postsynaptic thickening and barely discernible dense projections and cleft material (Jones, 1973c; compare Plates 1.25 and 1.26). Further work is required to elucidate this problem, and decide the selectivity of the PTA staining in early development (Woodward, Hoffer, Siggins and Bloom, 1971; Del Cerro and Snider, 1972; West, 1974).

Chapter 2: The Preparation of Synaptosomes and Derivatives

2.1 THE DEVELOPMENT OF TECHNIQUES

2.1.1 Background

It is characteristic of the human enterprise that ideas in a particular realm do not develop in isolation from the currents of thought in neighbouring ones. Similarly, technical developments have a way of influencing more than one sphere of activity. It is not surprising then to find that the emergence of subcellular fractionation (e.g. Bensley and Hoerr, 1934; Dounce, 1943; Claude, 1946) as a major technique of experimental biology should have resulted in the isolation of a wide range of subcellular organelles at much the same time.

Initial studies were directed towards distinguishing nuclear, mitochondrial and microsomal fractions (Schneider, 1946; Hogeboom, Schneider and Palade, 1948; Palade, 1951; Schneider and Hogeboom, 1951), with different workers concentrating upon the different fractions, that is, nuclei (Dounce, 1943), mitochondria (Berthet and De Duve, 1951; De Duve, Berthet, Berthet and Appelmans, 1951) and microsomes (Palade and Siekevitz, 1956a, b).

With progress underway on the basic components of the cell other workers turned their attention towards specialized particles, amongst which can be mentioned chromaffin granules (Blaschko and Welsch, 1953; Blaschko, Hagen and Welsch, 1955; Blaschko, Hagen and Hagen, 1957), lysosomes (De Duve, 1963a), glycogen granules (Drochmans, 1962), lipofuscin granules (Björkerud, 1963) and zymogen granules (Greene, Hirs and Palade, 1963). Meanwhile, other studies had as their prime objective the isolation of storage granules containing, for example, histamine (Hagen, Barnett and Lee, 1959), catecholamines (see Blaschko, 1959), and vasopressin and oxytocin (Weinstein, Malamed and Sachs, 1961; Sachs, 1961; LaBella, Beaulieu and Reiffenstein, 1962; Barer, Heller and Lederis, 1963; LaBella, Reiffenstein and Beaulieu, 1963; LaBella and Sanwal, 1965).

Using the techniques which had become part-and-parcel of such subcellular fractionation studies early attempts were made by Brody and Bain (1951) and Abood, Cavanaugh, Tschirgi and Gerard (1951) at fractionating nervous tissue. The principal interest of these early studies centred on the 'mitochondrial' fraction, and although the increased complexity and number of cell types in the CNS as compared with the liver for example were not overlooked, the brain fractions obtained were regarded as analogous to fractions from other tissues (Brody and Bain, 1952). The 'mitochondrial' fraction was so named because of its biochemical similarity to liver mitochondria, and on account of the cytochemical properties of its constituent particles (Brody and Bain, 1952). Homogenization was initially carried out in 0·7 or 0·88M sucrose but was reduced to 0·25M, as the resultant preparations using hyperosmotic sucrose were of low oxidative phosphorylative activity. In general terms these studies together with that of Abood, Gerard, Banks and Tschirgi (1952) demonstrated that the distribution pattern of enzymes in nervous tissue was the same as that in liver and kidney, the glycolytic enzymes were soluble, while the enzymes responsible for oxidative phosphorylation were associated with particles having histological and sedimentation characteristics similar to those of mitochondria.

2.1.2 Acetylcholine system and synaptosomes

It was not until 1956 that the distribution of a member of the ACh system was investigated in brain fractions. Directing their attention towards the fractions sedimenting at 12 000g and 15 000g, the 'mitochondrial' fractions, Hebb and Smallman (1956) noted that 52–69% of the choline acetyltransferase (choline acetylase; ChAc) was located in these fractions. Assuming that these fractions contained only mitochondria (cf. Brody and Bain, 1952), they concluded that this enzyme, which is responsible for synthesizing ACh, is firmly bound in mitochondria. In order to activate the enzyme Hebb and Smallman (1956) found it necessary to treat the crude mitochondrial fraction with ether or acetone, a finding consistent with the earlier experiments of Stedman and Stedman (1937, 1939), and Feldberg (1945), pointing to a localization of the enzyme within a membrane-bound compartment (see Whittaker, 1965).

In a follow-up study Hebb and Whittaker (1958) investigated the subcellular distribution of ACh and its relation to the distribution of ChAc. Both sedimented in the crude mitochondrial fraction and generally in the same subfractions. 70 to 75% of the total tissue ACh remained in the bound form on homogenization, while on differential centrifugation all the free ACh and the ChAc of the original homogenate were recovered in the high speed supernatant fraction. The bound ACh and occluded ChAc were recovered in the particulate fractions. They concluded therefore that both reside in the same subcellular particle although, on histological and enzymatic grounds, it was becoming evident that this particle while in the crude mitochondrial fraction was not synonymous with the mitochondria.

In an attempt to characterize this ACh-containing particle Whittaker (1959) refined the centrifugation procedures, extended the biochemical investigations and employed EM to identify the constituents of some of the fractions. In resolving the crude mitochondrial fraction into three distinct subfractions on a sucrose density gradient, he conclusively demonstrated the heterogeneity of the so-called mitochondrial fraction. Furthermore he was able to show by means of EM examination that the densest subfraction mainly consisted of mitochondria, an observation in agreement with the high level of succinate dehydrogenase (SDH) in this subfraction. The particles in the subfraction of intermediate density he readily distinguished from mitochondria, as they were vesicular in appearance and contained a significant proportion of the bound ACh, 5-hydroxytryptamine (5-HT) and acid phosphatase of the brain. Unfortunately, he underestimated their dimensions and mistakenly equated them with synaptic vesicles (40 to 50 nm in diameter) rather than the pinched-off nerve terminal itself (0·5 μm in diameter), an error rectified in subsequent work (Gray and Whittaker, 1960, 1962; Whittaker and Gray, 1962).

Another important point to emerge from Whittaker's study (1959), and one which laid the basis for future ideas, concerned the concept of bound ACh. Evidence was obtained for two forms – a *labile fraction* released by mildly disruptive techniques and behaving 'as though it were imprisoned in the free state inside a membrane which is readily damaged by osmotic dilution, and freezing and thawing', and a more *stable fraction* which is held by chemical forces, including ionic bonds, to the particle matrix.

The improved EM techniques necessary for accurate identification of the sub-fraction rich in bound ACh were provided by Gray and Whittaker (1962), who showed that it consisted principally of particles derived from nerve endings (Fig. 2.1). These

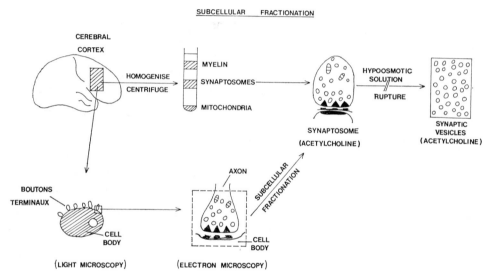

Fig. 2.1 A schematic diagram to illustrate the derivation of synaptosomes from brain tissue by subcellular fractionation. The relationship of synaptosomes to intact synapses is also depicted.

nerve ending particles or *synaptosomes* (Whittaker *et al.*, 1964; Section 3.1), as they were shortly to become known, were packed with synaptic vesicles and were extremely fragile, a property which probably accounted for the earlier difficulties experienced in identifying them. The subdivision of the crude mitochondrial fraction was now clear: the lightest subfraction (A) consisted largely of myelin fragments, the intermediate subfraction (B) was the synaptosomal fraction, while the densest subfraction (C) was confirmed as the mitochondrial element (Plates 2.1 to 2.3).

Gray and Whittaker (1962) also outlined the morphology of the nuclear and micro-somal fractions, describing nuclei and tissue fragments in the former and vesicular profiles and ribosomes in the latter. Only Hanzon and Toschi (1959) had previously described the ultrastructural features of a brain microsomal fraction with any accuracy, while Petrushka and Giuditta (1959) had failed to recognize synaptosomes isolated from rat cerebral cortex due to the hypertonic conditions (0·88M sucrose) of their homogenizing medium.

While Whittaker and his associates were defining the constituents and making a start on elucidating the biochemical properties of brain subcellular fractions, De Robertis and his colleagues (De Robertis, Pellegrino De Iraldi, Rodriguez and Gomez, 1961a; De Robertis et al., 1961b) working independently were arriving at similar, although not identical, results. It was clear to them that Whittaker's (1959) 'synaptic vesicles' could not be synaptic vesicles on account of their size and sedimentation properties, and they produced some remarkably good micrographs of synaptosomes containing synaptic vesicles, coated vesicles and mitochondria (De Robertis et al., 1961). On further centrifugation a 'microsomal' fraction was obtained, two subfractions of which were essentially composed of synaptic vesicles, although their purity and ultrastructural quality left much to be desired.

Refinement of centrifugation procedures (De Robertis, Pellegrino De Iraldi, Rodriguez De Lores Arnaiz and Salganicoff, 1962a) produced five subfractions from the mitochondrial fraction, the principal difference between this scheme and that proposed by Gray and Whittaker (1962) being a subdivision of the synaptosomal fraction into three (contrast Schemes 2.1 and 2.2). Two of the subfractions (C and D) contained synaptosomes, but differed in their content of bound ACh and acetylcholinesterase (AChE). On this basis De Robertis et al. (1962a) distinguished between cholinergic synaptosomes (C) and non-cholinergic ones (D).

The obvious next step was to devise a procedure for disrupting the synaptosomes and releasing their components, and of these isolating the synaptic vesicles as a separate subfraction. Whittaker et al. (1964) and Whittaker and Sheridan (1965) achieved this by suspending synaptosomes in media hypotonic to plasma and then subjecting them to differential density gradient centrifugation. Using their techniques fractions were obtained consisting of soluble cytoplasmic components, synaptic vesicles, microsomes, larger membrane fragments, partially disrupted synaptosomes and mitochondria (Fig. 2.5). Bound ACh was found partly in the synaptic vesicle fraction and partly in the fraction containing incompletely disrupted synaptosomes; lactate dehydrogenase (LDH), potassium and ChAc were recovered mainly in the soluble cytoplasmic fraction; SDH appeared in the mitochondrial fraction and AChE in the microsome and large membrane fractions. It is notable that the results of these workers suggest that the three components of the ACh system (ACh, ChAc, and AChE) have separate localizations within the synaptic region.

It is on this latter point that De Robertis's findings are in conflict with Whittaker's. De Robertis, Rodriguez De Lores Arnaiz and Pellegrino De Iraldi (1962) obtained a synaptic vesicle fraction without employing differential density gradient centrifugation and found that ChAc as well as bound ACh was concentrated in it. Although AChE was also concentrated in the vesicle fraction about 70% of it was in the fraction containing ruptured synaptosomes, pointing to its localization at synaptosomal membranes. Possible reasons for this disagreement concerning the distribution of ChAc will be discussed in a subsequent section (Section 2.4.2).

2.1.3 Synaptosomal derivatives

Over recent years a growing number of techniques has become available to neuro-biologists for the isolation of an ever-increasing range of components of the nerve terminal (Table 2.1). Starting with the isolation of the terminal itself – the synaptosome*

Table 2.1 Principal investigations aimed at isolating components of the nerve terminal from mammalian brain

Component separated	Investigators	Type of gradient/centrifugation
Synaptosomes	Gray and Whittaker, 1962	Discontinuous sucrose gradient
	De Robertis *et al.*, 1962a	Discontinuous sucrose gradient
	Kurokawa *et al.*, 1965a, b	Discontinuous Ficoll gradient
	Whittaker, 1968a	Continuous sucrose gradient
	Kornguth *et al.*, 1969	Discontinuous sucrose and continuous caesium chloride gradients
	Kornguth *et al.*, 1971	Discontinuous sucrose and continuous caesium chloride gradients/zonal centrifugation
	Lagercrantz and Pertoft, 1972	Continuous Ludox and discontinuous sucrose gradients
	Baldessarini and Vogt, 1971	Ultrafiltration
Synaptic vesicles	De Robertis *et al.*, 1963	Discontinuous sucrose gradient
	Whittaker *et al.*, 1964	Discontinuous sucrose gradient
	Vos *et al.*, 1968	Sucrose gradient electrophoresis
	Ryan *et al.*, 1971	Free-flow electrophoresis
	Kadota and Kanaseki, 1969	Differential centrifugation and DAEA-Sephadex column chromatography
Synaptic plasma membranes	Rodriguez de Lores Arnaiz *et al.*, 1967	Discontinuous sucrose gradient
	Cotman and Matthews,1971	Discontinuous Ficoll and discontinuous sucrose gradients
	Cotman *et al.*, 1968a	Continuous sucrose gradient/zonal centrifugation
	McBride *et al.*, 1970	Continuous sucrose gradient/zonal centrifugation
Synaptic (junctional) complexes	De Robertis *et al.*, 1967a	Continuous Ficoll gradient/Triton X-100
	Cotman *et al.*, 1971b	Discontinuous Ficoll and discontinuous sucrose gradients/Triton X-100
	Cotman and Taylor, 1972	Discontinuous sucrose gradient/Triton X-100
	Davis and Bloom, 1973	Discontinuous sucrose gradient/Triton X-100
Postsynaptic membranes	Garey *et al.*, 1972	Continuous Ficoll and continuous sucrose gradients

(Whittaker, 1959; Gray and Whittaker, 1960, 1962; De Robertis *et al.*, 1961a, b, 1962a) – attention was quickly directed towards the isolation of synaptic vesicles (De Robertis *et al.*, 1963; Whittaker *et al.*, 1964; Whittaker and Sheridan, 1965). Following the successful preparation of highly enriched fractions of these constituents of the nerve terminal, interest was directed towards other components of the terminal, namely the synaptic membrane (Rodriguez de Lores Arnaiz, Alberici and De Robertis, 1967; De Robertis, Rodriguez de Lores Arnaiz, Alberici, Butcher and Sutherland, 1967b; Cotman, Mahler

* The term *synaptosome* was originated by Whittaker and co-workers (Whittaker *et al.*, 1964; Whittaker, 1965) and refers to the nerve-ending particle or simply nerve ending of earlier studies (e.g. Gray and Whittaker, 1962; De Robertis *et al.*, 1962a). See Section 3.1 for further discussion.

and Anderson, 1968a; Cotman, Mahler and Haga, 1968b; Koch, 1969; Cotman and Matthews, 1971; Morgan, Reith, Marinari, Breckenridge and Gombos, 1972), the synaptic (or junctional) complex (De Robertis, Azcurra and Fiszer, 1967a; Kornguth, Anderson and Scott, 1969; Kornguth, Flangas, Siegel, Geison, O'Brien, Lamar and Scott, 1971; Sellinger, Lodin and Azcurra, 1972) and the postsynaptic membrane (Garey et al., 1972).

Accompanying this expanding range of interest there has been a proliferation in the range of techniques at the disposal of workers. Consequently, while initial and many later studies employed only discontinuous sucrose gradients (e.g. Gray and Whittaker, 1962; De Robertis et al., 1962a; 1963), a wealth of additional techniques have been adapted for use with brain tissue. Among these can be mentioned continuous sucrose gradients (Whittaker, 1968a), continuous and discontinuous Ficoll gradients (Kurokawa, Sakamoto and Kato, 1965a; Abdel-Latif, 1966; De Robertis et al., 1967a; Autilio, Appel, Pettis and Gambetti, 1968; Flexner, Gambetti, Flexner and Roberts, 1971; Cotman and Matthews, 1971; Haga, 1971; Garey et al., 1972), caesium chloride gradients (Kornguth, Anderson, Scott and Kubinski, 1967; Kornguth et al., 1969, 1971; Kornguth, Flangas, Geison and Scott, 1972) and colloidal silica gradients (Lagercrantz and Pertoft, 1972). Other techniques include zonal centrifugation (Mahaley, Day, Anderson, Wilfong and Brater, 1968; Cotman et al., 1968a, b; Mahler and Cotman, 1970; Festoff, Appel and Day, 1971), various forms of electrophoretic separation (Hannig, 1967; Vos, Kuriyama and Roberts, 1968; Sellinger and Borens, 1969; Ryan, Kalant and Thomas, 1971) and the use of diethylaminoethyl (DAEA) – Sephadex column chromatography to purify vesicle fractions (Kadota and Kanaseki, 1969). In addition methods have been devised for preparing subcellular fractions using Millipore filters (Baldessarini and Vogt, 1971) and from small amounts of tissue by a microscale modification of conventional techniques (Giacobini, Hökfelt, Kerpel-Fronius, Koslow, Mitchard and Noré, 1971).

2.1.4 Neurons and glia

Although outside the immediate scope of this book reference must be made to fractionation procedures directed towards separating neurons from glia, and the subsequent studies on the morphological and biochemical characteristics of these elements and their constituent organelles. The importance of these studies for synaptosomal investigations lies in the possibility of contamination of synaptosomal fractions by one or more of these elements, a factor largely ignored in much synaptosomal work.

Attempts at isolating neurons and glia from central nervous tissue have employed a number of approaches. In one approach single cells are micro-dissected in the presence of isotonic solutions (Hydén, 1959; Roots and Johnston, 1965; Bondareff and Hydén, 1969), or they may be disrupted by sieving (Roots and Johnston, 1964; Johnston and Roots, 1965). Although a number of these preparations are morphologically homogeneous the quantity of tissue is insufficient for routine biochemical investigations. A second approach therefore, producing neuronal and glial enrichments on a bulk scale

(Rose, 1965, 1967, 1969; Satake and Abe, 1966; Fewster, Scheibel and Mead, 1967; Satake, Hasegawa, Abe and Tanake, 1968; Blomstrand and Hamberger, 1969; Henn and Hamberger, 1972), appeared to offer considerable advantages to the biochemist. This type of approach however, also has deficiencies, one of the chief ones being that of morphological heterogeneity. In this respect the procedure of Rose (1965, 1967) has been severely criticized (Cremer, Johnston, Roots and Trevor, 1968; Johnston and Roots, 1970, 1972), criticisms which to an extent have been acknowledged (Rose, 1968; Rose and Sinha, 1969) and which may have contributed to modifications of the original technique. A modification of the Rose technique by Flangas and Bowman (1968) using zonal centrifugation has been claimed to produce intact neuronal perikarya, although the number of intact cells so produced is unknown, and detailed ultrastructural studies were not performed.

The technique of Norton and Poduslo (1970) for the isolation of neurons, astroglia and oligodendroglia involves trypsinization and fractionation of the brain tissue on sucrose gradients (see also Poduslo and Norton, 1972). Although trypsin has an adverse effect on the properties of neural membranes (Somogyi, 1968) on ultrastructural study of the isolated neurons and glia has shown that a triple-layered plasma membrane is constantly present, while the fractions are essentially free of contaminants (Raine, Poduslo and Norton, 1971).

It is wise to bear in mind that, as Johnston and Roots (1970) point out in their review of this literature, one of the difficulties in assessing work in this field is the definition of the term 'isolated neuronal and glial perikarya', let alone the meaning of 'pure' and 'enriched' when referring to the morphological and biochemical assessment of fractions. Furthermore, as Johnston and Roots also stress 'it is imperative that questions regarding the cellular integrity of these fractions be answered *before* they are extensively used for postulations regarding the chemical events . . .' (italics are mine). In line with Bocci (1966) they draw attention to the fact that slight glial contamination of a neuronal environment may lead to erroneous evaluation of enzyme content. These strictures are timely, and should be heeded as much in synaptosomal studies as in neuronal–glial investigations.

Allied to the above investigations are the studies of Henn, Hansson and Hamberger (1972), designed to isolate neuronal plasma membranes; of Kuenzle, Pelloni and Kistler (1972) to isolate neuronal membranes rich in AChE; and at a different level the subfractionation by Cotman, Herschman and Taylor (1971a) of a clonal line of glial cells. Within neurons, a certain amount of interest has been shown in preparing enriched fractions of nonmyelinated axons (Lemkey-Johnston and Larramendi, 1968; Lemkey-Johnston and Dekirmenjian, 1970; De Vries, Norton and Raine, 1972), as this opens the way to biochemical characterization of otherwise inaccessible axons from the mammalian CNS. Taking fractionation further a start has been made in separating neuronal (and perhaps glial as well) organelles, such as microtubules (Kirkpatrick, 1969) and filaments (Shelanski, Albert, De Vries and Norton, 1971), from mammalian brain. Both procedures offer promising methods of isolating and purifying these organelles, and hence of studying their function and dynamics.

2.1.5 Non-mammalian synaptosomes and synaptic vesicles

A limited number of fractionation studies have been carried out on invertebrate and *Torpedo* nervous tissue, and have employed either discontinuous density gradients or zonal centrifugation to isolate the synaptosomes and synaptic vesicles. Synaptosomes have been characterized morphologically and biochemically from ganglia of *Octopus* (Jones, 1967; Florey and Winesdorfer, 1968; Martin *et al.*, 1969) and *Loligo* (Heilbronn, Hause and Lundgren, 1971; Welsch and Dettbarn, 1972; Dowdall and Whittaker, 1973) and from the electric organ of *Torpedo* (Frontali and Toschi, 1958; Sheridan, Whittaker and Israël, 1966; Israël and Gautron, 1969). Disruption of synaptosomes to release the synaptic vesicles has proved a more difficult task, although varying degrees of success have been achieved in obtaining enriched vesicular fractions from octopus (*Eledone*) brain (Jones, 1970c) and *Torpedo* electric organ (Israël and Gautron, 1969; Israël, Gautron and Lesbats, 1970; Heilbronn, 1972; Whittaker, Essman and Dowe, 1972; Soifer and Whittaker, 1972; Morris, 1973). With the increasing sophistication of preparative techniques, these cholinergic systems are proving almost ideal experimental models by which ideas formulated on mammalian brain can be tested. Concepts analysed in this way in these systems include the compartmentation of ACh in the nerve-ending (Dunant, Gautron, Israël, Lesbats and Manaranche, 1972), the localization of AChE in the ending (Morris, 1973), and the choline-uptake potential of synaptosomes (Dowdall and Simon, 1973). For a fuller discussion of these studies see Sections 2.3.7 and 2.4.5.

2.2 PRINCIPLES AND METHODS OF FRACTIONATION

2.2.1 Methods of centrifugation

Cell fractionation can be viewed as a three step progression (De Duve, 1963b). The existing structure is destroyed in the first when the homogenate is produced. Following this, cell components are regrouped according to their physical properties. This is the function of the centrifugation procedures employed. The third step involves analysis, the building-up of concepts about cell function from a knowledge of the isolated cell components. The first of these steps is considered in a following section (2.3.1), while the third forms an integral part of the continuing discussion. This present section therefore is principally concerned with centrifugation procedures.

The centrifugation techniques applied to the separation and isolation of brain subcellular particles fall into two principal categories, *rate or differential* centrifugation and *isopycnic, equilibrium* or *buoyant density* centrifugation (see for example Spanner, 1972). These procedures owe their effectiveness to differences in the *sedimentation rates* and *buoyant densities* of the particles respectively. In practice, preliminary separation of heavy and light particles is achieved using rate centrifugation, and is possible because of differences in the density, size and shape of particles. Further separation on density gradients is accomplished by isopycnic centrifugation (Cotman, 1972).

Rate centrifugation is effective because populations of subcellular particles have variable sedimentation rates (Cotman, Brown, Harrell and Anderson, 1970; Kuhar, Green, Snyder and Gfeller, 1970; Kuhar, Shaskan and Snyder, 1971). There is nevertheless overlap in the rates of different particles, and in practice it is the fractions which are the last to come down in a centrifugation procedure that are the most highly enriched. During homogenization, membranes shear into vesicles of a size determined by the conditions of shear. As rate separations are in general based on the size of particles, the conditions under which homogenization is carried out are critical. One further factor influencing rate centrifugation is the washing of fractions. This increases the separation between fractions, although this in turn may be counteracted by any decrease in synaptosomal size resulting from osmotic damage caused by resuspension and recentrifugation (Cotman, 1972).

During rate centrifugation nuclei and whole cells are brought down by a gravitational force of the order of 4×10^4 g min, and remaining cellular debris by a force of 2.4×10^5 g min. Cell sap and microsomes require a greater force – approximating 6×10^6 g min – for their isolation. The crude mitochondrial fraction (P_2 of Whittaker; Section 2.1.2; Scheme 2.1) sediments between $4-5 \times 10^4$ and $2.4-3.6 \times 10^5$ g min, but in order to separate its myelin, synaptosomal and mitochondrial components isopycnic centrifugation must be resorted to (Spanner, 1972: Ansell and Spanner, 1972). Overall therefore, rate centrifugation has an apparently low resolution. Nevertheless it has proved extremely useful, principally because it has most often been applied to the separation of particles whose sedimentation coefficients differ by orders of magnitude (Anderson, 1966).

When isopycnic centrifugation is carried out using sucrose density gradients, complete separation of the principal brain particles is not possible on the basis of their densities alone. This is because glial and neuronal membranes, mitochondria, synaptosomes, lysosomes and a part of the microsome fraction band close together (Cotman, 1972; Table 2.2). Partial separation of the particles is possible however (Fig. 2.2). For instance, because synaptosomes are isopycnic at 36% sucrose (w/w) while most non-synaptosomal

Table 2.2 Isopycnic banding densities of some brain particles (modified from Cotman, 1972)

Brain particle	Density gradient	Density (g/ml)	Investigators
Synaptosomes	Sucrose	1·141–1·182	Cotman, 1968
	Sucrose	1·14 –1·17	Whittaker, 1968a
	Ficoll–sucrose	1·063–1·090	Autilio et al., 1968
	Caesium chloride–sucrose	1·175–1·190	Geison et al., 1972
Synaptic plasma membranes	Sucrose	1·120–1·161	Cotman et al., 1968a
	Sucrose	1·130–1·157	Rodriguez de Lores Arnaiz et al., 1967
	Caesium chloride	1·150	Cotman, 1968
Synaptic vesicles	Sucrose	1·08	Cotman, 1968
	Sucrose	1·056	Whittaker et al., 1964
	Caesium chloride–sucrose	1·15	Cotman, 1968
Glial membranes	Sucrose	1·121–1·167	Cotman et al., 1970, 1971a
Mitochondria and whole brain	Sucrose	1·141–1·192	Cotman, 1968
			Hamberger et al., 1970
			Whittaker, 1968
	Ficoll–sucrose	1·116	Cotman, 1968
			Autilio et al., 1968

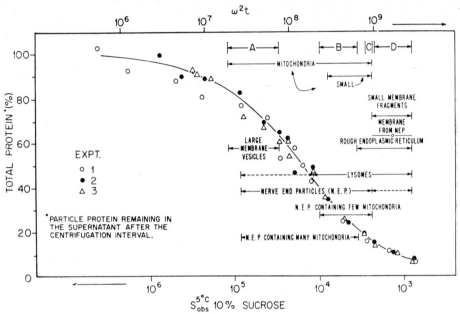

Figure 2.2 Summary of morphological and enzymatic analyses on the sedimentation of particles from brain homogenates. (From Cotman *et al.*, 1970.)

mitochondria sediment through 36% sucrose, these two particles can be largely separated by taking the leading edge of the synaptosomal fraction and the trailing edge of the mitochondrial fraction. When this procedure is combined with preliminary rate centrifugation, highly enriched fractions are obtained.

2.2.2 Homogenization conditions

The disruption of cells with the consequent separation of cell constituents may be accomplished by a number of means, including shearing, shocking, swelling and sonicating. As no single disruption technique will yield all particles intact, some particles may have to be sacrificed depending upon the nature of the investigation. In practice those aspects of the homogenization procedure of critical importance are: the clearance of the homogenizer, the speed of rotation of the pestle, the number of up-and-down strokes, the viscosity of the medium and in some instances the bivalent cation concentrations and pH (Appel, Day and Mickey, 1972).

Initial homogenization has the object of separating tissues into a few major categories, in readiness for centrifugation. This step is dependent upon the size and density of the constituents, and as shown in Fig. 2.3 subcellular constituents within a suspension of disrupted brain cells may be ordered according to their sedimentation coefficients and intrinsic densities (Appel *et al.*, 1972). This lays the basis for rate or differential centrifugation, with its initial separation of nuclear, crude mitochondrial and microsomal subdivisions.

A consequence of homogenization with its release of subcellular particles into a suspending medium is the change of particle properties through solvation, osmotic action and ion effects. The sedimentation coefficient of particles will therefore reflect in part the environment under which they are separated.

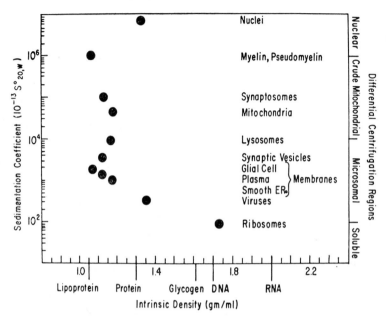

Figure 2.3 Size and density of subcellular particles in a typical brain homogenate as ordered by sedimentation coefficient and intrinsic density. (From Appel *et al.*, 1972.)

The principal criterion used to determine optimum conditions of shear in synaptosomal studies is the yield of bound ACh, which is an important marker substance for synaptosomes (Whittaker, 1965). The homogenization conditions originally selected by Whittaker (Gray and Whittaker, 1962) involve the use of a smooth-walled Perspex and glass homogenizer of the type devised by Aldridge, Emery and Street (1960). This has a clearance of 0·25 mm and a speed of rotation of the pestle of 840 rev/min. A later investigation by Whittaker and Dowe (1965) confirmed the suitability of these conditions, in that more vigorous conditions reduced the yield of ACh and therefore presumably of synaptosomes. Milder conditions did not affect the yield of bound ACh, but a higher proportion sedimented in the P_1 fraction suggesting a less complete disintegration of brain tissue (Whittaker, 1969b). These investigations however, do not constitute an adequate systematic study of the optimum conditions for synaptosomal formation. This empirical approach to the separation of synaptosomes is typical of practically all studies in this area (cf. Hughes, Wimpenny and Lloyd, 1971). Attempts at formulating theoretical principles for the optimization of centrifugation conditions by Cotman and co-workers (Cotman *et al.*, 1970; Cotman, 1972) have not as yet influenced significantly centrifugation schedules.

An attempt to quantify the yield of synaptosomes, and compare this with estimates of the number of nerve terminals in intact tissue, was made by Clementi, Whittaker and Sheridan (1966b) in Whittaker's laboratory. Using polystyrene bead 'tagging' procedures (Plate 2.9) they calculated that the number of synaptosomes/g guinea-pig cerebral cortical tissue was of the same order of magnitude as the 4×10^{11} and 8×10^{11} for the number of nerve endings/g whole tissue in rat and mouse visual cortex respectively (Gray and Cragg, quoted by Clementi et al., 1966). While undue reliance should not be placed on these figures as they involve a number of approximations and assumptions, they suggest that the synaptosomal yield is reasonable.

The suspension medium initially adopted by Whittaker (1959) and employed in most laboratories today is 0·32M sucrose which is isotonic for the osmotically sensitive synaptosomes. This molarity is not of universal applicability as some lower organisms such as Octopus and Torpedo require a suspension medium of much higher molarity to match that of the organism's environment (Section 2.3.7). In mammals however, 0·32M has proved generally successful.

It has been estimated that the threshold concentration for coacervation of synaptosomes is 0·5 mg–atoms/litre for calcium and 20 mg–atoms/litre for sodium (Whittaker, 1969b). Calcium may be present in sucrose and water, but the use of analytical grade sucrose and double distilled water results in a calcium level of about 12 μg–atoms/litre. Unbuffered 0·32M sucrose is routinely used in most laboratories, with perhaps a pH adjustment to 6·5 or 7·4 (Marchbanks, 1967, 1968b). The addition of magnesium to the sucrose has also been advocated (Hajós, Tapia, Wilkin, Johnson and Balázs, 1974).

Sucrose has established for itself an almost unchallenged reputation as the homogenizing medium of first choice. Alternatives such as glucose (Cottrell, 1966; Jones, 1971), sucrose–saline (Florey and Winesdorfer, 1968; Israël et al., 1970; Whittaker et al., 1972; Dowdall and Whittaker, 1973) or sucrose–urea (Sheridan et al., 1966; Jones, 1967) mixtures have only been resorted to when high molar media have been required as in molluscs, Octopus and Torpedo. In spite of its almost universal acceptance however, it all too readily damages synaptosomes when hypertonic, a disadvantage which has led to the development of alternative density gradients (Section 2.3.2).

Minor variations on the above scheme include a homogenizer clearance of 0·15 mm (Giacobini et al., 1971), rotation speeds of up to 900 rev/min and the use of 0·25M sucrose as the homogenizing medium (e.g. Abdel-Latif and Abood, 1964; Abood, Kurahasi and Del Cerro, 1967; Del Cerro, Snider and Oster, 1969). Other homogenizers such as a glass homogenizer with a motor driven teflon pestle (Potter-Elvehjem) or a Dounce homogenizer are also widely used. For instance Hajós et al. (1974) adapted the Dounce homogenizer for the gentle disruption of cerebellar tissue and the consequent separation of relatively intact mossy fibre terminals (Section 3.3.5). In other instances a modified Potter-Elvehjem homogenizer for hand homogenization (Jacob and Bhargava, 1962) has been found satisfactory for synaptosomal separation (Lagercrantz and Pertoft, 1972). Comparing hand and motor homogenization, Coakley (1974) noted that the principal difference between the two lies in the time of exposure of the tissue to the shearing force.

One constant factor throughout fractionation schemes is the tissue concentration of the homogenate, namely a 10% w/v of brain tissue (Gray and Whittaker, 1962; De

Robertis *et al.*, 1962a). If a tissue concentration of 20% or 30% w/v is initially required, it is diluted to 10% w/v prior to fractionation (e.g. Michaelson and Dowe, 1963: Cotman and Taylor, 1972) in order to facilitate satisfactory fractionation.

2.3 SEPARATION OF SYNAPTOSOMES

2.3.1 Discontinuous sucrose gradients (Schemes 2.1 and 2.2)

In spite of the diversity of fractionation procedures employed by neurochemists to obtain synaptosomes, the majority are derived from schemes originally developed by Whittaker and De Robertis.

The steps of the homogenization procedure outlined in the previous section (2.2.2) are similar in the Whittaker and De Robertis schemes, as well as in the majority of schemes based on them. The actual fractionation procedures are also similar as demonstrated by Schemes 2.1 and 2.2., although both are flexible in order to adapt the routines to meet different requirements. For instance Whittaker's schedule may be modified in a

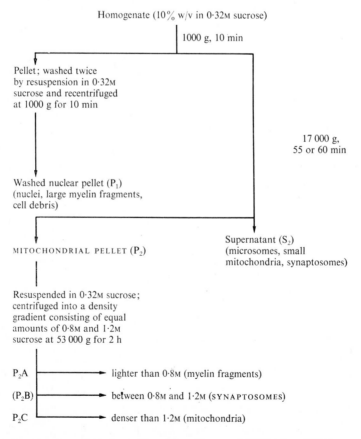

Homogenate (10% w/v in 0·32M sucrose)

1000 g, 10 min

Pellet; washed twice by resuspension in 0·32M sucrose and recentrifuged at 1000 g for 10 min

17 000 g, 55 or 60 min

Washed nuclear pellet (P_1) (nuclei, large myelin fragments, cell debris)

MITOCHONDRIAL PELLET (P_2)

Supernatant (S_2) (microsomes, small mitochondria, synaptosomes)

Resuspended in 0·32M sucrose; centrifuged into a density gradient consisting of equal amounts of 0·8M and 1·2M sucrose at 53 000 g for 2 h

P_2A → lighter than 0·8M (myelin fragments)

(P_2B)   → between 0·8M and 1·2M (SYNAPTOSOMES)

P_2C → denser than 1·2M (mitochondria)

Scheme 2.1   Preparation of synaptosomes after Gray and Whittaker (1962)

number of ways depending on the biochemical aspect of synaptosomes under investigation (e.g. Michaelson and Dowe, 1963; Nyman and Whittaker, 1963; Michaelson and Whittaker, 1963; Eichberg, Whittaker and Dawson, 1964; Marchbanks, 1967). Alternatively, when the synaptosomes serve as a source of synaptic vesicles an abbreviated scheme is sometimes employed (Whittaker *et al.*, 1964; Whittaker and Sheridan, 1965).

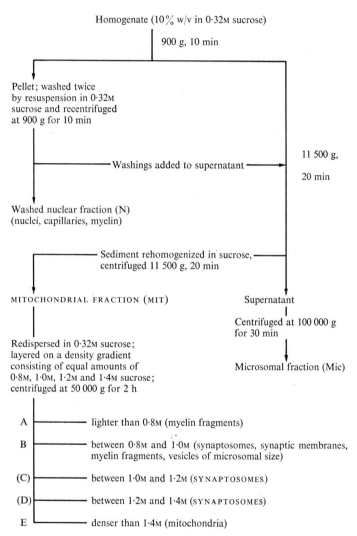

Scheme 2.2   Preparation of synaptosomes after De Robertis *et al.* (1962a)

The rationale of the schemes stems from the fact that the sedimentation properties of synaptosomes are similar to those of myelin fragments and isolated mitochondria (Section 2.2). Consequently the P_2 pellet of Whittaker and the Mit fraction of De Robertis, the mitochondrial fractions of earlier terminology, consist of these three constituents. It was in order to separate them that discontinuous sucrose density gradients were employed, by making use of differences in their sedimentation curves. While the degree of separation of the particles is significant, morphological evidence demonstrates that each fraction may be contaminated by particles of the others (Plates 2.2 and 2.3). Furthermore, the higher the gravitational field used to prepare the P_2 fraction as in Scheme 2.1, the greater its microsomal contamination. Consequently when synaptosomes are prepared prior to isolating synaptic vesicles (e.g. Scheme 2.3), a lower gravitational field is employed.

In an attempt to quantify the conditions under which brain subcellular particles are prepared, and to elucidate optimum conditions, Cotman *et al.*, (1970) analysed their sedimentation characteristics using an analytical differential centrifugation procedure (Fig. 2.2). The large majority of mitochondria appeared homogeneous with respect to their sedimentation characteristics, being completely removed from the supernatant after 4×10^8 w^2t or $5\cdot7 \times 10^5$ g min. The remaining mitochondria were not completely sedimented until 1×10^9 w^2t. By contrast, synaptosomes constituted a heterogeneous population, 55% of the particulate ChAc sedimenting with the mitochondrial population. Of direct relevance to other fractionation studies is their calculation that 80% of synaptosomes are sedimented at forces up to 100×10^7 w^2t, the use of higher forces resulting in the inclusion of broken synaptosomal membranes and quantities of rough endoplasmic reticulum. The forces used by other groups to obtain the mitochondrial pellet are 768×10^7 w^2t (Gray and Whittaker, 1962), 147×10^7 w^2t (Whittaker *et al.*, 1964) and 169×10^7 w^2t (De Robertis *et al.*, 1962). However, as these refer to the mitochondrial rather than a specific synaptosomal fraction their relevance to contamination of the latter is open to question.

The density gradient procedure adopted by Whittaker employs layers of 0·8M and 1·2M sucrose, with the P_2 pellet resuspended in 0·32M sucrose as the top layer (Scheme 2.1). Centrifugation at 53 000 g for 2 h results in two bands, P_2A and P_2B, and a pellet, P_2C, consisting respectively of enriched fractions of myelin fragments, synaptosomes and mitochondria (Plates 2.1–2.3). De Robertis's scheme, by contrast, utilizes a gradient consisting of 0·8M, 1·0M, 1·2M and 1·4M sucrose which, after comparable centrifugation conditions, yields four bands, A–D, and a pellet, E (Scheme 2.2). The interesting feature about the resulting fractions is that the three intermediate ones contain synaptosomes, which are largely confined to C and D, the two synaptosomal fractions. The high levels of bound ACh, AChE (De Robertis *et al.*, 1962a) and ChAc (De Robertis *et al.*, 1963) in C led De Robertis *et al.* (1962a) to postulate that this fraction contains cholinergic nerve endings, in contrast to D with its low levels of these substances and therefore non-cholinergic nerve endings.

Such a separation of synaptosomes into two distinct subpopulations raises exciting possibilities if it is a valid one. On checking this separation, Inouye, Katuoka and Shinagawa (1963) and Bradford, Brownlow and Gammack (1966) obtained results supporting De Robertis's general contentions. It has been criticized by Whittaker on the grounds that the lighter synaptosome fractions, while relatively rich in ChAc, are contaminated with synaptosome ghosts and membrane fragments (Whittaker, 1968a), with the result that the separation of cholinergic from non-cholinergic endings may be more apparent than real (Whittaker, 1969b). Furthermore, Whittaker and co-workers (Michaelson and Whittaker, 1963; Fonum, 1968) have been unable to confirm the finding.

Further investigations by De Robertis's group have tended to confirm the subdivision of synaptosomes into cholinergic and non-cholinergic populations. Salganicoff and De Robertis (1963) demonstrated that the two main enzymes of the γ-aminobutyric acid (GABA) system have different submitochondrial localizations, with glutamic acid decarboxylase (GAD) in the non-cholinergic (D) fraction and γ-aminobutyric acid aminotransferase (GABA-AT) in neuronal mitochondria (E). From this it was postulated that the non-cholinergic nerve endings also contain GABA (Salganicoff and De Robertis, 1963, 1965; De Robertis, 1967). Other biogenic amines, namely 5-HT (Zieher and De Robertis, 1963), NE and dopamine (Zieher and De Robertis, 1964) and histamine (Kataoka and De Robertis, 1967) were found preferentially in the B and C fractions, suggesting that the C fraction not only consists of cholinergic nerve endings but the more general category of aminergic nerve endings. Conversely, the non-cholinergic D fraction may be referred to as the non-aminergic fraction.

The effect of these diverse biochemical studies was to consolidate the concept of synaptosomal subdivision, already an established fact in De Robertis's writings. The presence of GAD in the D fraction suggested that these synaptosomes were derived from inhibitory nerve endings, and the cholinergic synaptosomes in C from excitatory ones. In view of this, the two populations should be capable of separation on morphological grounds, the inhibitory synaptosomes containing ellipsoidal vesicles after aldehyde fixation and the excitatory ones spherical vesicles (Section 1.2.1). This is precisely what De Robertis (1968) found on fractionating cat cerebral cortex and examining synaptosomes in fractions C and D, as well as isolated vesicles in fraction M_2.

Two further pieces of evidence bearing on this problem should be mentioned. The subfractionation of synaptosomes to give synaptic membranes has, in De Robertis's hands (Rodriguez de Lores Arnaiz et al., 1967), produced two main types of synaptic membranes, one rich in AChE and the other not (Scheme 2.7). The convulsant drug, methionine sulphoximine, which acts on several enzymes related to the glutamine–glutamate–GABA system, is reported to produce structural alterations in the non-aminergic synaptosomes (fraction D) but not in those of the aminergic system (De Robertis, Rodriguez de Lores Arnaiz and Sellinger, 1966b; De Robertis, Sellinger, Rodriguez de Lores Arnaiz, Alberici and Zieher, 1967c).

There have been many strands of evidence therefore from De Robertis's laboratory in support of his contention that cholinergic (aminergic) synaptosomes can be distinguished from non-cholinergic (non-aminergic) ones.

Evidence in support of the general concept of two or more synaptic populations has been forthcoming from a variety of sources as discussed in other sections (1.2.1; 2.3.4; 3.4). The separation of cholinergic and non-cholinergic synaptosomes has, however, proved a more formidable task. The most direct evidence in favour of such a separation is that of McGovern, Maguire, Gurd, Mahler and Moore (1973), with their demonstration that the cerebral cortices of 15-day-old rats can be separated on Ficoll gradients into two fractions, P_2B_2 and P_2B_3, the former having adrenergic characteristics and the latter cholinergic.

The scheme of McGovern *et al.* (1973) has two key steps, namely, the use of a flotation gradient for the isolation of crude synaptosomes (P_2B_2), and the separation of two discrete subpopulations banding sharply at the 6%–11·5% interface for P_2B_2 and the 11·5%–18% interface for P_2B_3. Of these subfractions, P_2B_2 demonstrates a preferential uptake of dopamine relative to choline compared with P_2B_3, while the adrenergic transmitters (dopamine, NE and 5-HT) are concentrated in P_2B_2 and ACh in P_2B_3. Enzyme assays confirm this subdivision of transmitters.

These results, while tending to confirm De Robertis's general contention, differ in details. For instance, the distribution of the transmitter substances in the respective 'lighter' and 'heavier' fractions is different, in addition to which De Robertis's lighter 'cholinergic' fraction contains a mixture of catecholamines, histamine and ACh. The GABA-related enzymes in De Robertis's experiments are principally found in the heavier 'noncholinergic' fraction. Furthermore, Synder, Kuhar, Green, Cole and Shaskan (1970) have provided evidence that synaptosomes labelled by GABA sediment with others labelled by catecholamines, and not separately as would be anticipated in terms of De Robertis's results.

2.3.2 Ficoll (Ficoll–sucrose) gradients

As pointed out above a disadvantage of sucrose gradients is the damage they may cause to osmotically sensitive particles such as synaptosomes. An alternative is to substitute the high molecular weight polysaccharide Ficoll for sucrose, in an attempt to reduce the osmotic damage to vulnerable structures (Plate 2.4). Consequently gradients consisting of Ficoll dissolved in 0·32M sucrose are now used extensively in the preparation of synaptosomes (Kurokawa, Sakamoto and Kato, 1965a, b; Abdel-Latif and Abood, 1964, 1965; Abdel-Latif, 1966; Abood *et al.*, 1967; Autilio *et al.*, 1968; Diamond and Kennedy, 1969) and as a preparatory step in the isolation of synaptic membranes (Cotman and Matthews, 1971), junctional complexes (De Robertis *et al.*, 1967a) and postsynaptic membranes (Garey *et al.*, 1972).

A number of advantages are claimed for Ficoll gradients over sucrose ones. Firstly, separation of synaptosomes and free mitochondria is said to be improved because synaptosomes undergo a greater density decrease in Ficoll gradients than do mitochondria (Cotman, 1972). No comparable disparity is observed in sucrose gradients. Secondly, according to Morgan *et al.* (1972) synaptosomes prepared on Ficoll gradients are much less contaminated with myelin, glial membranes and axonal fragments than are synaptosomes prepared on sucrose gradients (see also Section 2.6.2). A disadvantage noted by these workers is a greater contamination with free mitochondria, an observation difficult to reconcile with the theoretical postulate of Cotman referred to previously. Appel *et al.* (1972), by contrast, found minimal contamination by mitochondria or myelin, but as much as 20% contamination by membranes of unknown origin. Lastly, synaptosomes prepared on Ficoll gradients are prepared under isotonic conditions, whereas those prepared on sucrose gradients are hypertonic. A consequence of this is that the former synaptosomes are more sensitive to osmotic shock, a property of importance when synaptic vesicles or plasma membranes are being prepared (Morgan et al., 1972).

The biochemical and morphological results obtained with Ficoll gradients may be comparable to those obtained by the sucrose method. For example Autilio et al. (1968) found that the distributions of AChE and SDH were in essential agreement with those obtained using sucrose gradients, while the synaptosomal fraction was relatively pure on EM examination. Abdel-Latif (1966) has claimed that synaptosomes prepared in Ficoll retain most of their ACh, their LDH and AChE activities and 90% of their capability for oxidative phosphorylation. Studies by Kurokawa et al. (1965a, b) have also provided fractions comparable to those produced on sucrose gradients, although Whittaker (1969b) reports his dissatisfaction with the homogeneity of the fractions obtained in his laboratory.

De Belleroche and Bradford (1973b) have argued that, while hypertonic sucrose does cause shrinkage of synaptosomes, this may actually prove an advantage by increasing the viscosity of the cytoplasm. Consequently synaptosomes prepared in hypertonic sucrose can be repeatedly sedimented and resuspended without considerable loss of ACh, unlike those prepared in isotonic sucrose (Potter, 1968).

It is difficult to compare the homogeneity of the fractions or the preservation of the synaptosomes from published reports, although a number of points can be made about the use of Ficoll density gradients. Thus, in order to take full advantage of the negligible osmotic pressure exerted by Ficoll, the lower molecular weight contaminants of the commercial product must be removed before use (Garey et al., 1972; Appel et al., 1972). In addition, a precisely constructed continuous linear gradient is essential, with care being taken to prevent over-loading of the gradient and consequent failure of the gradient to achieve optimum separation of the particles (Garey et al., 1972). Differences between workers therefore may result from variations in constructing the gradients, although if care is taken with regard to the above points an improvement in resolutional efficiency is undoubtedly possible.

Synaptosomal morphology following separation on Ficoll density gradients requires further investigation. The micrographs of Autilio et al. (1968), Garey et al. (1972) and Morgan et al. (1972) contain many synaptosomes which closely resemble those separated on sucrose density gradients and subsequently incubated in physiological media (Jones and Bradford, 1971a). They are comparatively spherical, with well-preserved mitochondria, synaptic vesicles and frequently vacuoles within a limiting membrane (Plate 2.4). In the study of Garey et al. (1972) however, there are two synaptosomal fractions, one with synaptosomes of the type just described and the other containing synaptosomes with a dark appearance resulting from their dense cytoplasmic matrix. The latter may represent degenerative nerve endings, although such a large percentage of degenerating endings is unlikely in normal tissue; alternatively they may be the result of an unexpected osmolarity artefact.

2.3.3 Continuous sucrose gradients

Continuous gradients were developed as a means of achieving greater separation of particles than was possible with discontinuous gradients. In the case of synaptosomes they have been employed, for instance, in studies of the intracellular localization of GAD and GABA-AT (Van Kempen, Van Den Berg, Van Der Helm and Veldstra, 1965; Balázs, Dahl and Harwood, 1966; Fonnum, 1968), while Whittaker (1968a) used them in an attempt to resolve synaptosomes into morphologically distinct fractions (Section 3.5.1).

The advantages claimed for continuous gradients are: (a) the elimination of the tendency for material to layer at interfaces and hence retard the movement of denser particles; (b) their stability, thereby allowing the adoption of abbreviated fractionation procedures; and (c) their potential for separating particles over a wide density range (Balázs et al., 1966). In general they give a clear separation of subcellular structures and good recoveries of enzymic activities, and have proved useful in substantiating and clarifying results previously obtained using discontinuous sucrose gradients, for example, concerning glutamate metabolism. In spite of these arguments in their favour, synaptosomes prepared in continuous sucrose gradients sediment at greater densities than in discontinuous sucrose gradients, and so are not well separated from microsomes and mitochondria (Whittaker, 1968a). According to Day, McMillan, Mickey and Appel (1971) this is due to myelin coalescing at 0·8M sucrose and its interaction with synaptosomes. Furthermore, the opinion has been expressed that when used in zonal rotors continuous gradients give rise to ill-defined fractions (Ansell and Spanner, 1972; Spanner, 1972) and are inferior to shallow discontinuous gradients (Spanner and Ansell, 1971).

Used alone they have not proved sufficiently powerful to separate different populations of synaptosomes (Whittaker, 1968a). However, when used in conjunction with the radioactive labelling of brain slices prior to homogenization and centrifugation they have led to remarkable advances in our understanding of neurotransmitter mechanisms. In these instances linear continuous sucrose gradients ranging from about 1·5M to about 0·32M are used, following preparation with a triple outlet mixer and peristaltic pump. Detailed results of these studies will be considered in a subsequent section (4.3.4), but an idea of their potential is relevant at this point. Most of the work has come from the laboratories of Snyder and Iversen, the initial studies being concerned with the separation of synaptosomes storing catecholamines from those binding GABA (Iversen and Synder, 1968; Kuhar et al., 1970). Related to this was the finding that catecholaminergic synaptosomes constitute a heterogeneous population, each synaptosomal type being distinguished by its equilibrium density (Green, Snyder and Iversen, 1969). In parallel with these pharmacological studies, efforts were made to characterize the different synaptosomal fractions morphologically, and relate any observed variations to the different neurotransmitter-specific terminals in the brain (Kuhar et al., 1970; Gfeller, Kuhar and Snyder, 1971). While these latter findings are not conclusive, they point to the potential value of continuous gradients as a tool for separating morphologically distinct nerve endings.

An allied approach to the localization of transmitter or potential transmitter substances in synaptosomes has been employed to localize glutamic and aspartic acids in a particular synaptosomal fraction (Wofsey, Kuhar and Snyder, 1971) and to detect a synaptosomal fraction that selectively accumulates glycine in spinal cord (Arregui, Logan, Bennett and Snyder, 1972).

2.3.4 Zonal centrifugation

The principles of zonal centrifugation have been known for some time and have been incorporated in the design of a number of different zonal rotors (Anderson, Price, Fisher, Canning and Burger, 1964; Anderson, 1966; Anderson, Waters, Fisher, Cline, Nunley, Elrod and Rankin, 1967; Anderson, Nunley and Rankin, 1969). In spite of this, the application of zonal centrifugation to the separation of the subcellular components of brain tissue is in its infancy. Amongst the studies to have utilized it in tackling a variety of neurochemical problems can be mentioned those by Cotman *et al.* (1968a), Mahaley *et al.* (1968), Rodnight, Weller and Goldfarb (1969), Barker, Dowdall, Essman and Whittaker (1970), Mahler, McBride and Moore (1970), Shapira, Binkley, Kibler and Wundram (1970), Spanner and Ansell (1970), Day *et al.* (1971), Kornguth *et al.* (1971, 1972), Ansell and Spanner (1972), and Churchill and Cotman (1973).

Of the zonal rotors developed the one which has been used almost exclusively for the separation of brain tissue is the B-type. As with analytical centrifugation techniques, the same range of gradients is available with zonal rotors. Consequently sucrose and Ficoll gradients are employed, the gradients themselves being either of the continuous or discontinuous varieties. Furthermore, both rate–zonal and isopycnic–zonal separations are possible. No attempt is made here to consider the principles of zonal centrifugation. For discussions of these, reference should be made to Anderson (1966) and Cotman (1972).

The studies referred to above have had as their targets the isolation of membranes (Cotman *et al.*, 1968a; Rodnight *et al.*, 1969; Mahler *et al.*, 1970) and myelin (Shapira *et al.*, 1970) as well as of synaptosomes (Ansell and Spanner, 1972; Spanner, 1972), while Kornguth and co-workers (1971, 1972) have used zonal centrifugation in the preparation of what they refer to as 'synaptic complexes' (Section 2.3.5). Our attention in this section is limited to the synaptosomal studies.

Using a B-XIV zonal rotor and discontinuous sucrose gradients, Ansell and Spanner (1972) were able to subfractionate the P_2 fraction from rabbit cerebral cortex into six peaks, A–F (Fig. 2·4). This followed initial removal of the myelin by centrifugation for 8×10^6 g min. Peak A is rich in myelin and also contains a high concentration of membranous material (plasma membranes and endoplasmic reticulum; high concentration of AChE). The myelin and membranous material can be largely separated by two combined zonal fractionations of the P_2 fraction. In addition, two myelin fractions can be isolated by zonal fractionation, one between 0·4 and 0·6M and the other between 0·6 and 0·8M sucrose (Spanner, 1972; see also Autilio, Norton and Terry, 1964 using analytical centrifugation).

Peak B also demonstrates some AChE activity and it has been suggested that it contains fragments of synaptosomes and axons (Spanner, 1972). This will be more fully discussed in Section 2.6.2.

Peaks C and D contain what appear to be synaptosomes on EM examination and are rich in occluded LDH. The latter is a cytoplasmic marker and in its occluded form it is a good enzyme marker for synaptosomes (Marchbanks, 1967). This, plus the high AChE activity in these fractions, considerably strengthens the case for a synaptosomal identity. The existence of two synaptosomal peaks could point towards the existence of two

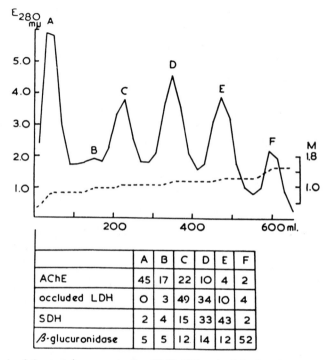

	A	B	C	D	E	F
AChE	45	17	22	10	4	2
occluded LDH	O	3	49	34	10	4
SDH	2	4	15	33	43	2
β·glucuronidase	5	5	12	14	12	52

Figure 2.4   Graph of the protein concentration (O.D. 280 nm) of the fractions separated from the P_2 fraction by zonal centrifugation. The dotted line gives the sucrose concentration. Below the graph is a table giving the activity of the various enzyme markers, with the results expressed as a percentage of the total P_2 fraction. (From Spanner, 1972.)

distinct synaptosomal populations. The chief differences between the two peaks are that peak C has higher AChE and occluded LDH levels than D, but a lower SDH level (Ansell and Spanner, 1972). In line with this was the observation that fraction D is capable of taking up α-methyl-NE, unlike fraction C. This evidence for more than one synaptosomal population must be viewed alongside that of Iversen and Snyder (1968), Kuhar *et al.* (1970) and Gfeller *et al.* (1971) (see Section 4.3.4).

Peak E is characterized by a high level of SDH and monoamine oxidase, suggesting that it is almost exclusively mitochondrial. Peak F, by contrast, has a high percentage of β-glucuronidase pointing towards a lysosomal content.

Cotman *et al.* (1968) in an earlier series of experiments had come to substantially similar conclusions although in less detail. Centrifugation of the P_2 fraction in a B-XV zonal centrifuge yielded two major bands, the one at 23% sucrose (w/w) consisting of myelin and membrane fragments and the other at 35% sucrose (w/w) consisting of synaptosomes and a few free mitochondria. The shoulder at 38–41% sucrose consisted of free mitochondria.

A number of advantages are generally ascribed to the zonal rotor: (a) its large capacity means that very large volumes of material can be handled at any one time, with the corollary that a very small proportion of the total gradient can be collected without disturbing the gradient *in toto*; (b) the wall effects characteristic of centrifuge tubes are absent, with the result that clumping, premature sedimentation of particles and convective disturbances are minimized (Anderson, 1966); (c) as the gradient is always under the influence of the centrifugal field it is stable, with the result that the diffusional forces which lead to band broadening are opposed at all times by a centrifugal field (Cotman, 1972; Spanner, 1972); and (d) the geometry of the zonal gradient is claimed to be nearer optimal for resolution than the geometry of gradients in centrifuge tubes (Cotman, 1972).

In the light of these considerations zonal centrifugation is most useful as an experimental tool when maximum resolution in a gradient is required and when it is important to increase the amount of sample that can be handled in a single run (Cotman, 1972).

Against these advantages of zonal centrifugation some disadvantages need to be mentioned. It is not as time-saving as was once imagined; it can be very expensive on account of the volume of samples involved; and each run is confined to one experimental approach. The temptation to use large areas of brain or even whole brain in order to provide the large amount of tissue necessary for zonal centrifugation is a real one. It would be a pity if this were to override the use of more specific fractions and hence limit the potential of this method for solving specific problems.

2.3.5 Caesium chloride gradient (Scheme 2.3)

This gradient was developed in Kornguth's laboratory as a means of (a) decreasing the contamination of synaptosomal preparations with myelin and mitochondria, and (b) preserving the morphological characteristics of the complete synaptic junction (Kornguth *et al.*, 1967, 1969, 1971, 1972; Wannamaker, Kornguth, Scott, Dudley and Kelly, 1973). The technique which involves centrifugation using a discontinuous sucrose density gradient followed by a continuous caesium chloride (CsCl) gradient, is directed towards the preparation of *synaptic complexes*, which may be defined as 'pinched off nerve endings with synaptic junctions and containing entrapped mitochondria and synaptic vesicles' (Geison, Flangas and Kornguth, 1972). They are not to be confused with synaptic or junctional complexes of other workers (Section 2.5.2). The expectations behind this preparation are that it provides an experimental system for the study of the macromolecular components of the pre- and postsynaptic membranes as well as of filaments between them (Kornguth *et al.*, 1969).

Details of the experimental procedure are outlined in Scheme 2.3. The centrifugation of the mitochondrial pellet in the discontinuous sucrose density gradient differed from the Whittaker and De Robertis methods mainly in that the gradient contained 0·01M-MgCl$_2$ as opposed to 0·001M-MgCl$_2$. The effect of this was to increase the clarity and bulk of the C (synaptosome) band.

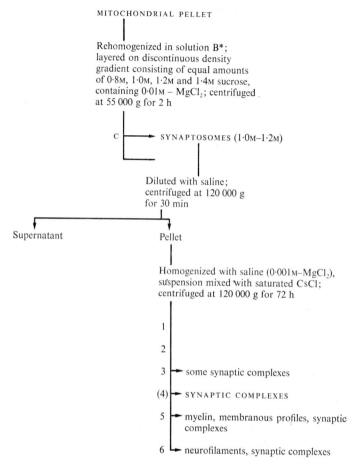

MITOCHONDRIAL PELLET

Rehomogenized in solution B*; layered on discontinuous density gradient consisting of equal amounts of 0·8M, 1·0M, 1·2M and 1·4M sucrose, containing 0·01M – MgCl$_2$; centrifuged at 55 000 g for 2 h

C ——→ SYNAPTOSOMES (1·0M–1·2M)

Diluted with saline; centrifuged at 120 000 g for 30 min

Supernatant   Pellet

Homogenized with saline (0·001M–MgCl$_2$), suspension mixed with saturated CsCl; centrifuged at 120 000 g for 72 h

1

2

3 ├—► some synaptic complexes

(4) ├—► SYNAPTIC COMPLEXES

5 ├—► myelin, membranous profiles, synaptic complexes

6 └—► neurofilaments, synaptic complexes

Scheme 2.3   Isolation of 'synaptic complexes' (synaptosomes) in a caesium chloride density gradient after Kornguth *et al.* (1969)

* Initial homogenization was carried out in solution A, that is, 0·32M sucrose, 0·001M MgCl$_2$, 0·0004M phosphate pH 7·0. Solution B contained 0·32M sucrose, 0·01M -MgCl$_2$, 0·0004M phosphate pH 7·0.

Of the six bands resulting from the CsCl gradient, synaptic complexes occur in bands 3–6 with a preponderance in band 4. On EM examination of this band the pre- and post-synaptic terminals of the complexes are often relatively complete with synaptic vesicles presynaptically, a prominent dense postsynaptic thickening and cleft material between the terminals (Plate 2.5). When compared with the synaptosomes and synaptosomal fractions of most other workers, a number of distinguishing features become evident. The percentage of profiles in Kornguth's band 4 recognizable as complete synaptic complexes appears fairly low on visual inspection of EMs. However, it has been estimated from serial section work that of the membranous elements banding between ρ 1·178–1·190, 85% of them belong to synaptic complexes (Kornguth et al., 1972; cf. Kornguth et al., 1967). It would be interesting to know how this compares with the percentage of intact synaptic junctions discernible in routine synaptosomal preparations. The profiles in Kornguth's synaptic complex fractions are very closely packed together, far more so than in most synaptosomal preparations (cf. Figs. 3 and 6 in Kornguth et al., 1971; Fig. 3 being of material from a gradient containing no sucrose and Fig. 6 from a sucrose-containing gradient). One wonders therefore, to what extent the apparent integrity of the synaptic complexes is a function of the tight packing of the brain particles in general. The enveloping membrane of both terminals, especially the presynaptic one, often appears irregular in outline, following the contours of neighbouring profiles. This appearance is quite unlike that of synaptosomes.

The band pattern outlined above was obtained only from fractions C or D prepared in a sucrose gradient containing 0·01M-MgCl$_2$ (Kornguth et al., 1969). When 0·001M-MgCl$_2$ was substituted, the pre- and postsynaptic terminals were present but frequently were separated from each other. Whether the difference between the two situations is a qualitative one is difficult to determine on the available evidence, and hence the significance of the MgCl$_2$ is open to question. It would also be interesting to know the effect of 0·01M-MgCl$_2$ during homogenization, as Kornguth's scheme utilizes only 0·001M at this stage.

Fluorescent immune studies demonstrated that the major antigenic components of band 4 are situated within the synaptic complexes, while neither myelin nor free mitochondria are present as major antigens (Kornguth et al., 1969). The principal synaptic complex fraction (band 4) is largely devoid of myelin and free mitochondria, thereby justifying one of the main reasons for using a CsCl gradient.

In further studies, Kornguth and his group (1971, 1972) have modified the technique as outlined in Scheme 2.3, replacing the continuous generated CsCl gradient with large scale preparation in a zonal rotor. This produced three major density bands, at 1.16, 1·17 or 1·18, and 1·21 (or 1·19, depending respectively on the presence or absence of sucrose in the CsCl gradient). The band at 1·16 contained membranes of undetermined origin and myelin fragments, the 1·17 or 1·18 band synaptic complexes or separated pre- and postsynaptic terminals (depending on the presence or absence of sucrose), and the 1·19 or 1·21 band free mitochondria, filamentous structures, synaptic complexes, unidentifiable membranes and parts of dendrites (Kornguth et al., 1971).

The lipid composition of the synaptic complex fraction fell within the range determined for synaptosomes. In particular this applied to the phospholipid to cholesterol molar ratios (e.g. Seminario, Hoen and Gomez, 1964; Eichberg et al., 1964; Cuzner and Davison, 1968), the phospholipid to protein ratios and the cholesterol to protein ratios (Seminario et al., 1964; Lapetina, Soto and De Robertis, 1968). Levels of NE in the synaptic complex fraction were also similar to that in synaptosomal fractions prepared on sucrose gradients (Zieher and De Robertis, 1963; Whittaker, 1965).

Comparing synaptic complexes from a number of brain regions, and also comparing foetal and adult brains, Kornguth et al. (1972) noted a remarkable similarity in their isopycnic density in these diverse situations (1·178–1·190). This finding was unexpected as there is evidence to suggest a variability in the number of mitochondria and neuro-filaments per unit volume between complexes (cf. Gray and Guillery, 1966). Another notable factor about the banding density is its level. It is relatively high compared with synaptosomes prepared in isotonic Ficoll-sucrose gradients and which also separate into two bands (1·072 and 1·152 g/ml–Day *et al.*, 1971; also Table 2.2). As the isopycnic density of particles in CsCl is inversely related to lipid content, the high banding density may result from loss of, or dissociation of, lipids from the complexes. It may also be due in part to differences in centrifugal conditions. Separation in Ficoll-sucrose is dependent upon rate zonal conditions and therefore involves mass-density relationships, while separation in CsCl is effected only by the buoyant density of the particles (Kornguth *et al.*, 1972).

2.3.6 Additional methods

The use of Ficoll as an alternative to sucrose in density gradients has already been discussed in Section 2.3.2 above. Another low osmotic gradient medium that has been tried is Ludox, a colloidal silica sol (Lagercrantz and Pertoft, 1972). The Ludox was either mixed with polyethylene glycol or isotonic sucrose was added to it; it was incorporated into a continuous gradient and its efficacy compared with discontinuous and continuous sucrose gradients. The three fractions obtained by centrifugation corresponded to Whittaker's A–C fractions, the most apparent difference being the much higher densities of the corresponding fractions in the sucrose gradients as opposed to the silica gradients. According to Lagercrantz and Pertoft this high density of the synaptosomes in the sucrose gradients is probably due to their dehydration in hypertonic sucrose. This, in turn, may be responsible for the lower catecholamine and cytochrome oxidase levels recorded in the main synaptosomal fraction prepared on the sucrose compared with the silica gradient. An interesting feature of this study is that the partial separation of NE- and dopamine-containing synaptosomes in sucrose gradients (Green *et al.*, 1969) was not obtained with silica gradients. In view of the potential importance of techniques for distinguishing between synaptosomal populations, this latter observation has far-reaching consequences if valid. Studies are urgently required to investigate further the comparative merits of sucrose and silica gradients.

Baldessarini and Vogt's (1971) use of ultrafiltration techniques to isolate synaptosomes is interesting as it provides a very simple and rapid method of synaptosomal preparation. The resulting synaptosomes appear to be metabolically active, to be capable of accumulating and releasing labelled NE and to possess monoamine oxidase activity. The use of ultrafilters with a variety of pore sizes may form the basis of future attempts at separating different subpopulations of synaptosomes.

The fractionation of peripheral nerve tissues presents difficulties not encountered with CNS tissues. One of these is the toughness of the material resulting from its collagen content and leading to problems with tissue fragmentation. Sympathetic ganglia for instance are potentially rich sources of cholinergic synaptosomes and synaptic vesicles provided they can be satisfactorily fragmented and the synaptosomes obtained in sufficient quantities. The difficulties of fractionation however, are compounded because (a) the ratio of nerve endings to cell bodies is much lower in ganglia than in the CNS, (b) the appearance of axon terminals and the structural relationship between neuron and neuronal processes differ in ganglia and CNS tissue (cf. Elfvin, 1963; Grillo, 1966; Hökfelt, 1969), leading possibly to the fragmentation rather than 'pinching-off' of nerve endings during homogenization (Giacobini et al., 1971), and (c) non-cholinergic inter-neurons are present in the cervical ganglia of some species (see discussion by Wilson and Cooper, 1972).

Giacobini et al. (1971) devised a microscale procedure for the preparation of sub-cellular fractions from one or two pooled ganglia (mg amounts), applying micromethods of analysis to characterize enzymatically the fractions obtained. While they were partially successful in their endeavour, their 'synaptosomal' fractions were heavily contaminated and hardly distinguishable as such. Few well-preserved synaptosomes were obtained in those fractions showing the highest activities of AChE and ChAc.

Wilson and Cooper (1972), unlike Giacobini et al. (1971), were successful in achieving tissue dispersion with collagenase. Using bovine superior cervical ganglia these workers incubated sliced ganglia in a modified Krebs solution, and then dispersed the tissue by adding 0·15 (w/v) collagenase and 0·15% hyaluronidase (or simply 0·3% collagenase) to the incubation medium. Differential centrifugation procedures yielded a crude synapto-somal fraction (P_2) which was further purified by centrifugation on sucrose-tris or Ficoll density gradients. Assay of ACh and ChAc plus EM confirmed that presynaptic nerve endings had survived the incubation procedure, appearing in the P_2 fraction and sedi-menting to a density of 1·13 in sucrose and 1·06 in Ficoll. The washed P_2 fraction had an ACh content of 2·3 nmol/mg protein, compared with corresponding levels of 0·08 in rat brain (De Robertis et al., 1962a), and 0·19 (Kurokawa et al., 1965b) and 0·6 (Richter and Marchbanks, 1971b) in guinea-pig cerebral cortex.

2.3.7   Non-mammalian techniques

Detailed morphological and biochemical studies of non-mammalian synaptosomes have been largely confined to two experimental situations, cephalopod brain (head ganglion) and *Torpedo* electric organ, both of which have relatively high concentrations of ACh. They are useful situations therefore, in which to study cholinergic systems, and while investigations of them are still in their infancy their potential value is considerable. They are considered together because their fractionation presents similar problems and because they are both good examples of cholinergic systems.

(i) *Cephalopod brain.* The first attempts at isolating synaptosomes from *Octopus* brain were made by Jones (1967) and Florey and Winesdorfer (1968), and have more recently been supplemented by the work of Heilbronn et al. (1971) and Dowdall and Whittaker (1973) on *Loligo*. It soon became obvious to these workers that the most critical aspect of the fractionation procedures was the tonicity of the homogenization medium. The use of 0·32M sucrose severely damaged the material, producing mainly empty profiles and badly distorted mitochondria (Jones, 1967). A few synaptosomes did survive even these hypotonic conditions however, as demonstrated by EM and by the distribution of ACh, fumarase and LDH (Dowdall and Whittaker, 1973). There can be no doubt that condiions as hypotonic to sea water as these cause considerable osmotic damage to membrane-bound structures with subsequent loss of constituents. For instance, in Dowdall and Whittaker's experiments only 5% of the ACh survived the homogenization.

The question is whether a medium isotonic to sea water (1·1M) is the ideal one. In order to answer this, Dowdall and Whittaker (1973) measured the yield of bound ACh as a function of the osmolarity of various homogenization media. They found that the yield of bound ACh is increased when the osmolarity of the medium is raised from 0·32M to 1·1M, while sucrose alone is more effective at preserving bound ACh than NaCl of equivalent osmolarity (Table 2.3). The most effective medium appears to be a mixture of

Table 2.3   Acetylcholine content of homogenates and extracts of squid head ganglia (from Dowdall and Whittaker, 1973)

| Homogenization medium | | ACh *content of tissue preparation* |
Solute	Concentration (M)	(nmol/g *of tissue*)
Homogenates:		
Sucrose	0·32	443
	0·70	715
	1·10	743
NaCl	0·35	520
	0·55	520
Sucrose	0·35	800
plus NaCl	0·17	
Whole tissue:		
Trichloroacetic acid extract		2090 ± 220 (4)

0·35M sucrose and 0·17M-NaCl, with which approximately 40% of the ACh survives homogenization. A little less effective are 1·1M sucrose (36%) and 0·7M sucrose (34%). Before deciding on the most satisfactory medium a number of other factors require consideration. The higher the osmotic pressure of a sucrose solution the greater its density and the slower the sedimentation of particulate material. This would favour the use of a medium of intermediate osmolarity. Mixtures of sucrose and NaCl, while combining high osmotic pressure and relatively low density, may cause coacervation of particles of different sizes, thereby militating against their suitability. In view of these diverse factors Dowdall and Whittaker (1973) selected 0·7M sucrose as the homogenization medium of choice. This compares with Jones's (1967) use of either 0·7M sucrose containing 0·33M urea or 0·8M sucrose alone, the latter giving comparable morphological results to the former, Florey and Winesdorfer's (1968) use of a 1:1 mixture of saline and 1M sucrose and the use of a 0·2M sucrose–0·3M-NaCl mixture by Heilbronn *et al.* (1971). In empirical terms there is little to choose between these media, while those with high sucrose concentrations suffer from the disadvantage that in the presence of such high sucrose concentrations negative staining is virtually impossible due to sucrose contamination (Jones, 1967). It was for this reason that Jones (1970c) resorted to glucose as a homogenization medium when negative staining of synaptosomes was desired (Section 3.1.3).

The centrifugation techniques used are essentially similar to those designed for the fractionation of mammalian brain, those of Jones (1967) and Dowdall and Whittaker (1973) closely following the Gray and Whittaker (1962) schedule. The P_2 fractions of both sets of workers are dominated by well-preserved synaptosomes, the main contaminants being small vesicular structures of unknown origin and occasionally nuclei (Plate 2.6). Synaptosomes also occur in the other primary fractions, P_1 and P_3. This wide distribution of synaptosomes is in contrast to that of their mammalian counterparts, and was also noted by Florey and Winesdorfer (1968). Of the six subfractions of the latter workers' crude mitochondrial fraction (M), four contained synaptosomes, their densities ranging from 0·7M–1·3M sucrose. The ultrastructural appearance of these subfractions is very similar to that of the Jones (1967) and Dowdall and Whittaker (1973) P_2 fractions.

These studies clearly confirm those earlier ones (Bacq, 1935; Bacq and Mazza, 1935; Florey, 1963; Loe and Florey, 1966) which demonstrated that the cephalopod brain contains high levels of ACh. While one cannot be certain about the location of this ACh it seems reasonable to assume that much of it is located within neurons and hence synaptosomes. It may be that, as first suggested by Loe and Florey (1966), the distinction between cholinergic and non-cholinergic neurons in cephalopods lies in their relative concentrations of ACh. Other putative transmitters have also been detected in many parts of cephalopod CNS (5-HT, Welsh and Moorhead, 1959; Juorio, 1971; dopamine and NE, Juorio, 1970, 1971), and while their levels are low in comparison to ACh they should dispel any illusions about the CNS being entirely cholinergic. ChAc and AChE also occur in high concentrations in cephalopod synaptosomes (Welsch and Dettbarn, 1972),* which contain a high-affinity choline uptake system capable of transporting choline 60 times more rapidly than that of mammalian synaptosomes (Whittaker *et al.*, 1972; Dowdall and Simon, 1973). Even if not entirely cholinergic, it would appear that cephalopod neurons are primarily and predominantly cholinergic.

This conclusion is supported by the specific concentrations of ACh found in synaptosomes, the highest reported values ranging from 15 nmol/mg protein in *Loligo* (Dowdall and Whittaker, 1973) to 23 nmol/mg protein in *Octopus* (Florey and Winesdorfer, 1968). These compare with values in the vicinity of 0·35 nmol/mg protein in mammalian brain. By contrast, the maximum yield of bound ACh is of the order of 40–45% of the total ACh in cephalopods (Dowdall and Whittaker, 1973 and Florey and Winesdorfer, 1968 respectively) compared with about 70% in mammalian brain (Hebb and Whittaker, 1958). This suggests that cephalopod synaptosomes are more fragile than mammalian ones, although the comparative osmotic conditions during homogenization may have a role to play in this discrepancy.

(ii) Torpedo *electric organ.* The principal goal of subfractionation studies of *Torpedo* electric organ has been the isolation of highly enriched fractions of vesicles, the separation

---

* Welsch and Dettbarn (1972) working with the optic lobes of the squid, *Loligo*, homogenized them in 0·82M sucrose but were only able to obtain a small percentage of the bound ACh in the mitochondrial fraction. Homogenization in 1·5M sucrose and direct centrifugation resulted in 3 fractions, one of which contained large amounts of bound ACh ('total' ACh–19 nmol/mg protein).

of synaptosomes taking a subsidiary place. The fractionation procedures used in *Torpedo* investigations will be described in detail therefore in Section 2.4.5.

Investigations on *Torpedo* synaptosomes by Frontali and Toschi (1958), Sheridan *et al.* (1966), Israël and Gautron (1969) and Israël *et al.* (1970) have not been particularly successful in producing highly enriched fractions of undamaged synaptosomes. This may in part be due to the predominant interest of these workers in isolating vesicles. The osmolarity of the homogenization medium presented similar difficulties to those experienced in the cephalopod work described above, and the same principles apply. Sheridan *et al.* (1966) used 0·5M sucrose containing 0·33M urea, although the mixture of 0·2M sucrose–0·3M-NaCl adopted by Israël and co-workers (Israël and Gautron, 1969; Israël *et al.*, 1970), is now accepted as a more useful one (Whittaker *et al.*, 1972).

Sheridan *et al.* (1966) modified the fractionation procedures then current for mammalian tissue, using a combination of rate and isopycnic centrifugation schemes. The primary fraction P_2 was heterogeneous, although it contained vesicular profiles (0·2–1·0 μm across) some of which resembled synaptosomes. Fractions S_1 and P_{23} were similar, having compositions equivalent to a mixture of P_2 and P_3.

Homogenization in 0·2M sucrose–0·3M-NaCl, and similar centrifugation conditions (Israël and Gautron, 1969), yields heterogeneous vesicular fractions. The synaptosomes are readily recognizable although frequently damaged, the enveloping membranes having ruptured releasing many vesicles. Fragments of the non-innervated face of the electroplaque are also common constituents of these fractions.

The electric tissue of the eel *Electrophorus electricus* was the subject of a study by Karlin (1965), whose principal interest lay in correlating AChE levels with cell membranes. His fractionation procedures therefore were directed towards isolating membrane fragments rather than synaptosomes.

(iii) *Mussel CNS.* Another situation of interest is the CNS of the fresh water mussel, *Anodonta.* Isotonic conditions in this instance are the converse of those found in *Octopus* or *Torpedo*, a satisfactory homogenization medium being 0·05M sucrose (Potts, 1954; Hiripi, Sálanki, Zs-Nagy and Muskó, 1973). The misleading results of earlier subcellular fractionation studies were undoubtedly due in large part to the use of 0·25M sucrose, leading to the excessive disruption of tissue and a failure to produce synaptosomes (e.g. Zs-Nagy, Rózsa, Salánki, Földes, Perényi and Demeter, 1965).

Hiripi *et al.* (1973), starting from a conventional mitochondrial (P_2) fraction, adopted three fractionation schemes to produce synaptosomes. In the first, the P_2 fraction was resuspended in 0·05M sucrose and placed on a discontinuous gradient. The resulting synaptosomes sedimented in a hypertonic solution (1·2–1·5M) and were severely shrunken and frequently distorted. In the second scheme, the P_2 fraction was osmotically shocked in distilled water and the resulting synaptosomes sedimenting between 0·4 and 0·8M sucrose were better preserved, containing numerous DCV. Also in this fraction were cytosomes and heterogeneous membrane fragments. The third scheme employed the same density gradient as the second, but the osmotic shock was omitted.

Overall, 90% of the 5-HT, dopamine and NE present in the CNS is bound to particles,

60–70% of the bound monoamines being localized in the mitochondrial fraction and 15–20% in the microsomal fraction. The synaptosomal fractions display a high relative specific activity of the three monoamines, the relative specific activity of 5-HT being particularly high in them.

2.4 ISOLATION OF SYNAPTIC VESICLES

The early attempts at isolating synaptic vesicles followed closely on the separation of synaptosomes, which naturally provided the source of the vesicles. The principal workers involved were therefore Whittaker and co-workers (Whittaker *et al.*, 1964; Whittaker and Sheridan, 1965) and De Robertis and his co-workers (De Robertis, Rodriguez de Lores Arnaiz and Pellegrino de Iraldi, 1962b; De Robertis *et al.*, 1963).

The type of gradient used by these investigators was a discontinuous sucrose one (Table 2.1), although as is made clear by Schemes 2.4 and 2.5 this gradient played a much larger part in Whittaker's procedures than in those of De Robertis. While other methods have since been employed to obtain synaptic vesicle fractions in mammalian tissues (see below), those originated by Whittaker and De Robertis remain the principal ones and still constitute the basis of the majority of vesicle studies. The electric organ of *Torpedo* has more recently proved an excellent source of synaptic vesicles; the techniques and results of these studies are considered in Section 2.4.5.

2.4.1 Whittaker's procedure (Scheme 2.4)

Synaptosomes are osmotically sensitive structures and can therefore be disrupted either by resuspending in distilled water (Johnson and Whittaker, 1963) or by successively freezing-and-thawing a number of times. As the former method is more amenable to accurate reproduction than the latter, it is more reliable and therefore the method of choice. The addition of eserine sulphate to the water preserves the 50% of the ACh present in the P_2 fraction, by preventing its destruction by AChE (Whittaker *et al.*, 1964). Disruption of the synaptosomes produces a mixture of synaptic vesicles, external membranes, intraterminal mitochondria, partially disrupted synaptosomes and soluble cytoplasmic constituents, which are susceptible to separation by centrifuging into a 5-layered discontinuous density gradient. The resulting fractions are depicted in Fig. 2.5 and schematically in Scheme 2.4.

According to Whittaker *et al.* (1964) LDH, potassium and ChAc are recovered mainly in the soluble cytoplasmic fraction (O), SDH in the mitochondrial fraction (I), and AChE in the microsome and large membrane fractions (E–G). Bound ACh has a bimodal distribution, occurring in the synaptic vesicle fraction (D) and in the partially disrupted synaptosomal fraction (H). This distribution is depicted diagrammatically in Fig. 4.2.

Morphological investigation of fraction D using negative staining (Section 3.3.3) shows that it consists of numerous synaptic vesicles plus a few larger vesicular profiles, probably microsomal in origin, and some larger membrane fragments (Plate 2.7). Vesicles also occur to a limited extent in fraction E.

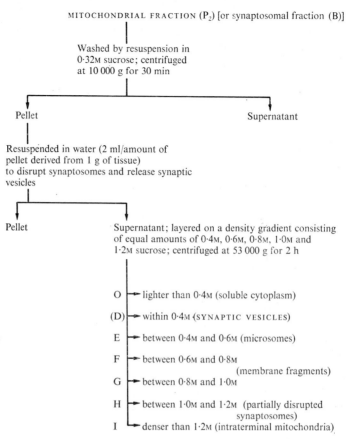

MITOCHONDRIAL FRACTION (P₂) [or synaptosomal fraction (B)]

Washed by resuspension in
0·32M sucrose; centrifuged
at 10 000 g for 30 min

Pellet   Supernatant

Resuspended in water (2 ml/amount of
pellet derived from 1 g of tissue)
to disrupt synaptosomes and release synaptic
vesicles

Pellet

Supernatant; layered on a density gradient consisting
of equal amounts of 0·4M, 0·6M, 0·8M, 1·0M and
1·2M sucrose; centrifuged at 53 000 g for 2 h

O → lighter than 0·4M (soluble cytoplasm)

(D) → within 0·4M (SYNAPTIC VESICLES)

E → between 0·4M and 0·6M (microsomes)

F → between 0·6M and 0·8M
                        (membrane fragments)
G → between 0·8M and 1·0M

H → between 1·0M and 1·2M (partially disrupted
                        synaptosomes)
I → denser than 1·2M (intraterminal mitochondria)

Scheme 2.4   Separation of synaptosomes into component organelles after Whittaker *et al.*
(1964) and Whittaker and Sheridan (1965)

An abbreviated procedure developed by Whittaker and Sheridan (1965) consists of
centrifuging the synaptosomal suspension into a partially continuous sucrose density
gradient to obtain four fractions, one of which (D_1) contains monodispersed synaptic
vesicles. Micrographs of a sectioned pellet of isolated vesicles prepared by the method
of Whittaker *et al.* (1964) demonstrate the relative homogeneity of the fraction, although
a number of microsomal-like vesicles are also present in the field (Plate 2.7).

A further aspect of Whittaker and Sheridan's (1965) work involved 'tagging' a synaptic
vesicle suspension with polystyrene latex beads (Plate 2.9). In this way they calculated
that the number of synaptic vesicles in a homogeneous fraction of isolated vesicles is
$3·84 \times 10^{12}$/volume of fraction equivalent to 1g of cerebral cortex. The isolated vesicle
fraction accounted for about 35% of the bound ACh recovered in the various fractions
derived from the disrupted synaptosomes, this parent fraction accounting for about 45%
of the ACh of the original homogenate. In all therefore the yield of isolated vesicles was
roughly 15–16% of that in the original homogenate. From this they concluded that there
are of the order of $2·4 \times 10^{13}$ synaptic vesicles/g cortex.

A minor modification of the Whittaker and Sheridan technique has more recently been employed by Johnson, Boukma, Lahti and Mathews (1973) working with mouse whole brain. The difference introduced by these workers is an abbreviated density gradient and a higher centrifugal force to remove ghosts, membranes and intact synaptosomes from vesicles after the hypotonic shock. The resulting fraction at 0·4M sucrose appears as a

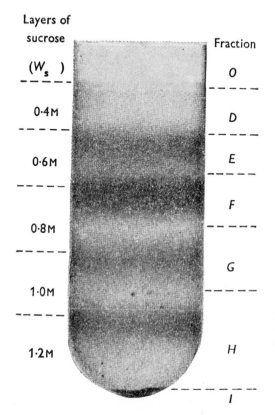

Layers of sucrose

(W_s)

0·4M

0·6M

0·8M

1·0M

1·2M

Fraction

O

D

E

F

G

H

I

Figure 2.5 Appearance of centrifuge tube after layering the osmotically shocked P_2 fraction (Ws) on a discontinuous sucrose density gradient and centrifuging at 53 500 *g* for 2h. This is the final stage in Whittaker's procedure for isolating synaptic vesicles (Scheme 2.4). (From Whittaker *et al.*, 1964.)

very homogeneous vesicle fraction which, by applying virus counting techniques (Mathews and Buthala, 1970) contains approximately $3·4 \times 10^9$ vesicles/ml (compared with Whittaker and Sheridan's estimate using a 'tagging' procedure of about $1·36 \times 10^{12}$ vesicles/ml).

2.4.2 De Robertis's technique (Scheme 2.5)

In order to minimize the time the tissue is in contact with sucrose, the primary mito-chondrial fraction (Mit) is treated rapidly with sucrose. Towards this end a discontinuous density gradient is dispensed with, the synaptosomes being disrupted by treatment with distilled water and briefly centrifuged. The pellet (M_1) removed the myelin fragments, mitochondria and ruptured synaptosomes, leaving the supernatant which was further centrifuged to yield another pellet (M_2) and supernatant (M_3). M_2 served as the source of synaptic vesicles, although larger membranous profiles also occurred in it (De Robertis *et al.,* 1963). Negative staining of this fraction clearly revealed coated vesicles (termed annular synaptic vesicles by De Robertis), DCV and some membranous profiles, in addition to the more usual agranular synaptic vesicles (Plate 2.8).

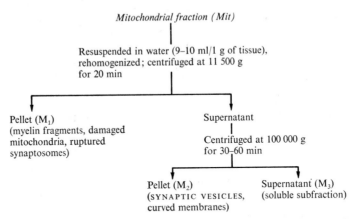

Scheme 2.5   Separation of synaptosomes into component organelles after De Robertis *et al.* (1963)

A point in the technique stressed by De Robertis was the presence of $CaCl_2$ in the distilled water used to rupture the synaptosomes. The amount of Ca^{2+} in the distilled water was 10 μmol/litre of Ca^{2+} to bring the concentration of the solution to 0·32M. The value of Ca^{2+} is to avoid clumping of the subcellular particles and to bring about retention of the vesicles, together with soluble proteins and enzymes, in the synaptosomes prior to their distribution. Its concentration however, is critical if it is to act in this way and not prevent liberation of the vesicles once the endings are torn (see also Whittaker *et al.*, 1964).

The biochemical estimations carried out by De Robertis *et al.* (1963) suggested that ChAc and ACh are concentrated in the vesicular fraction (M_2). AChE is also present in this fraction, although its principal location is in M_1 presumably associated with the membranes of the damaged synaptosomes. SDH is chiefly localized in M_1, reflecting the presence of mitochondria.

The details of the conflicting results between the Whittaker and De Robertis groups concerning the localization of ChAc will be considered in Section 4.1.1. What is of relevance at this juncture is the degree of enrichment of the vesicular fractions of the two groups, because if there is a significant difference between the two methods this in itself may account for variations in the level of enzymes.

The published micrographs of the two groups are remarkably similar considering the differences in preparation and the diverse interpretations placed on the results. The discrepancy between the reported distributions of ChAc can be largely accounted for in other terms as will be argued later (Section 4.1.1) On the assumption that the published micrographs are representative of the fractions as a whole, the vesicle fractions of both groups are good workable preparations of isolated synaptic vesicles.

2.4.3 Electrophoretic separation

Vos *et al.* (1968), using sucrose gradient electrophoresis (Svensson, 1960), were able to obtain the electrophoretic mobilities of subcellular particles of brain, including synaptosomes and synaptic vesicles (Table 2.4). All particles tested were negatively charged with

Table 2.4 Electrophoretic mobilities and binding properties of brain synaptic vesicles, synaptosomes, and mitochondria (Modified from Vos *et al.*, 1968)

Fraction	Electrophoretic mobility (u/sec/V/cm)	% total counts bound/mg protein			
		GABA	ACh	NE	5-HT
Synaptic vesicles	− 0·96	7·39	8·45	7·76	21·32
Synaptosomes	− 1·68	13·55	5·94	6·02	18·82
Mitochondria	− 1·58	6·21	0·93	7·08	6·56

isoelectric points around 4. GABA was well bound by the vesicles, synaptosomes and mitochondria, as was NE. ACh and 5-HT however, were bound to vesicles and synaptosomes, but only slightly to mitochondria.

In a follow-up to this study Kuriyama, Roberts and Vos (1968b) attempted to characterize further the binding of GABA and ACh to the vesicle fraction from mouse brain, to determine whether the same or different binding sites were being utilized. In terms of their requirements of Na^+, the authors concluded that the binding of GABA and ACh takes place by different mechanisms and at different sites. Separation of this heterogeneous vesicle population into sub-groups with regard to GABA content, GAD activity and binding capacity for GABA and ACh was not as successful. Discontinuous density gradient centrifugation and the electrophoresis of vesicles in a continuous sucrose gradient both produced subfractions, but failed to yield significant fractionation of the vesicles in terms of either the variables being measured or morphological features. Kuriyama *et al.* (1968b) conclude: 'It is possible that several vesicle types are present, each specializing in different transmitters, but that the densities and distribution of surface charges on the vesicles are sufficiently similar so that our procedures were not capable of obtaining clean separations.'

Although not yet applied to vesicle separation, the technique of zonal density gradient electrophoresis deserves mention in this section. Sellinger and Borens (1969) in a study of membrane fractions isolated from rat cerebral cortex determined the electrokinetic profiles of the membranes in each fraction. This approach revealed marked differences in electrophoretic mobility between the fractions, correlating directly with their membrane-bound *N*-acetylneuraminic acid (NANA) content and their AChE activity. As the latter components are preferentially located in membranes of synaptic origin, it is significant that the fraction in which they predominate was isolated as a single, homogeneous electrophoretic peak.

Continuous free-flow electrophoresis, originally described by Hannig (1967) has been used by Ryan *et al.* (1971) to obtain enriched preparations of synaptosomes and synaptic vesicles from crude fractions of guinea-pig brain homogenates. For instance Whittaker's synaptosomal preparation P_2 and synaptic vesicle fraction D_1 were subfractionated by electrophoresis in order to produce purified versions of the original fractions. EM evidence of the degree of purity of the electrophoretic subfraction of D_1 shows that some of the membranous contaminants have been removed but, in addition to readily recognizable synaptic vesicles, small white profiles (10 nm across) are present in large numbers. The identity of these profiles is far from clear, although they may be sucrose artifacts. The synaptosomal fraction purified by electrophoresis of P_2 contains synaptosomes plus a few isolated mitochondria and membrane fragments.

The mobilities of synaptosomes, synaptic vesicles and mitochondria are in the same relative order as those reported by Vos *et al.* (1968), although their absolute values in the present study are twice those of Vos and co-workers. Free-flow electrophoretic separation reduces the time required for preparation when compared with the more usual density centrifugation techniques. It is also useful in that it allows the electrokinetic interpretation of data obtained during the separation steps. The claims made by Ryan *et al.* (1971) regarding the purity of the fractions require confirmation by other workers.

A non-electrophoretic method of value in the separation of synaptic vesicles into subpopulations was that adopted by Kadota and Kanaseki (1969) and Kanaseki and Kadota (1969) to separate agranular synaptic vesicles from coated vesicles. In an effort to prepare a large quantity of vesicles, and also to eliminate contaminating membrane fragments, they used a combination of techniques involving differential centrifugation and Sephadex column chromatography. In essence the synaptosomal fraction (P2) was washed (P3), subjected to hypotonic treatments and centrifuged (precipitate, P4). The resulting supernatant was again centrifuged, and the precipitate resuspended in Tris-maleate (P5). This was applied to a DEAE–Sephadex column, which was eluted and centrifuged to give the final precipitate (P6). Different layers of P6 are occupied by synaptic or coated vesicles (Plate 2.10). Marchbanks (1968a) had earlier noted that synaptic vesicles retain their characteristic morphology after passing through Sephadex columns, as well as their ACh content when the columns are equilibrated and eluted with 0·4M sucrose. A refinement of the Kadota and Kanaseki (1969) and Kanaseki and Kadota (1969) technique is described in the following section (2.4.4).

2.4.4. Coated vesicles (Scheme 2.6)

In an attempt to investigate the structure and function of coated vesicles in nervous tissue, Kanaseki and Kadota (1969) followed by Kadota and Kadota (1973b, c) have devised subcellular fractionation techniques for their isolation and separation from plain synaptic vesicles. An outline of the Kadota and Kadota (1973 b, c) technique, which is a refinement of that proposed earlier by Kanaseki and Kadota (1969) is illustrated in Scheme 2.6.

Following homogenization in 0·32M sucrose using a Potter-Elvehjem homogenizer with a clearance of 0·01 mm, brain tissue is centrifuged approximately according to the Gray and Whittaker (1962) schedule. The P_1 pellet is the nuclear fraction, and the P_2 the crude synaptosomal one. Washing of the P_2 fraction produces another synaptosomal pellet (P_3) which is the starting point for the isolation of the vesicular structures (Kadota and Kadota, 1973c). The remaining steps in the fractionation procedure are shown in Scheme 2.6, from which it can be seen that three fractions of note are produced.

78

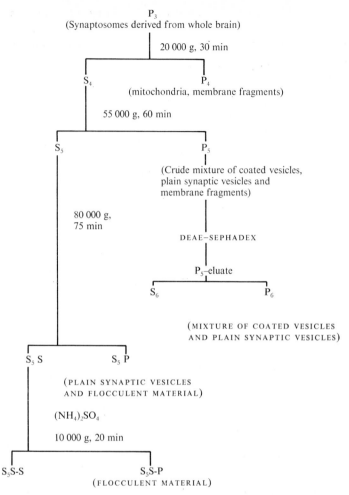

P$_3$
(Synaptosomes derived from whole brain)

20 000 g, 30 min

S$_4$ P$_4$
(mitochondria, membrane fragments)

55 000 g, 60 min

S$_5$ P$_5$
(Crude mixture of coated vesicles,
plain synaptic vesicles and
membrane fragments)

80 000 g,
75 min

DEAE–SEPHADEX

P$_5$–eluate

S$_6$ P$_6$

(MIXTURE OF COATED VESICLES
AND PLAIN SYNAPTIC VESICLES)

S$_5$ S   S$_5$ P

(PLAIN SYNAPTIC VESICLES
AND FLOCCULENT MATERIAL)

(NH$_4$)$_2$SO$_4$

10 000 g, 20 min

S$_5$S-S   S$_5$S-P
(FLOCCULENT MATERIAL)

Scheme 2.6   Isolation of coated vesicles after Kadota and Kadota (1973b, c)

The P$_6$ precipitate is in two layers, a bottom layer containing coated vesicles, shell fragments, plain synaptic vesicles and membrane fragments, and an upper layer with plain synaptic vesicles and flocculent material.* Attempts to obtain separate fractions of coated vesicles and plain synaptic vesicles proved unsuccessful. Resuspension of the P$_6$ precipitate in Tris-maleate gave the fraction P$_6$, a mixture of coated and plain synaptic vesicles.

The S$_5$ P precipitate contains principally plain synaptic vesicles, with some flocculent material and very few contaminating membrane fragments. The synaptic vesicles occur mainly in the lower part of the pellet and the flocculent material in the upper part. Attempts at removing the flocculent material proved unsatisfactory with the result

* This is the diffuse material within the cytoplasm of synaptosomes, particularly when an unbuffered fixative has been employed. It can also be recognized as isolated profiles in fractions (Fig. 1.7). It may be irregular in size and shape, with a string-like or mesh-like appearance and may correspond to the cytonet of Gray (1972).

that the S_5 P fraction consists of a mixture of plain synaptic vesicles and flocculent material.

The S_5 S-P precipitate was obtained from the S_5 S supernatant by the addition of ammonium sulphate, and contains aggregates of the flocculent material (Plate 2.11).

One of the chief characteristics of this fractionation scheme is the use of a medium consisting of 10mM Tris-maleate (pH 6·5) and 10mM-KCl for resuspension of precipitates, and subsequent passage through Sephadex columns. The aim of this combination is to preserve presynaptic fine structure while eliminating as far as possible contaminating particles.

Although the procedure of Kadota and Kadota failed to separate coated vesicles from plain synaptic vesicles, fractions P_6 and S_5 P are sufficiently different to allow preliminary conclusions. For instance, S_5 P (plain synaptic vesicles) has a higher ACh content than P_6 (coated vesicles), whereas choline is only associated with P_6 (Kadota, Kamiya and Kumegawa, 1970; Kamiya, Kadota and Kadota, 1972). It remains to be seen if this means that coated vesicles are confined to an involvement in the synthesis of ACh, with the agranular or plain synaptic vesicles alone participating in the release of transmitter substance into the cleft.

2.4.5 Non-mammalian techniques

The problems associated with finding a suitable homogenization medium for the fractionate of cephalopod and elasmobranch tissues have been discussed in a previous section (2.3.7). These issues will be taken as read in the present section.

(i) *Cephalopod brain.* Synaptic vesicles have been isolated from octopus (*Eledone*) brain by Jones (1970c), and from the head ganglion of the squid (*Loligo*) by Heilbronn *et al.* (1971) and Dowdall and Whittaker (1973). In each case synaptosomes were disrupted using a hypotonic shock, and the resulting suspension layered on a discontinuous sucrose density gradient. Disruption of the synaptosomes was achieved with distilled water, while the density gradient consisted of sucrose steps ranging from either 0·4 or 0·6M to 1·2M.

A noteworthy feature of Jones's (1970c) morphological study is that synaptic vesicles were present in four of the five fractions resulting from isopycnic centrifugation. Although synaptic vesicles constituted the primary component of the three lightest fractions, they could not be separated from other components such as larger nonspecific vesicular profiles, some containing vesicular inclusions, and a smaller number of synaptosome ghosts and intact synaptosomes (Plate 2.12). In view of these findings it is not surprising that Dowdall and Whittaker (1973) recovered ACh from all their fractions, some fractions demonstrating considerable enrichment of ACh. Unfortunately they were unable to examine these fractions morphologically with the exception of one, which revealed numerous synaptic vesicles together with larger vesicular membrane fragments.

The vesicular fractions in Dowdall and Whittaker's (1973) experiments had a specific concentration of ACh about twice that of intact synaptosomes, that is, 30 nmol/mg protein. Compared with a corresponding value of 570 nmol/mg protein for pure preparations of cholinergic vesicles from *Torpedo* electroplaque tissue (Whittaker *et al.*, 1972), this low figure suggests that the number of intact vesicles isolated in cephalopods is very small indeed. This is borne out by the morphological controls. In spite therefore of the potential of this tissue for the study of cholinergic vesicles, a number of technical problems will have to be overcome before it can be exploited.

(ii) Torpedo *electric organ*. The isolation technique devised by Israël and co-workers (Israël and Gautron, 1969; Israël *et al.*, 1970) utilizes preliminary rate centrifugation followed by isopycnic density gradient centrifugation. Rate centrifugation of the 20% homogenate results in a pellet containing the non-innervated elements of the electroplaque, unbroken or half-broken synaptosomes and empty profiles, and a supernatant which is rich in synaptic vesicles and membrane fragments. Density gradient centrifugation, with its upper fractions being brought to 0·8M by the addition of NaCl to the sucrose, produces four fractions. Fraction 1 consists of soluble proteins and is free of particulate material, fraction 2 is the vesicle fraction, fraction 3 consists of large membrane fragments, while fraction 4 comprises large empty profiles.

Fraction 2 is an excellent example of a highly enriched vesicle fraction, the vast majority of the profiles conforming to the criteria demanded of synaptic vesicles (Plate 2.13). Only a very limited amount of membranous contamination is evident in the published micrographs, an observation confirmed by the low activity in this fraction of 5′-nucleotidase, a membrane marker. This fraction contains 85% of the ACh activity layered on the gradient, and this is 150–300 times more ACh than found in the vesicular fraction prepared from guinea-pig cerebral cortex (Israël, 1969). ChAc and LDH behave as soluble cytoplasmic enzymes, 78% and 80% of their activities respectively being recovered in fraction 1. Of the AChE recovered, 87% is in fraction 4, with a further preponderance in the primary membrane-containing fraction.

The principal modification to Israël and Gautron's (1969) technique by Whittaker *et al.*, (1972) was the use of zonal centrifugation. Initial homogenization of the tissue was also modified in that it was first frozen with liquid Freon 12 and then crushed to a coarse powder. After warming to 0° C the tissue was homogenized in 0·2M sucrose–0·3M-NaCl using an Aldridge homogenizer. Initial centrifugation removed coarse membrane fragments, nuclei and mitochondria, and the supernatant (S_{12}) was layered against a continuous sucrose density gradient containing 0·2M–1·4M sucrose in a zonal centrifuge. Centrifugation was carried out at 115 000 *g* for 3 h, or its equivalent, and recoveries averaged 71% ACh and 75% protein.

Zonal centrifugation caused the bound ACh to migrate as a sharp peak with a density at the peak (VP) equivalent to 0·37–0·39M sucrose containing 0·225–0·215M-NaCl. The peak ACh fractions are rich in monodisperse synaptic vesicles (Soifer and Whittaker, 1972) with little large membranous contamination. The ACh content of these fractions was estimated by Whittaker *et al.* (1972) to be of the order of 570 nmol/mg protein, with values ranging up to 680 nmol/mg protein or even higher. On the basis of these values and by 'tagging' vesicle suspensions with polystyrene beads of known diameter and number (Whittaker and Sheridan, 1965; Sheridan *et al.*, 1966), the number of ACh molecules/vesicle was calculated. The mean figure obtained, 66 000 molecules/vesicle (360 nmol ACh/μl), compares with the earlier estimate of 40 000 molecules/vesicle by Sheridan *et al.* (1966).

Before these figures can be accepted, two points require consideration. The initial freezing and comminution of the tissue may have damaged or even destroyed the vesicles. Anticipating this possibility, Soifer and Whittaker (1972) examined them morphologically and found that even after temperatures of $-20°$ C to $-60°$ C vesicles were still intact. It is not clear what proportion of vesicles survive these extreme conditions, although those that do appear normal on negative staining. A second query concerns the high degree of variabiliy of the results, the ACh content of vesicles ranging from 8 000 to 137 000 molecules, with a mean of 66 000. Whittaker *et al.* (1972) ascribe this variability to the need for repeated application of suspensions to the grids, this being necessitated by the low concentration of vesicles (Soifer and Whittaker, 1972). It would be hazardous therefore to place undue emphasis on the reliability of the resulting estimates, and the appropriateness of zonal centrifugation as applied to *Torpedo* tissue may be questioned.

A figure of the order of 40 000–70 000 molecules ACh/synaptic vesicle for *Torpedo* tissue must be compared with 2000 molecules/cholinergic vesicle for guinea-pig cerebral cortex. The latter estimate by Whittaker and Sheridan (1965) was derived using polystyrene beads and is considered by them a reasonable estimate of the number of molecules to fill a 31 nm diameter vesicle core with isotonic ACh (Section 5.2.2). Even allowing for the larger diameter of *Torpedo* synaptic vesicles (30–120 nm – Sheridan, 1965; 84 nm, S.D. $\pm$ 30 nm, as the true mean diameter – Sheridan *et al.*, 1966), the vastly higher estimates of ACh content in *Torpedo* vesicles call for a revised concept of the method of accommodating the ACh molecules within vesicles.

2.5 FURTHER DISSECTION OF THE SYNAPTOSOME

2.5.1 Synaptic plasma membranes (Schemes 2.7 and 2.8)

Following the isolation of synaptosomes and synaptic vesicles the next step was to dissect the synaptosome further and analyse the synaptic membrane (Fig. 2.6c). The approaches adopted by workers to achieve this end mirrored the expanding array of experimental tools employed in synaptosomal studies. These are outlined in Table 2.1, from which it is evident that whereas De Robertis's group relied on its previous experience with discontinuous sucrose gradients (De Robertis, Alberici, Rodriguez de Lores Arnaiz and Azcurra, 1966a), other workers placed greater emphasis upon a variety of techniques including Ficoll gradients (Cotman and Matthews, 1971; Morgan, Wolfe, Mandel and Gombos, 1971; Morgan *et al.*, 1972), zonal centrifugation (Cotman *et al.*, 1968a; McBride Mahler, Moore and White, 1970) and the French press (Austin, Rostas, Livett and Jeffrey, 1973).

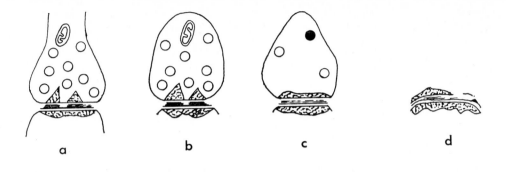

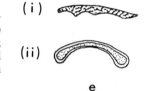

Figure 2.6 A schematic diagram illustrating the derivation of nerve-ending components from an intact synapse. (a) *in situ* synapse; (b) synaptosome; (c) synaptic plasma membrane plus junctional region; (d) synaptic complex; (e, i) postsynaptic membrane with anticipated characteristics; (e, ii) profile described as a postsynaptic membrane in studies of Garey *et al.* (1972). For discussion of details see text.

Rodriguez de Lores Arnaiz *et al.* (1967) used their M_1 fraction as the starting point for the separation of synaptic membranes (Scheme 2.7). Containing as it does myelin fragments, swollen mitochondria and numerous additional membranes, its heterogeneity is a distinct drawback when it comes to identifying the origin of any resulting membrane fractions. On the assumption that all nondescript membranes are synaptic in origin, a hazardous one in view of the similar morphological and sedimentation characteristics of axonal, synaptosomal and glial membranes (Lemkey-Johnston and Dekermenjian, 1970; Cotman *et al.*, 1971a), this technique can probably separate the bulk of these

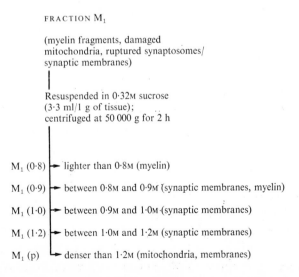

FRACTION M_1

(myelin fragments, damaged
mitochondria, ruptured synaptosomes/
synaptic membranes)

Resuspended in 0·32M sucrose
(3·3 ml/1 g of tissue);
centrifuged at 50 000 g for 2 h

M_1 (0·8) — lighter than 0·8M (myelin)

M_1 (0·9) — between 0·8M and 0·9M (synaptic membranes, myelin)

M_1 (1·0) — between 0·9M and 1·0M (synaptic membranes)

M_1 (1·2) — between 1·0M and 1·2M (synaptic membranes)

M_1 (p) — denser than 1·2M (mitochondria, membranes)

Scheme 2.7 Isolation of synaptic membranes after Rodriguez de Lores Arniaz *et al.* (1967)

83

membranes from myelin and mitochondrial fragments. There is however, no certainty regarding the identity and homogeneity of the plasma membranes, as a variety of vesicular elements may be bound by a plasma membrane (Cotman and Matthews, 1971).

According to Rodriguez de Lores Arnaiz *et al.* (1967) two subfractions of the M_1 fraction appeared to consist principally of synaptic membranes. These were the M_1 (1·0) and M_1 (1·2) subfractions and were characterized by EM and by the presence of membrane-bound enzymes, namely AChE, (Na^+–K^+)-activated ATPase, K^+-activated *p*-nitrophenylphosphatase and glutamine synthetase.

Morphologically the two subfractions are similar, with round or oval membranous profiles corresponding in size to synaptosomes (Plate 2.14). Thickened and dense areas are evident on some of the profiles, especially where membranes are juxtaposed (see also De Robertis *et al.*, 1967a). A number of these resemble the paramembranous densities of synaptic junctions, although others are difficult to categorize. A few synaptic vesicles and small mitochondria were also described in the M_1 (1·2) fraction, trapped within the membranes.

The principal biochemical difference observed by the authors between the two subfractions was in the distribution of AChE, 40% of which was detected in the M_1 (1·0) subfraction with a relative specific activity of 2·96. By contrast 13·7% occurred in M_1 (1·2) its relative specific activity in this subfraction being 0·80. Their general conclusion therefore, regarding the distribution of AChE was that AChE-rich membranes remain mainly about the 1·0M sucrose concentration, a conclusion in accord with De Robertis's views on the localization of this enzyme in subcellular fractions (De Robertis *et al.*, 1962a; Rodriguez de Lores Arnaiz, 1964).

In an attempt to overcome the difficulties inherent in preparing synaptic plasma membranes from a crude mitochondrial fraction, Cotman and Matthews (1971) prepared them directly from synaptosomes. In view of the experience of a number of other workers that synaptosomal preparations isolated on Ficoll–sucrose gradients are purer and better preserved than those isolated on sucrose gradients (Autilio *et al.*, 1968), 60–80% of the profiles being synaptosomes (Autilio *et al.*, 1968; Flexner *et al.*, 1971), Cotman and Matthews (1971) employed a Ficoll–sucrose gradient for preparing their synaptosomal fraction (Scheme 2·8). Furthermore they achieved optimal osmotic shock by employing alkaline conditions.

The synaptosomal fraction which served as the basis of their membrane isolation procedure consisted of approximately 60–75% synaptosomes, with free membranes, mitochondria and membrane vesicles as the principal contaminating elements. The problem of isolating a synaptic plasma membrane fraction under these conditions therefore, becomes one of separating synaptosomal membranes, which are clearly in the majority, from mitochondria and synaptic vesicles (Cotman and Matthews, 1971). They must also be obtained in sufficiently high yield, thereby minimizing the chances of obtaining plasma membranes from non-synaptosomal sources.

In order to separate effectively the membrane and mitochondrial fractions in the subfractionation of synaptosomes, Cotman and Matthews (1971) found that the more alkaline the conditions during osmotic shock the more complete the separation. For instance, at pH 8·5, 95% of the cytochrome oxidase separates from approximately 85% of the (Na+–K+)-ATPase; by contrast at pH 7·1, 50% of the cytochrome oxidase overlaps 89% of the (Na+–K+)-ATPase. As cytochrome oxidase is a mitochondrial marker (Parsons, Williams and Chance, 1966), and (Na+–K+)-activated ouabain-sensitive ATPase a membrane marker with a high specific activity in synaptosomal membranes (e.g. Hosie, 1965; Bradford *et al.*, 1966; Rodriguez de Lores Arnaiz *et al.*, 1967), the

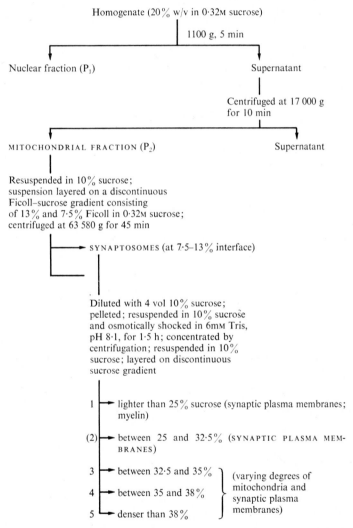

Scheme 2.8   Isolation of synaptic plasma membranes after Cotman and Matthews (1971)

degree of separation of the mitochondrial and membrane subfractions differs considerably depending on pH.

The discontinuous sucrose density gradient selected by Cotman and Matthews (1971) and illustrated in Scheme 2·8 was designed to prepare relatively large quantities of membrane. Fraction 2 collected at the 25% and 32·5% sucrose interface contained 50% of the (Na+–K+)-ATPase activity and also had the highest relative specific activity for this enzyme. By contrast only 7% of the total cytochrome oxidase of the gradient was recovered in it. On morphological examination this fraction consisted largely of plasma membranes of variable shape, although generally the size of synaptosomes (Plate 2.15)· As with the membrane fractions of Rodriguez de Lores Arnaiz et al. (1967), many of the membranes were thickened in places suggesting the presence of junctional regions. The principal contaminants of Cotman and Matthews's membrane fraction were a few synaptic vesicles and small dark structures tentatively identified as lysosomal or cytoplasmic in nature (Plate 2.15).

Enzymatic analysis of the synaptosomal subfractions demonstrated the localization in the synaptic plasma membrane fraction of (Na+–K+)-ATPase, an alkaline phosphatase and β-N-acetylglucosaminidase, while 5'-nucleotidase and AChE sedimented at lighter densities although with considerable overlap. (Na+–K+)-ATPase in this fraction was enriched 5-fold after correction for enzyme inactivation, from which Cotman and Matthews (1971) concluded that 10–20% of particulate material in a brain homogenate is neuronal plasma membrane.

Gurd, Jones, Mahler and Moore (1974) have prepared synaptic plasma membranes in the presence of PO_4/EDTA and find that the resulting membrane fraction exhibits a ten-fold enrichment of (Na+–K+)-ATPase. They further estimate that its microsomal contamination is less than 15% and its mitochondrial contamination less than 10%.

A complementary approach to the isolation of a synaptic plasma membrane fraction utilizes procedures using continuous density gradient ultracentrifugation in zonal rotors (Cotman et al., 1968a; McBride et al., 1970). Cotman et al. (1968a) employing a 15–50% sucrose gradient in a zonal rotor, noted that when a crude brain mitochondrial fraction was subjected to osmotic shock and resolved on a linear sucrose gradient, a particulate band was observed at the 29–32% (w/w) sucrose level. EMs of this zone, which was not present following centrifugation of an isotonically prepared crude mitochondrial fraction, showed that it contained free membranes with some synaptic thickenings. (Na+–K+)-activated ATPase was concentrated in this fraction, while the levels of mitochondrial and microsomal marker enzymes were low. Cotman et al. (1968) estimated that the assayable contamination of this fraction was in the neighbourhood of 10–20%.

Basing their studies on the procedures of Cotman et al. (1968a), McBride et al. (1970) compared the peaks obtained on fractionation of a crude mitochondrial pellet (P_2) and an osmotically-lysed crude mitochondrial pellet (P_2L). Membrane fragments only appeared as subfractions of P_2L, the principal membrane subfractions occurring in P_2L-F (28–29% sucrose) and P_2L-G (30–31% sucrose). (Na+–K+)-activated ATPase exhibited a bimodal distribution, the first peak occurring between 23–26% sucrose (corresponding to nondescript membrane fragments) and the second between 29–31% sucrose.

Cytochemical analyses of the membrane fraction at 29·0–30·5% sucrose substantiated its membranous nature. Positive results were obtained using the periodic acid – silver methenamine (PAS) stain for glycoproteins (Rambourg and Leblond, 1967), colloidal iron hydroxide for acidic carbohydrates (Mowry, 1963; Benedetti and Emmelot, 1968) and PTA for proteins containing a preponderance of basic amino acids (Bloom and Aghajanian, 1966).

2.5.2 Synaptic (junctional) complexes (Scheme 2.9)

The synaptic complex is best regarded as the synaptic junctional region, which itself has been isolated from the remaining membranes of the synaptic terminal (Fig. 2.6d). For this reason De Robertis and co-workers adopt the term *junctional complex* which they define as 'a unit composed of the two synaptic membranes, the cleft with the inter-synaptic filaments and the subsynaptic web' (De Robertis *et al.*, 1967a). The junctional complex of De Robertis therefore, and the synaptic complex of certain other workers (Davis and Bloom, 1970, 1973; Cotman, Levy, Banker and Taylor, 1971b; Cotman and Taylor, 1972), refers specifically to that area of the synaptic terminal consisting of pre- and postsynaptic membrane, plus the intervening synaptic cleft together with associated paramembranous densities. This corresponds to the contact region of synaptosomes (Jones, 1967).

By contrast, Kornguth and co-workers who also use the term *synaptic complex* are concerned with the synaptic terminal as a whole. Consequently, this term according to them 'refers to the synaptosome attached to the postsynaptic membrane, with retention of the subsynaptic web and intervening filaments' (Kornguth *et al.*, 1969; also Geison *et al.*, 1972). Clearly they are considering complete synaptosomes, bearing in mind that synaptosomes consist of pre- and postsynaptic components together with the intervening contact or junctional region (Jones, 1972; Section 3.1). The term as used by them there-fore would appear to be superfluous, although it must be admitted their principal concern is with the junctional region (Kornguth *et al.*, 1969, 1971, 1972). For the sake of clarity however, the synaptic complexes described by Kornguth's group are treated as synapto-somes in this book and have been considered in detail in Section 2.3.5.

The demonstration by Fiszer and De Robertis (1967) that Triton X-100, a non-ionic surface-active agent, disrupts most of the limiting membrane of synaptosomes while leaving the junctional region intact, opened the way for the isolation of synaptic com-plexes. In particular these authors noted that the most dramatic effect of $0 \cdot 1$–$0 \cdot 5 \%$ Triton X-100 was on AChE levels in crude mitochondrial, synaptosomal and synaptic mem-brane fractions, as little as $13 \cdot 7$–$23 \cdot 4 \%$ remaining in the crude mitochondrial pellet. The solubilization of AChE is higher than that of protein, leading therefore to a concentration of this enzyme in the supernatant (also Cotman *et al.*, 1971b). There is however, no activation or inactivation of this enzyme by the detergent, a point noted previously by other workers (Lawler, 1964; Ord and Thompson, 1951) and in contrast to the action of anionic and cationic detergents, both of which produce considerable inactivation (Lawler, 1964).

Triton X-100 also had a solubilization effect on protein in the fractions studied, although this was less marked than with AChE (Fiszer and De Robertis, 1967). Mono-amine oxidase was minimally affected, while ChAc was practically unaffected by the action of the detergent in the synaptosomal fraction. (Na^+-K^+)-ATPase, on the other

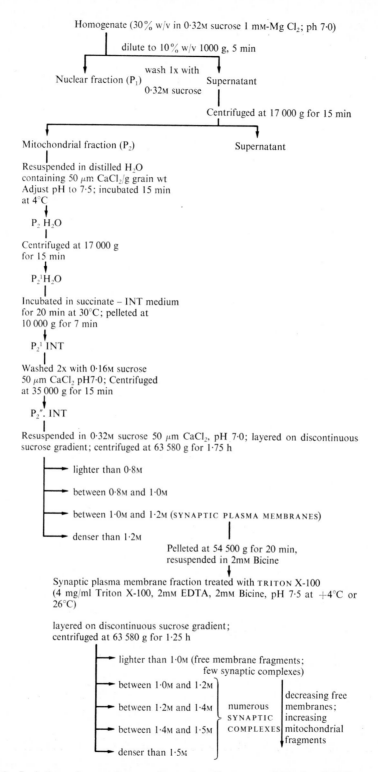

Homogenate (30% w/v in 0·32M sucrose 1 mM-Mg Cl₂; ph 7·0)

dilute to 10% w/v 1000 g, 5 min

wash 1x with

Nuclear fraction (P₁)   Supernatant

0·32M sucrose

Centrifuged at 17 000 g for 15 min

Mitochondrial fraction (P₂)   Supernatant

Resuspended in distilled H₂O
containing 50 μm CaCl₂/g grain wt
Adjust pH to 7·5; incubated 15 min
at 4°C

P₂ H₂O

Centrifuged at 17 000 g
for 15 min

P₂¹H₂O

Incubated in succinate – INT medium
for 20 min at 30°C; pelleted at
10 000 g for 7 min

P₂¹ INT

Washed 2x with 0·16M sucrose
50 μm CaCl₂ pH7·0; Centrifuged
at 35 000 g for 15 min

P₂″. INT

Resuspended in 0·32M sucrose 50 μm CaCl₂, pH 7·0; layered on discontinuous
sucrose gradient; centrifuged at 63 580 g for 1·75 h

→ lighter than 0·8M

→ between 0·8M and 1·0M

→ between 1·0M and 1·2M (SYNAPTIC PLASMA MEMBRANES)

→ denser than 1·2M

Pelleted at 54 500 g for 20 min,
resuspended in 2mM Bicine

Synaptic plasma membrane fraction treated with TRITON X-100
(4 mg/ml Triton X-100, 2mM EDTA, 2mM Bicine, pH 7·5 at +4°C or
26°C)

layered on discontinuous sucrose gradient;
centrifuged at 63 580 g for 1·25 h

→ lighter than 1·0M (free membrane fragments;
                     few synaptic complexes)

→ between 1·0M and 1·2M ⎫
                        ⎪   decreasing free
→ between 1·2M and 1·4M ⎪ numerous   membranes;
                        ⎬ SYNAPTIC   increasing
                        ⎪ COMPLEXES   mitochondrial
→ between 1·4M and 1·5M ⎪   ↓ fragments
                        ⎪
→ denser than 1·5M   ⎭

Scheme 2.9   Isolation of synaptic complexes after Cotman and Taylor (1972) hand, behaved differently undergoing considerable activation at certain concentrations of Triton X-100, confirming previous work on brain microsomes (Swanson and McIlwain, 1963; Swanson, Bradford and McIlwain, 1964). Activation of the (Na^+-K^+)-ATPase was observed by Fiszer and De Robertis (1967) at low Triton concentrations in their synaptosomal fraction and in their bulk submitochondrial fraction. By contrast, in their membrane fractions no activation occurred, only solubilization of the enzyme taking place.

Morphological examination of the various fractions after treatment with 0·05–0·1% Triton X-100 revealed marked disruption of synaptosomal membranes, liberating the axoplasm and synaptic vesicles, but leaving the junctional zone intact (Fiszer and De Robertis, 1967). The loss of AChE from the Triton-treated membranes is not accompanied, as demonstrated below, by a corresponding loss in the binding capacity of the membranes to cholinergic blocking agents. This suggests that the cholinergic receptor also escapes destruction by the detergent.

In a further investigation of synaptic complexes, De Robertis et al. (1967) studied the binding capacity of the membrane fractions for certain cholinergic blocking agents. The uptake of dimethyl-[^{14}C]-D-tubocurarine and methyl-[^{14}C]hexamethonium was noted before and after treatment with Triton X-100. Whereas the membrane-bound enzymes studied by Fiszer and De Robertis (1967) were greatly reduced following Triton treatment the binding capacity for these two cholinergic blocking agents was practically unaffected. From this they concluded that whereas the receptor properties are localized in the isolated junctional complexes, the enzymes have a much wider distribution (De Robertis et al., 1967a).

The synaptic complexes isolated by De Robertis et al. (1967a) from their membrane fractions are found in the midst of membranous debris. The Triton treatment appears to have increased the thickness and electron density of the subsynaptic web, while many of the complexes are curved with the convexity directed towards the synaptic membranes. Although the presynaptic membrane is evident in association with some synaptic webs, many of the profiles consist of subsynaptic webs alone suggesting that the integrity of the synaptic complex is lost in many instances. The cleft region with its distinctive cleft material is not visible in most profiles, and as this is perhaps the most characteristic feature of the intact synaptic complex, the majority of complexes isolated by De Robertis and co-workers appear to be predominantly postsynaptic. Cotman et al. (1971b) go further than this with their contention that the densities may be artefactually produced by detergent action on non-junctional membranes, close packing of the profiles leading to the apposition of these densities with membrane fragments.

Cotman et al. (1971) in a similar study concluded that, on the basis of morphological evidence, the most favourable conditions for the preservation of synaptic complexes are relatively low Triton concentrations (Triton: protein ratio of 1:2) and the presence of Ca^{2+} (Fig. 2.7). Furthermore, the solubilization of membrane protein is pH dependent, doubling between pH 6·0 and pH 10·0. In contrast, membrane phosphate is little affected by pH changes, as is the solubilization of sialic acid.

Ultrastructurally the synaptic complexes of Cotman et al (1971b) are similar to those of

De Robertis and co-workers, in so far as the postsynaptic thickening predominates (Plate 2.16). An additional component of the synaptic junction is recognizable in some profiles, and while it is difficult to label this component with certainty it is probably cleft material. PTA staining of these complexes again highlights the postsynaptic thickening, giving a faint impression of the presynaptic paramembranous densities (Section 1.3.1). Dense projections however, are not readily identifiable suggesting that even with these isolation procedures the presynaptic terminal is being underrepresented in the resulting synaptic complexes.

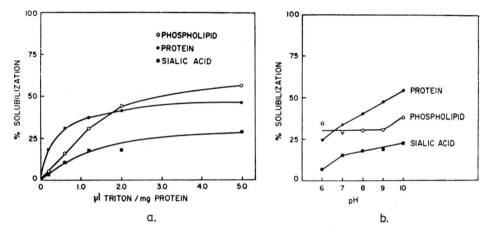

Figure 2.7 (a) Solubilization of synaptic plasma membrane protein, phospholipid phosphate and sialic acid with increasing amounts of Triton X-100. Solubilization was carried out in 3mM-Tris, pH 8·0 with 3mM-CaCl$_2$; membrane protein concentration was 2 mg/ml. (b) Effect of pH on the Triton solubilization of synaptic plasma membrane protein, phospholipid phosphate and sialic acid. Solubilization was carried out at a Triton-to-protein ratio of 1.2. Other conditions as for a. (From Cotman *et al.*, 1971b)

A modification of the preceding techniques for isolating synaptic complexes proposed by Cotman and Taylor (1972) is outlined in Scheme 2.9. The synaptic plasma membrane fraction was prepared from the crude mitochondrial fraction using the succinic dehydro-genase–iodonitroneotetrazolium (succinate–INT) procedure described by Davis and Bloom (1970). This increases the buoyant density of mitochondria so that the isolated membranes can be collected at heavier densities essentially free of mitochondrial con-tamination.

High resolution morphological examination of isolated synaptic complexes by Cotman and Taylor (1972) emphasized once again the prominence of the postsynaptic thickening, with cleft material at a majority of junctions and, less frequently, sections of presynaptic membrane (Plate 2.16). The postsynaptic plasma membrane is often vesicularized into a small closed vesicle just large enough to enclose the postsynaptic density, which often appears rigid. Detailed examination of these complexes also revealed projections within the cleft, possibly associated with the postsynaptic membrane, and globular and fibrous elements (7–9 nm across) within and subjacent to the postsynaptic thickening. They also noted that during isolation the synaptic complexes display a high degree of adhesiveness, sticking to each other and resisting easy resuspension. The intracleft projections are regularly spaced and extend 7–10 nm inwards from the postsynaptic membrane. They may be associated with fibrous extensions from the presynaptic membrane. While the exact details of these structures are not of paramount concern here they demonstrate the morphological integrity of these isolated synaptic complexes.

Cytochemical procedures carried out by Cotman and Taylor (1972) revealed that proteolytic enzymes at very low concentrations selectively destroyed the postsynaptic thickening, while at high concentrations they removed this thickening and opened the cleft. By contrast, treatment with sodium chloride, ethylene glycol bis(β-aminoethyl ether) [EGTA], and low concentrations of urea did not have a noticeable effect either on the structural integrity of the postsynaptic thickening or of the cleft region. The significance of these and other cytochemical studies for our knowledge of the structure and properties of the junctional region is discussed more fully in Section 4.4.

The procedures of Cotman and Taylor (1972) have been substantiated by Davis and Bloom (1973), employing similar techniques. The greater susceptibility of the presynaptic dense projections to disruption was commented upon by Davis and Bloom, who also stressed the protective effect of calcium on the synaptic complexes.

2.5.3 Postsynaptic membranes (Scheme 2.10)

Garey *et al.* (1972), employing continuous Ficoll gradients to separate synaptosomes, followed by continuous sucrose gradients for further subfractionation, have obtained an enriched fraction of postsynaptic membranes (Fig. 2.6e; Scheme 2.10). A variety of preparative and cytochemical techniques was used for their identification and for a high resolution study of individual profiles. The principal contaminants of the postsynaptic membrane fraction are small unidentified membrane fragments, many of which are probably synaptosomal in origin.

The postsynaptic membrane profiles are generally dark staining, their free ends 'balling up' to give a dumb-bell profile (Plate 2.17). Those postsynaptic membranes unattached to a presynaptic synaptosomal component are often, in addition, folded back on themselves to present an overall C-shaped profile. Their selective staining with PTA and indium techniques is claimed to provide further evidence of their derivation from the junctional region of synaptosomes, and appears to discount Whittaker's (1969b) suggestion that they are nonspecific strands of macromolecular material.

A surprising side to this study by Garey and co-workers is the apparent ease with which postsynaptic membranes were isolated. This is especially notable in view of the absence of detergents to solubilize non-synaptic membranes and hence dissociate the synaptic region. Consequently mechanical shearing forces alone must have been adequate in this instance, as postsynaptic membranes similar in morphology to those described here have been recognized repeatedly in synaptosomal fractions (e.g. Gray and Whittaker, 1962). If this is the explanation, it is pertinent to query the degree of damage inflicted on the particles by the procedures employed.

The typical dumb-bell postsynaptic membrane obtained by *Garey et al.* (1972) bears little resemblance to the postsynaptic region of intact tissue or of conventional synaptosomal preparations with its membrane, thickening and subsynaptic organelles (contrast Plates 2.17 and 3.1). The contrast is a striking one both in aldehyde/OsO$_4$-fixed and in PTA-stained material (compare Figs. 13 and 15 and Figs. 20 and 21 in *Garey et al.*, 1972). Although the membrane can be identified with its trilaminar structure, the paramembranous densities have been largely obscured or lost.

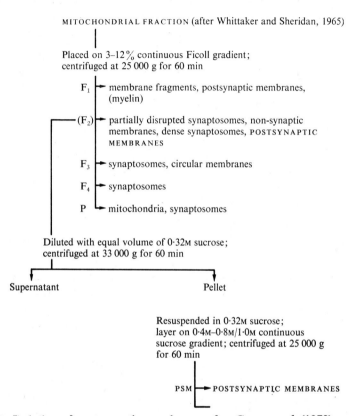

MITOCHONDRIAL FRACTION (after Whittaker and Sheridan, 1965)

Placed on 3–12% continuous Ficoll gradient; centrifuged at 25 000 g for 60 min

F$_1$ — membrane fragments, postsynaptic membranes, (myelin)

(F$_2$) — partially disrupted synaptosomes, non-synaptic membranes, dense synaptosomes, POSTSYNAPTIC MEMBRANES

F$_3$ — synaptosomes, circular membranes

F$_4$ — synaptosomes

P — mitochondria, synaptosomes

Diluted with equal volume of 0·32M sucrose; centrifuged at 33 000 g for 60 min

Supernatant   Pellet

Resuspended in 0·32M sucrose; layer on 0·4M–0·8M/1·0M continuous sucrose gradient; centrifuged at 25 000 g for 60 min

PSM — POSTSYNAPTIC MEMBRANES

Scheme 2.10   Isolation of postsynaptic membranes after *Garey et al.* (1972)

This raises the possibility that the profiles identified by these workers as postsynaptic membranes are, in fact, of nonsynaptic origin. Cohen and McGovern (1973), noting the similar appearance of these profiles to dumb-bell shaped mitochondria in some of their synaptosomal preparations, have tendered a cautionary note. According to them, the profiles described by Garey and co-workers may be mitochondria or, if this is not the case, mitochondria and postsynaptic membranes are being transformed into morphologically similar entities. Isolated dumb-bell mitochondria have also been seen by Jones (1974) in hypertonically prepared synaptosomes, these profiles being similar in appearance to those usually described as postsynaptic membranes (e.g. Plate 3.12).

2.6 CONTAMINATION OF FRACTIONS

2.6.1 Assessment of fractions

In early fractionation studies it was sufficient to identify the synaptosomes either in the crude mitochondrial (P_2 of Whittaker) fraction or in a specific subfractionated synaptosomal (P_2B) fraction (e.g. Gray and Whittaker, 1962; De Robertis et al., 1962a, 1963; Whittaker et al., 1964). Such identification provided adequate morphological background for the majority of biochemical studies, and while this remains true for synaptosomal studies in general the development of techniques aimed at further dissection of synaptosomes demands a more rigorous morphological analysis of fractions. This is because the contribution of other neuronal and also glial components of nerve tissue needs to be taken into account. Further stimuli to a more systematic assessment of fractions have accompanied the development of a theoretical basis for fractionation studies, and the increasing interest being shown in the separation of glia (Cotman et al., 1971a) and unmyelinated axons (Lemkey-Johnston and Larramendi, 1968).

Useful as the EM analysis of fractions is, a number of difficulties arise in practice. Chief among these is that of obtaining data representative of the entire fraction. This arises from the fact that an area of the order of only 200 μm^2 × 0·4 μm thick (total volume, 0·0008 mm^3) is examined (Cotman, 1972). On account of differences in the sedimentation coefficients of particles, a certain degree of layering occurs in pellets a factor which, taken in conjunction with the previous one, will result in unrepresentative EMs unless care is taken to avoid this pitfall.

In order to overcome this non-uniformity of pellets a number of elaborate techniques have been devised (Bandhuin, Evrard and Berthet, 1967; Worsfold, Dunn and Peter, 1969; Cotman and Flansburg, 1970; Grove, Bondareff and Veis, 1973), the aim of which is to section pellets incorporating the entire thickness of the pellet. These techniques vary in their degree of usefulness, and all suffer from being more complicated than routine procedures for embedding pellets or suspensions. For instance Grove et al. (1973) employ a sector-shaped analytical ultracentrifuge cell to prepare particulate layers of subcellular fractions after the stage of aldehyde fixation. Following this, they are poured out of the cell onto a millipore filter where the layers remain largely intact. These are then osmicated and embedded. With this method two to three EMs at × 37 000 span the entire thickness of the pellet. These workers found that synaptosomal volume percentages were consistent (41–47%) in widely separated regions of the layers.

In the absence of techniques such as the above the influence of non-uniformity can be minimized by sectioning pellets carefully at different depths and in different planes (cf. Gray and Whittaker, 1962). In this way it has been found that in 'typical' mammalian synaptosomal fractions there may be a transition between readily recognizable synaptosomes superficially and relatively empty membranous profiles deeper in a pellet (Jones, 1972). Serial sectioning can be used to determine the synaptosomal or non-synaptosomal nature of these membranous profiles (see below). Regardless of the method used however, care is required in obtaining and analysing representative micrographs of fractions.

93

Even with this proviso, one must agree with Cotman (1972) that the *quantitative* determination of the amount of contamination contributed by a particle remains a difficult one. It is essential to consider the net quantity of a particular material which may be contributed by each structure visualized in a particular field. A related point concerns the range of profiles present in fractions, mirroring all too closely the complexity of brain tissue itself. Besides readily identifiable profiles such as synaptosomes, synaptic or coated vesicles, mitochondria, myelin fragments and microsomes, a large variety of non-descript membrane fragments, membranous profiles and small vesicular profiles may also be seen, depending upon the fraction under examination. Without adequate marker techniques it is often virtually impossible to identify these with any degree of confidence.

In order to tackle this problem Jones and Brearley (1973) used serial sectioning, starting with unequivocal synaptosomal profiles and tracing them through adjacent serial sections (Plate 2.18 a–d). In this way those membranous profiles definitely belonging to synaptosomes could be analysed and distinguished from other profiles of non-synaptosomal origin, whether axonal, dendritic or glial. They found that synaptosomal profiles are characterized by their enclosed synaptic vesicles and possibly one or more mitochondria. They never occur as empty membranous profiles which therefore cannot be positively identified as synaptosomal solely on morphological grounds.

A related problem to which serial sectioning has made a contribution is the recognition of synaptic junctions in fractions. Kornguth *et al.* (1972) carried out limited serial sectioning to demonstrate that membranes which do not appear to be portions of synaptic complexes in a particular section are in fact part of the junctional unit on examination of adjacent sections. Jones and Brearley (1973) developed criteria for determining when the existence of a synaptic junction can be predicted in adjacent sections (Plate 2.19 a–d). These are the accumulation of synaptic vesicles at one locus within its presynaptic component, and the presence of a postsynaptic profile displaying at least two of the following features: a 20 nm gap, electron-dense material in the gap, a thickening of one or both adjacent membranes and parallelism of these membranes.

Whittaker (1969c), in an attempt to assess the degree of contamination of his B fraction with non-synaptosomal material, estimated the amount of nondiffusible dry solids in it. This is of the order of 22 mg/g of original tissue (Eichberg *et al.*, 1964), the total morphological synaptosomal volume being estimated as 36 mg/g of original tissue. These figures point to a water content of about 29% if all the dry solids originate from synaptosomes, compared with approximately 62% as the estimated content of the synaptosomes. Approximately 50% therefore of the material in this 'synaptosomal' B fraction could be nonsynaptosomal, although this does not specify the origin of this nonsynaptosomal material.

2.6.2 Axonal/glial contamination

(i) *Axonal contamination.* Lemkey-Johnston and Larramendi (1968) in a study of cerebellar fractions noted that this tissue yielded abundant segments of non-myelinated axons and that these axons sedimented predominantly in the crude mitochondrial fraction.

This finding raised the possibility that other parts of the CNS might, under appropriate fractionation conditions, also be induced to sediment non-myelinated axons and that, moreover, the presence of these axons may have been overlooked by previous workers in routine synaptosomal fractions. This contention received additional support from the biochemical studies of Dekirmenjian, Brunngraber, Lemkey-Johnston and Larramendi (1969) on cerebellum, and by biochemical and morphological studies on whole brain homogenates (Dekirmenjian and Brunngraber, 1969; Lemkey-Johnston and Dekirmenjian, 1970) and caudate-putamen (Lemkey-Johnston and Larramendi, 1970, 1973).

Using a conventional fractionation scheme Lemkey-Johnston and Larramendi (1968) isolated five subfractions (P_2A–P_2E) from a crude mitochondrial (P_2) fraction on density gradient centrifugation of cerebellar tissue. These are analogous to Whittaker's A–C subfractions, P_2A being the myelin subfraction and P_2D and P_2E the mitochondrial subfractions. P_2B and P_2C represent the 'synaptosomal' component of the fractionated tissue, P_2B containing tubular and oval profiles interpreted as non-myelinated axons, and P_2C synaptosomes with axonal attachments. In view of the morphology of these profiles, they were considered to have arisen from the parallel fibres of granule cells which fragment in a characteristic fashion to give chiefly intersynaptic and synaptic plus intersynaptic segments.

The point of general interest is whether the non-myelinated axonal subfraction is unique to cerebellar tissue or whether it has a homologue in other regions of the brain. In order to answer this Dekirmenjian and Brunngraber (1969), working with whole brain homogenates, devised a fractionation scheme to yield a similar fraction. A routine synaptosomal fraction was centrifuged at 100 000 g for 90 min, and the resuspended pellet layered on a discontinuous sucrose density gradient. After centrifuging for 6 h at 22 500 rev/min, five subfractions P_2B-a to P_2B-e eventuated. Careful EM examination of these subfractions by Lemkey-Johnston and Dekirmenjian (1970) revealed that layers a and b are most abundantly enriched in axonal segments (Plate 2.20), whereas the denser layers, c, d and e, have the highest concentration of synaptosomes. In quantitative terms axonal membranes contribute approximately 60% of membrane surface in layers a and b, 45% in c and d, and only 25% in e. Synaptosomal membranes contribute 35–40% in c, d and e. Besides these constituents all subfractions contain membranes of unknown origin while e contains significant numbers of free mitochondria.

In view of these findings Lemkey-Johnston and Dekirmenjian (1970) reach a conclusion of immense importance for synaptosomal investigations. They state that the main components of Whittaker's (1959) 'synaptosomal' fraction are, in decreasing order, axonal segments, synaptosomes and membranes of undetermined origin. Moreover, *axon segments free of synaptosomes* can be obtained in the two lightest layers, whereas there are *no* layers in which synaptosomes can be obtained free of axonal segments.

In assessing this conclusion a number of factors demand consideration. The first concerns the fractionation scheme used by them and developed originally by Dekirmenjian and Brunngraber (1969). Sedimentation of the synaptosomal fraction prior to density gradient centrifugation resulted in loss of part of this fraction, while the particles on the density gradient were exposed to hypertonic sucrose for as long as 6 h. These factors combined would undoubtedly have contributed to the low yield of synaptosomes coupled with the high yield and wide distribution of nonspecific membranes. These considerations in turn raise another difficulty, which is that of distinguishing morphologically between the various profiles in the subfractions, and thus of identifying axonal segments. Although synaptosomes are readily recognized in d and e, it is difficult to distinguish between them and axonal profiles in c, and between axonal profiles and some membrane fragments in a and b. Furthermore, as no information regarding the appearance of P_2B was given it cannot be compared with the synaptosomal fraction of other workers (Jones, 1972). The heterogeneity of routine synaptosomal fractions is not proved by these studies, although greater awareness of the possibility of axonal contamination is demanded.

Further evidence regarding synaptosomal and axonal subfractions has been of two kinds. Dekirmenjian and Brunngraber (1969) in whole brain homogenates and Dekirmenjian et al. (1969) in cerebellum measured the levels of gangliosides, glycoproteins, AChE and cytochrome oxidase in subfractions, and noted that whereas the amounts of AChE and gangliosides were highest in the axon-containing subfractions, cytochrome oxidase was lowest in these. The ratio of glycoprotein–NANA to ganglioside–NANA increased with increasing particle size.

The profiles interpreted as non-myelinated axons in subfractions generally have a shrunken appearance compared with the intact axons from which they are derived (e.g. Lemkey-Johnston and Larramendi, 1968). In an effort to discern the reason for this, Lemkey-Johnston and Larramendi (1973) examined intact brain tissue immersed for 2 h in either 0·32M or 1M sucrose before fixation. The resulting axons and synaptic terminals were shrunken and relatively electron-dense, resembling the equivalent fractionated profiles seen by them. While sucrose appears therefore to be a contributing factor to the shrivelled appearance of axonal segments, it is difficult to view it as a major factor in the ultrastructure of synaptosomes, which generally display a wide variety of appearances. The limited degree of shrinkage affecting certain synaptosomal indices (Jones and Brearley, 1972b; Section 3.3) does not noticeably increase the overall electron density of synaptosomes.

(ii) *Glial contamination.* The sedimentation properties of glial membranes are similar to those of synaptosomes (Cotman et al., 1970), raising the possibility that synaptosomal preparations may be contaminated by glia. Furthermore, it is possible to separate highly enriched fractions of glial membranes (Cotman et al., 1971a) and characterize them morphologically as well as biochemically. One subfraction of the glial cell crude mitochondrial fraction sediments to the same isopycnic density as synaptosomes (Table 2.2). This fraction consists of numerous membrane structures resembling plasma membranes on morphological examination (Plate 2.21), and containing 20% of the protein and 50% of the (Na^+-K^+)-ATPase and acid phosphatase of the crude mitochondrial fraction. Unlike brain membranes, this glial membrane fraction does not contain detectable quantities of ChE.

It is argued by these workers that because the sedimentation properties of the glial membranes are so similar to synaptosomes, synaptosomes prepared on sucrose gradients are probably contaminated by glial fragments. By contrast, when the separation is carried out on Ficoll gradients most of the glial membrane is found at densities lighter than that of synaptosomes. It may be therefore that Ficoll gradients are preferable to sucrose gradients for obtaining synaptosomes free of contaminating glial membranes (Section 2.3.2). Any contamination of synaptosomal fractions with glia has considerable repercussions as one of the significant features of these fractions is the opportunity they present to study neuronal properties in isolation and without glial contamination (e.g. Appel et al., 1972).

Whittaker was well aware of the problem of the possible glial contamination of synaptosomal fractions in 1965, and recognized then that to settle the point conclusively a glial cell cytoplasmic marker is required. He argued however, that those glial cells or glial cell fragments incompletely disintegrated by homogenization are recovered in the P_1 fraction. Marchbanks and Whittaker (1969), using butyrylcholinesterase as a marker of glial elements found it localized principally in the myelin peak using zonal centrifugation. The results of Cotman et al. (1971a) point instead to the probability that some of the membranous contamination of synaptosomal fractions is glial in origin. The elimination of membranous profiles from synaptosomal preparations is an essential prerequisite therefore to obtaining glial-free preparations, a procedure aided by Ficoll gradient separation (Cotman et al., 1971a). The necessity of obtaining such preparations has been increased by the finding that isolated ganglia, and presumably glia, take up and release amino acids (Bowery and Brown, 1972).

Chapter 3: Synaptosomes as Structural Units

3.1 PREPARATION AND IDENTIFICATION OF SYNAPTOSOMES

3.1.1 Definition

An account has been given in Chapter 2 of the development of fractionation techniques aimed at obtaining enriched fractions of synaptosomes and synaptic vesicles. It was seen that the particles referred to as synaptosomes consist essentially of 'pinched-off' presynaptic endings (Gray and Whittaker, 1962) plus, in some instances, an adherent postsynaptic membrane. In the light of these observations the term *synaptosome*, when adopted by Whittaker and co-workers (Whittaker *et al.*, 1964; Whittaker, 1965), has sometimes referred to the 'detached presynaptic nerve terminal' (e.g. Marchbanks, 1968b; Whittaker, 1969b, c). It is often not clear in the literature however, whether the term embraces the junctional and postsynaptic elements in addition to the presynaptic terminal. Whittaker (1971b) fortunately made his own position crystal clear on one occasion when he wrote: 'The term synaptosome has always been used to refer to the whole particle irrespective of whether postsynaptic adhesions are present or not, and has not been restricted to the presynaptic part of the structure . . .'

A postsynaptic membrane, either in isolation or as part of a more complete postsynaptic process, is commonly observed in routine sections of synaptosomal fractions (Plates 3.1–3.6). In these cases the junction between the presynaptic terminal and the postsynaptic membrane or process parallels remarkably closely corresponding junctions in synapses from non-fractionated, intact tissue (Jones and Brearley, 1972a, b). This implies that the intimate association of the presynaptic membrane, cleft material and postsynaptic membrane, essential to the integrity of the synaptic junction, is maintained in fractionated junctions (De Robertis *et al.*, 1963; Jones, 1968, 1969, 1970a). It follows that the presynaptic terminal can no more be viewed in isolation from its associated cleft and postsynaptic components in fractionated than in intact material.

The term *synaptosome* therefore should not be confined to the presynaptic terminal, but rather employed in a general way to include presynaptic, cleft and postsynaptic components (Jones, 1972.) Only in this way is justice done to the morphological evidence. Accordingly, this is the manner in which the term is used throughout the present text.

Synaptosomes are formed during tissue homogenization by the nerve terminal being torn away from the distal end of the axon, and the postsynaptic membrane from adjacent parts of the dendritic spine, dendrite, axon or soma. The ruptured membranes are drawn together and sealed during the process of vesiculation, resulting in the discrete entity which is the synaptosome. Once formed, synaptosomes, which have a high surface to

PLATES

Plate 1.1 Two types of synapses can be distinguished, both making contact with a common dendrite (d). Terminal *a* consists of round synaptic vesicles (rv) and contacts the dendrite by way of a junction with asymmetrical membrane differentiations. By contrast, terminal *b* displays many flattened vesicles (fv) in addition to round vesicles and has a symmetrical junction. mit, mitochondria. Rat lateral geniculate nucleus; aldehyde–OsO₄ fixation. $\times$ 42 750 (*By courtesy of Dr. A. R. Lieberman*)

Plate 1.2 The synaptic terminals displayed in this field are making contact with small dendrites and dendritic spines (ds). These axodendritic synapses contain round vesicles (rv) and have asymmetrically thickened junctions. A spine apparatus (sa) is well displayed in one of the dendritic spines. mit, mitochondria; mt, microtubules; my, myelin. Cat putamen; aldehyde–OsO₄ fixation. $\times$ 28 975 (*From Adinolfi, 1971a*)

Plate 1.3 Of the round vesicles shown in these synaptic terminals two size ranges can be distinguished: large (51 nm) synaptic vesicles (1v) and smaller (31 nm) synaptic vesicles (smv) in adjacent terminals. Cat putamen; aldehyde–OsO₄ fixation. $\times$ 29 350 (*From Adinolfi, 1971a*)

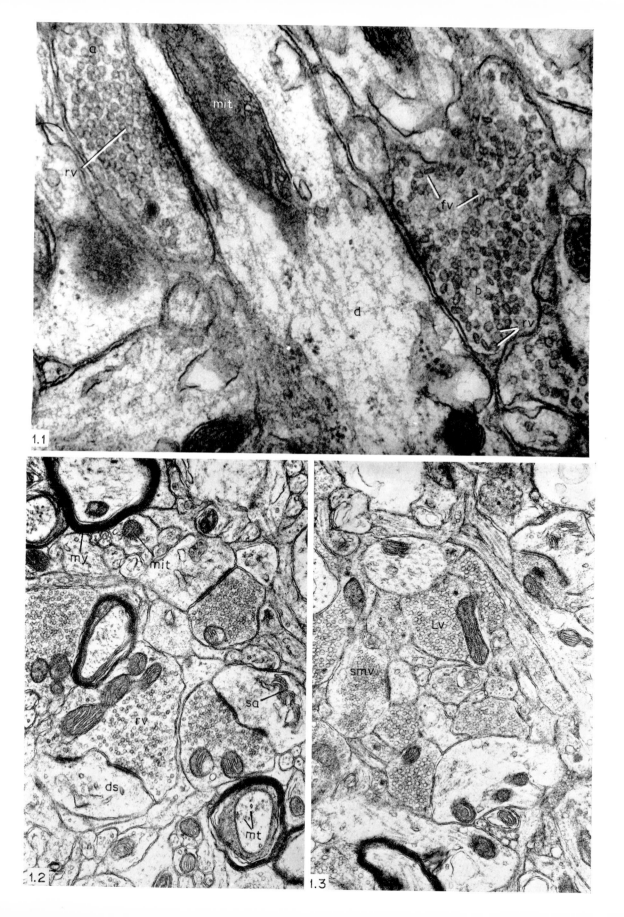

Plate 1.4 A row of subjunctional bodies (sb) is prominent, subjacent to an asymmetrical membrane differentiation. Synaptic vesicles (sv) are clearly demonstrated in the terminal itself. mit, mitochondria; my, myelin. *Echidna* inferior olivary nucleus; aldehyde–OsO_4 fixation. $\times$ 68 400

Plate 1.5 Crest synapse, in which two presynaptic terminals (pr_1 and pr_2) make contact with a common postsynaptic one (po). A row of subjunctional bodies (SB) is present in the postsynaptic terminal, and has fine weblike extensions running between individual subjunctional bodies and the postsynaptic thickenings. dp, dense projections. Cat subfornical organ; aldehyde–OsO_4 fixation. $\times$ 142 500 (*From Akert et al., 1967*)

Plate 1.6 A large subsynaptic cistern (SSC) lies subjacent to a synaptic terminal, *A*. No membrane differentiations are evident in the vicinity of the cistern. Glial lamellae are indicated by arrows. ER, endoplasmic reticulum. Frog oculomotor nucleus; aldehyde–OsO_4 fixation. $\times$ 47 500 (*From Pappas and Waxman, 1972*)

Plate 1.7 A subsynaptic formation (sf) lies in intimate apposition to a postsynaptic thickening (pt). The presynaptic component of this synaptic junction has disappeared as seven days have elapsed since section of the preganglionic fibres. Frog sympathetic ganglion; aldehyde–OsO_4 fixation. $\times$ 63 840 (*From Sotelo, 1971a*)

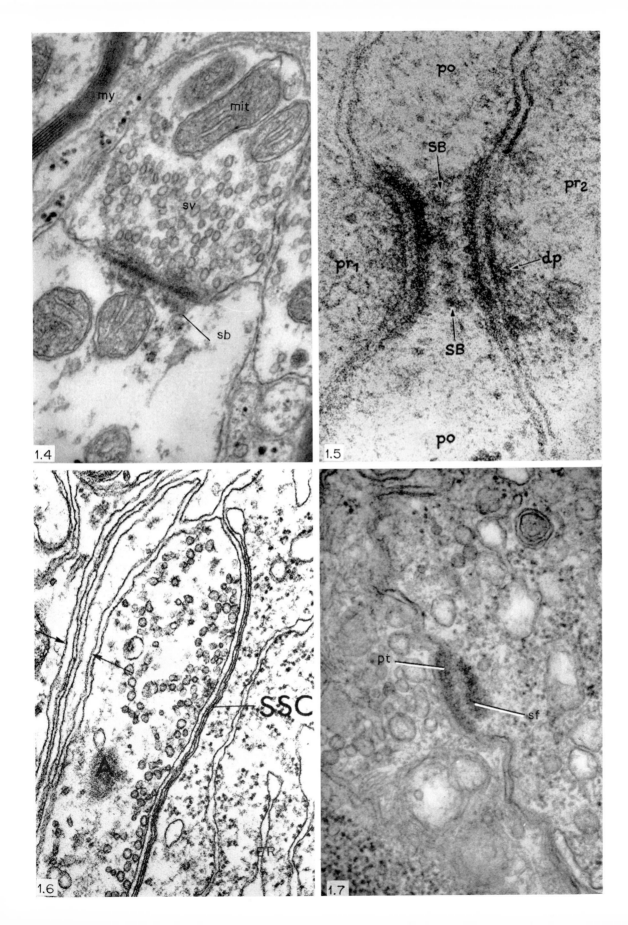

Plate 1.8 A low-power view of synaptic junctions stained with PTA. The presynaptic dense projections (dp) stand out as discontinuous, electrondense blobs, while the postsynaptic thickenings (pt) appear continuous and extend the length of the junctions. Cleft material can be recognized on careful examination of some of the junctions (arrows). Densities are also present postsynaptically in some instances, constituting part of the subsynaptic apparatus (ssa). The junctions, which vary in their degree of curvature, are readily distinguished from the nonsynaptic elements forming the background. Rat cerebellar cortex; glutaraldehyde fixed, PTA stained. $\times$ 26 300

Plate 1.9 The paramembranous densities are clearly depicted in this synaptic junction. Dense projections (dp) are present presynaptically, cleft densities (cd) in the cleft and a postsynaptic thickening (pt) postsynaptically. Rat hippocampus; glutaraldehyde fixed, PTA stained. $\times$ 105 200 (*From Jones, 1973a*)

Plate 1.10 A higher power view of paramembranous densities. In the presynaptic terminal (pr), dense projections and strands of the presynaptic network (pn) are evident. Each dense projection is drawn out at its periphery to form spikes, which may be continuous with the surrounding network (arrows). The dense projections are not homogeneously electron-dense, a dense framework (fr) intermingling with relatively electrontranslucent areas. *Setonix brachyurus* dorsal lateral geniculate nucleus; glutaraldehyde fixation, PTA staining. $\times$ 228 000 (*From Jones et al., 1972*)

Plate 1.11 An example of a synaptic junction prepared by the BIUL method. Intracleft lines (icl) occupy the cleft region. dcv, (?) dense-cored vesicle; pt, postsynaptic thickening. The arrow indicates a point at which the iodophilic cytoplasmic layer appears to be missing. Cat subfornical organ; glutaraldehyde fixation, BIUL staining. $\times$ 121 600 (*From Akert and Pfenninger, 1969*)

Plate 1.12 Dense projections (dp) and synaptic vesicles (sv) are visualized alongside each other in this terminal. *Echidna* inferior olivary nucleus; aldehyde–OsO$_4$ fixation. $\times$ 55 100

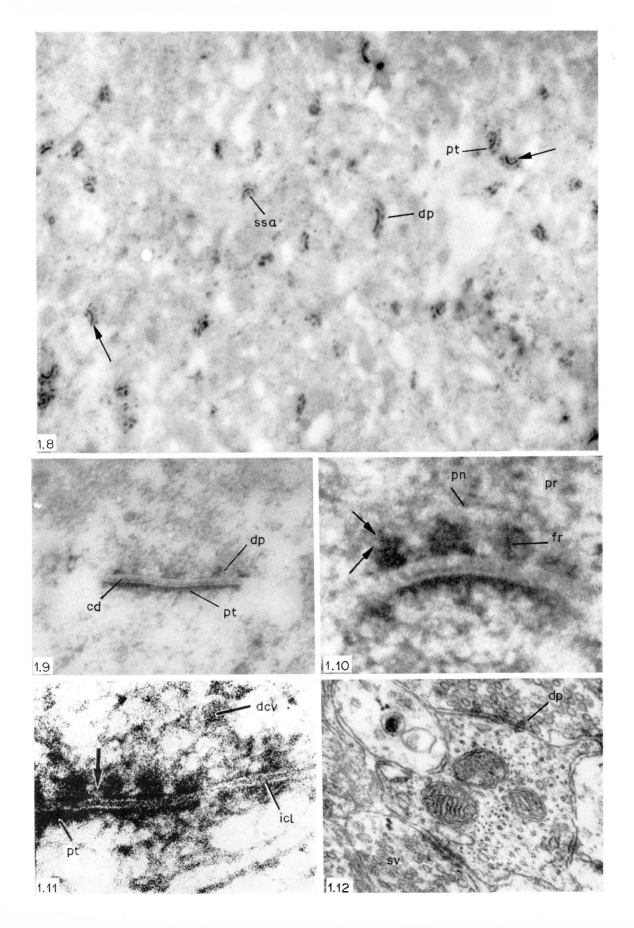

Plate 1.13 Tangential section through a synaptic terminal at the level of the presynaptic membrane. The dense projections (dp) are hexagonally arranged and are connected by spike-like processes (sp). The overall arrangement forms the basis of the presynaptic vesicular grid envisaged by Akert and co-workers. Cat subfornical organ; glutaraldehyde fixation, BIUL staining. $\times$ 163 400 (*From Akert and Pfenninger, 1969*)

Plate 1.14 Transverse section through the presynaptic network of a synaptic terminal. The hexagonal arrangement of some of the strands can be recognized (arrows). dp, dense projections. Rat cerebral cortex; glutaraldehyde fixation, PTA staining. $\times$ 209 000 (*From Jones and Brearley, 1972a*)

Plate 1.15 Screen equidensities (equidensitometry) of the synaptic junction shown in Plate 1.10. Substructural details of the dense projections (dp) are highlighted. cd, cleft densities; et, electron-translucent areas within the dense projections; g, globular opacities; pt, postsynaptic thickening; sp, spikes of dense projections. *Setonix brachyurus* dorsal lateral geniculate nucleus; glutaraldehyde fixation, PTA staining. $\times$ 888 250 (*From Nolan and Jones, 1974*)

Plate 1.16 Examples of coated vesicles (cv) and the empty shells (sh[1]) of coated vesicles in a synaptosome. The central vesicle (ce) is enclosed within a shell (sh) or basket which may be complete or only partially so. mit, mitochondrion; sv, synaptic vesicles. Rat cerebral cortex; unbuffered OsO_4 and unbuffered glutaraldehyde fixation. $\times$ 97 550 *Inset* A complete empty shell of a coated vesicle. $\times$ 182 400

Plate 1.17 A synaptosome containing a number of examples of coated vesicle shells in varying degrees of intactness. Details as for Plate 1.16. $\times$ 99 750

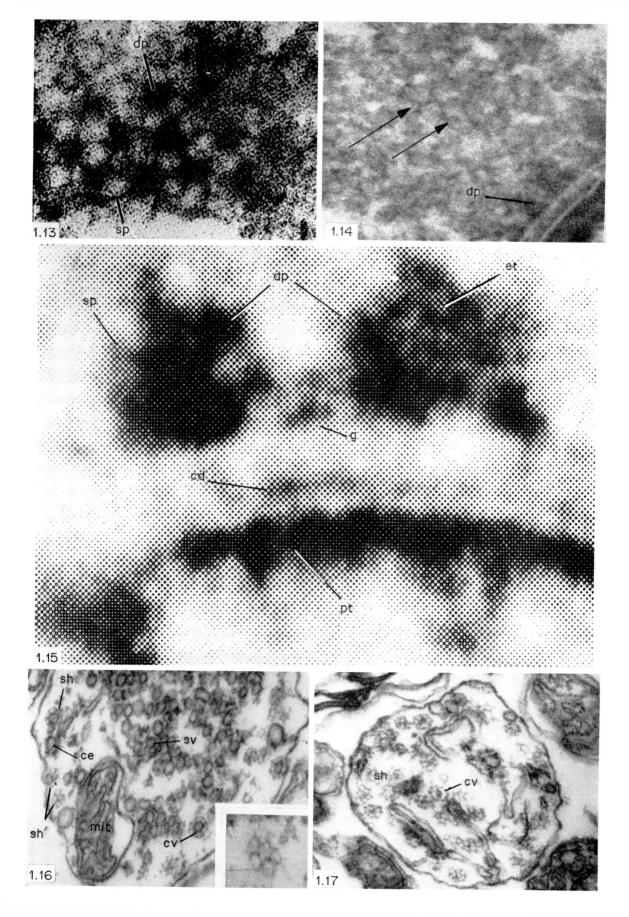

Plate 1.18 This, and the three succeeding plates are of freeze-etched preparations. This one shows a cross-fractured synapse with round synaptic vesicles (sv) of 48 nm outer diameter. The region of the synaptic cleft (c) is visible, while an outer face of a presynaptic active site (pr-of) can also be recognized. The circled arrow indicates the direction of shadowing. Rat cerebellar cortex; freeze-etched, following pentobarbital anaesthesia and aldehyde fixation. × 54 625

Plate 1.19 A cross-fractured presynaptic terminal is seen together with the outer face of a pre-synaptic inner membrane leaflet (pr-of). The cytoplasm is packed with vesicles (sv) of diameter less than 39 nm, while the particle studded outer face leaflet exhibits crater-like micropits (mp). Note the possible sites of surface vesicle activity adjacent to the active site on the inner leaflet of the axon membrane (arrow). mit, mitochondrion; po-of, outer face of the postsynaptic inner membrane leaflet. Details as for Plate 1.18. × 68 400

Plate 1.20 This is a view of the inner face of the outer leaflet of a presynaptic membrane (pr-if). Evidence is given in the text to suggest that this is a synaptic terminal. Note the central uplifting of the outer leaflet of the membrane, and the scattered particles (p) amongst which lie possible synaptopores (syp; or protuberances). There is no suggestion of particle or synaptopore organization. For details see Plate 1.18. × 87 400

Plate 1.21 The fracture in this instance has exposed the outer face of the inner leaflet of the pre-synaptic membrane (pr-of). Micropits (mp) indent the membrane concavity, and surface particles (p) abound. The latter is a characteristic of outer membrane faces. Note the possible presence of an adjacent active site (arrow). For details consult Plate 1.18 × 87 400

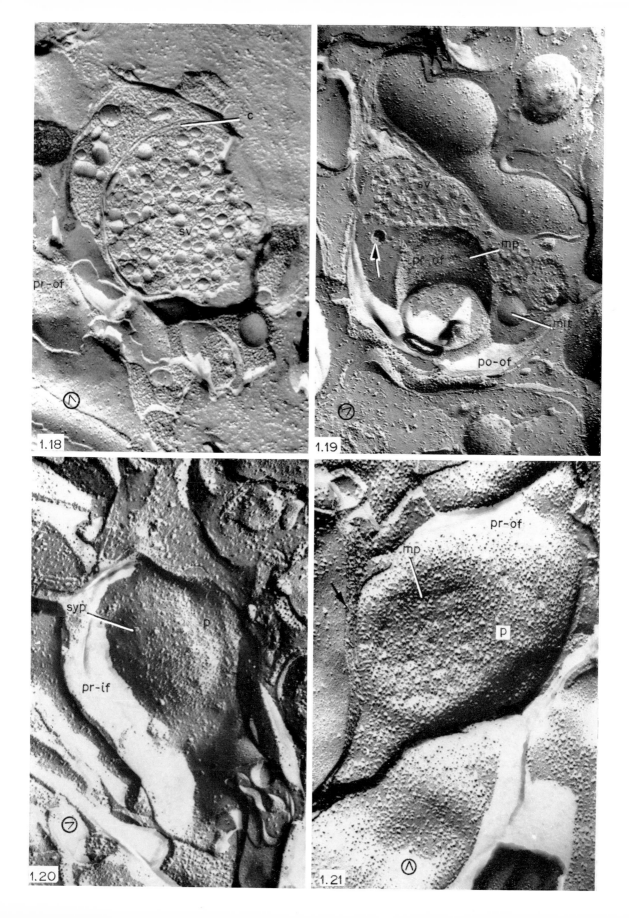

1.18

1.19

1.20

1.21

Plate 1.22 ZIO preparation. Two principal vesicle types are present, one in which the vesicles are filled with a dense precipitate (ZIO positive; ZIO+) and the other in which the vesicle cores remain electrontranslucent (ZIO negative; ZIO−). *Octopus* vertical lobe; aldehyde fixation, ZIO immersion. × 126 630 (*From Barlow and Martin, 1971*)

Plate 1.23 Synaptogenesis—10 days postnatal. An axosomatic synapse displays round vesicles (rv) and a symmetrical synaptic contact (arrow) at this stage. Cat somatic sensory cortex; aldehyde–OsO₄ fixation. × 31 350 (*From Adinolfi, 1972a*)

Plate 1.24 Synaptogenesis—21 days postnatal. The axosomatic synapse shown here is similarly situated to that shown in Plate 1.23. By this stage of maturation however, flattened vesicles (fv) have appeared. The membranes are symmetrically arranged at the junction. mit, mitochondria; r. ribosomes. Cat somatic sensory cortex; aldehyde–OsO₄ fixation. × 43 400 (*From Adinolfi, 1972a*)

Plate 1.25 Synaptogenesis—50 days gestation. This PTA stained synaptic junction is very immature, the most readily recognizable feature of it being the postsynaptic thickening (pt). Small dense globules (dg) are seen presynaptically, while cleft material is barely visible. Guinea-pig cerebral cortex; glutaraldehyde fixation, PTA staining. × 68 400 (*From Jones et al., 1974*)

Plate 1.26 Synaptogenesis—5 days postnatal. All the components of adult synaptic junctions are featured in this example, which should be compared with the preceding plate. cd, cleft densities; dp, dense projections; pfd, postsynaptic focal densities. Guinea-pig cerebral cortex; glutaraldehyde fixation, PTA staining. × 90 250 (*From Jones et al., 1974*)

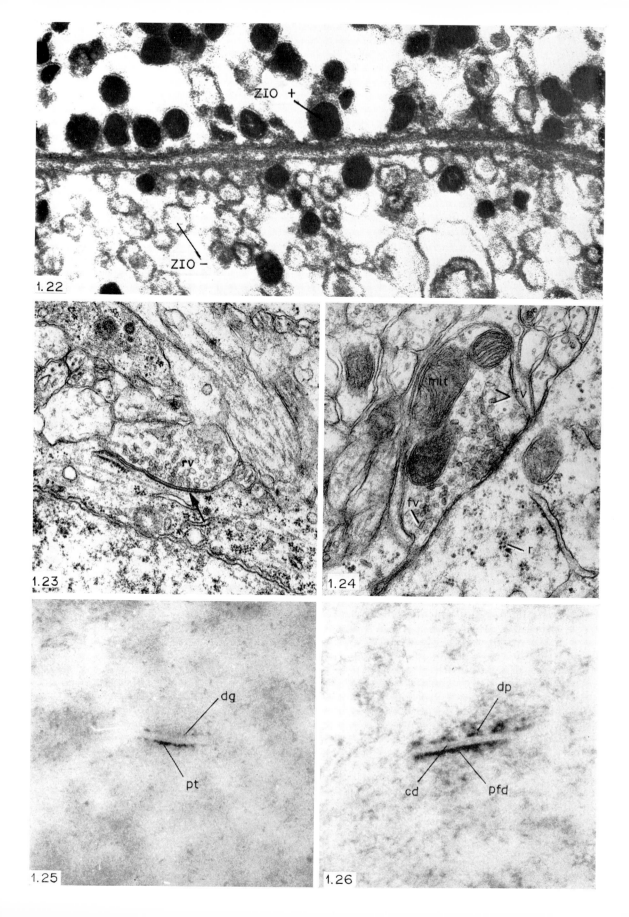

1.22

1.23

1.24

1.25

1.26

Plate 2.1 Myelin fraction (P₂A). A number of myelin balls (my) are present, each displaying axonal remnants (ax) surrounded by the myelin lamellae. Mouse cerebellum; permanganate fixation. × 35 340.

Inset. A higher-power view of a myelin fragment to show the axoplasm (ax) in greater detail. mit, mitochondria. Mouse cerebellum; permanganate fixation. × 20 900

Plate 2.2 Synaptosomal fraction (P₂B). Numerous synaptosomal profiles (s) are visible in this low power micrograph. Even at this magnification synaptic vesicles (sv) and mitochondria (mit) can be recognized within them, while a few attached postsynaptic membranes (pm) are visible. A few isolated mitochondria and heterogeneous membranous profiles (mem) are present as contaminants. Rat cerebral cortex; synaptosomes separated on a sucrose density gradient, and then resuspended and incubated at 37° C in a Krebs-phosphate medium prior to fixation in OsO₄. × 15 580.

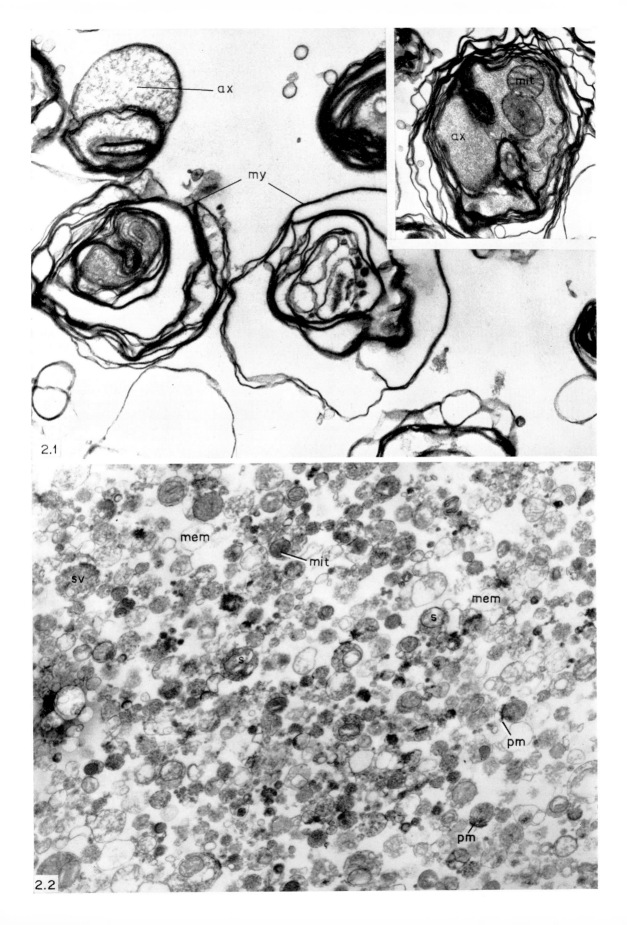

Plate 2.3 Mitochondrial fraction (P_2C). Numerous mitochondria (mit) are present with only limited contamination by nonspecific membranes (mem). Rat cerebral cortex; OsO_4 fixation. $\times$ 19 950

Plate 2.4 Synaptosomal fraction showing synaptosomes (s) separated on a Ficoll density gradient. In addition to the synaptosomes, membrane fragments (mem) and possibly postsynaptic synaptosomal components (po) are also seen. Rat cerebral cortex; aldehyde–OsO_4 fixation. $\times$ 19 950 (*From Garey et al., 1972*)

Plate 2.5 'Synaptic complex' (synaptosomal) fraction corresponding to the 1.17–1.18 band from a CsCl gradient containing 0.14M sucrose (Scheme 2.3). The presynaptic components of the complexes are labelled *s*. d, dendrites; jr, junctional regions. Pig cerebral and cerebellar cortices; OsO_4 fixation. $\times$ 23 650 (*From Kornguth et al. 1971*)

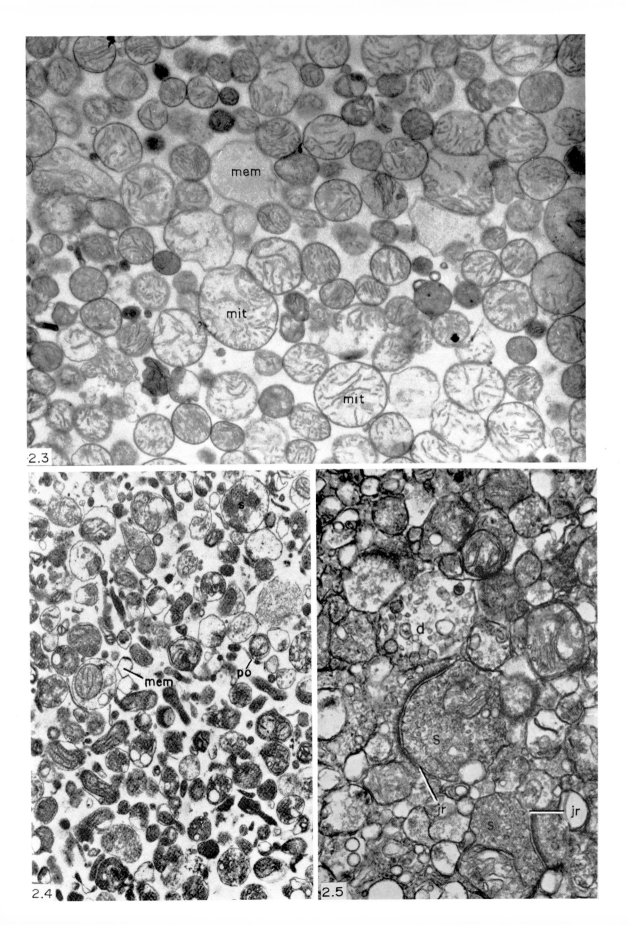

Plate 2.6 Synaptosomal fraction from *Octopus* brain. The synaptosomes (s) contain, besides agranular synaptic vesicles (sv) and mitochondria (mit), dense-cored vesicles (dcv) and occasional vacuoles (v). Vesicular profiles (ves) of varying sizes are interspersed between the synaptosomes. *Octopus vulgaris* supraoesophageal ganglia; permanganate fixation. $\times$ 16 625

Plate 2.7 Synaptic vesicle fraction (D) prepared by Whittaker's procedures (Scheme 2.4). The majority of the profiles are of synaptic vesicles with, infrequently, larger microsomal-sized vesicles (circled). Guinea-pig cerebral cortex; permanganate fixation. $\times$ 30 400 (*From Whittaker and Sheridan, 1965*)

Plate 2.8 Synaptic vesicle fraction (M_2) prepared by De Robertis's procedures (Scheme 2.5). The synaptic vesicles (sv) have a number of larger membranous profiles (mem) intermingled with them. Rat whole brain; negatively stained with phosphotungstate. $\times$ 59 850 (*From De Robertis et al., 1963*)

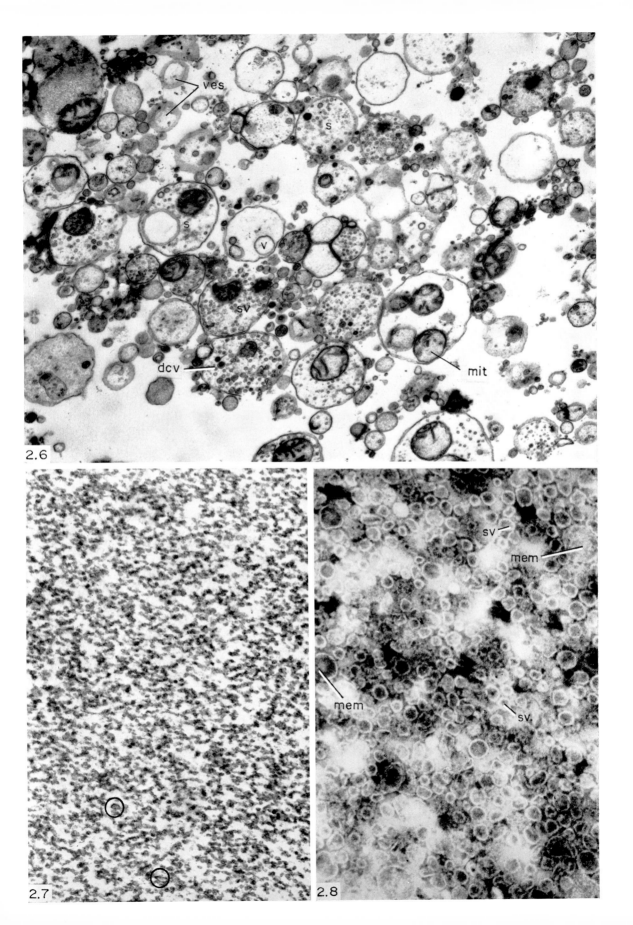

Plate 2.9 An example of the 'tagging' of a synaptic vesicle preparation using polystyrene beads (arrows.) The beads have a diameter of 88 nm and are interspersed with the synaptic vesicles (sv). Guinea-pig cerebral cortex; negatively stained with sodium phosphotungstate. × 66 500 (*From Whittaker and Sheridan, 1965*)

Plate 2.10 This is the C layer of the P6 fraction of Kanaseki and Kadota, and is enriched in coated vesicles (cv) and shell fragments (sh). Plain synaptic vesicles (sv) and membrane fragments (f) are the principal contaminants. Guinea-pig whole brain; unbuffered OsO_4 and unbuffered glutaraldehyde fixation. × 90 250 (*From Kadota and Kadota, 1973c*)

Plate 2.11 Contents of fraction S_5 S-P in the coated vesicle separation procedure of Kadota and Kadota (Scheme 2.6). This fraction consists essentially of flocculent material (arrow), which is variable in appearance and is diffusely scattered throughout the fraction. Guinea-pig whole brain; negatively stained with uranyl acetate. × 129 200 (*From Kadota and Kadota, 1973c*)

Plate 2.12 Synaptic vesicle fraction from octopus brain. This fraction contains numerous vesicles (sv) and a few synaptosome ghosts (sg) and synaptosomes (s). *Eledone* supraoesophageal ganglia; permanganate fixation. × 13 775 (*From Jones, 1970c*)

Plate 2.13 Synaptic vesicle fraction from *Torpedo* electroplaque. Vesicles of varying sizes are present, with remarkably little membranous contamination. *Torpedo marmorata* electroplaque; permanganate fixation. × 12 730 (*From Israël and Gautron, 1969*)

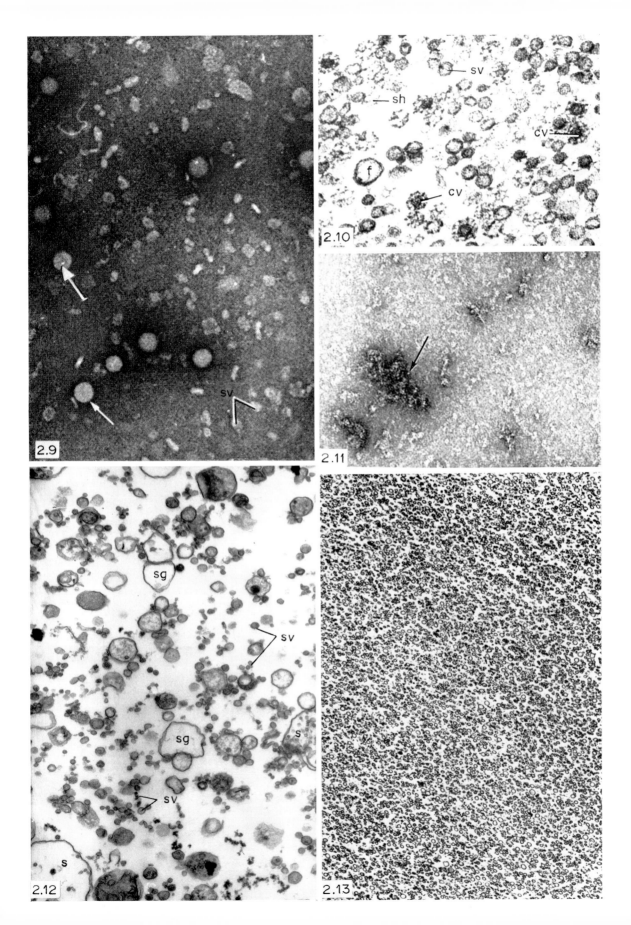

Plate 2.14 Synaptic membrane fraction (M_1 (1.0)) prepared by De Robertis's procedures (Scheme 2.7). The arrows point to profiles which may be synaptic junctional regions. Rat cerebral cortex; OsO_4 fixation. $\times$ 30 400 (*From Rodriguez de Lores Arnaiz et al., 1967*)

Plate 2.15 Synaptic membrane fraction following Cotman's procedures (Scheme 2.8). The arrow points to a synaptic junctional region recognizable by its thickened membranes. A few synaptic vesicles (sv) and dark staining bodies (d) are also present. Rat forebrain; aldehyde–OsO_4 fixation. $\times$ 38 000 (*From Cotman and Matthews, 1971*)

Plate 2.16 Synaptic complexes fraction (Scheme 2.9). The most readily recognizable part of the complexes is the postsynaptic thickening (pt). The whole of the junctional region is visible in places (arrows). The remnants of synaptosomal membranes (mem) are also seen. Rat forebrain; aldehyde–OsO_4 fixation. $\times$ 17 480 (*From Cotman and Taylor, 1972*)

Plate 2.17 Postsynaptic membrane fraction (Scheme 2.10). The profiles labelled *psm* are interpreted by Garey and coworkers as detached postsynaptic membranes. For comment on this, see text. Rat cerebral cortex; aldehyde–OsO_4 fixation. $\times$ 20 900 (*From Garey et al., 1972*)

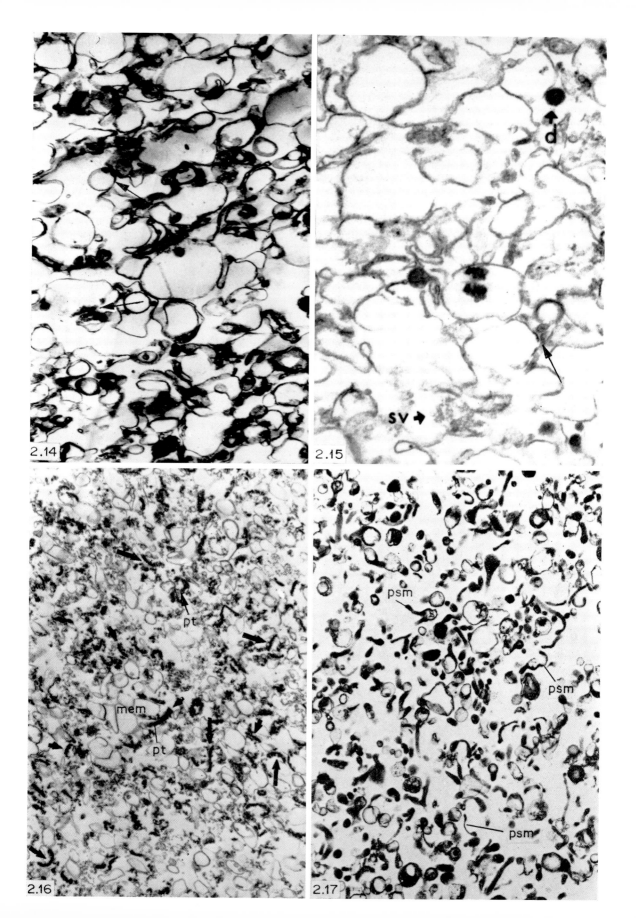

2.14

2.15

2.16

2.17

Plate 2.18 Serial sections through a synaptosome. a–d represent sections 1, 4, 6 and 10 respectively of a series of 10. The presynaptic component of the synaptosome contains synaptic vesicles (sv), coated vesicles (cv), the shell (sh) of coated vesicles and a mitochondrion (mit). A spine apparatus (sa) is present postsynaptically. Rat cerebellum; OsO_4 fixation. $\times$ 68 400. (*From Jones and Brearley, 1973*)

Plate 2.19 Serial sections through a synaptosome. a–d are sections through the pre- and postsynaptic components (pr and po respectively) of a synaptosome. They are sections 2, 4, 5 and 6 respectively of a series of 8. Emphasis in this series is on the synaptic junctional region (sj), in an attempt to develop criteria for recognizing this region. Rat cerebellum; OsO_4 fixation. $\times$ 16 530. (*From Jones and Brearley, 1973*)

Plate 2.20 Axonal profiles (ax) in P_2B–b subfraction of Dekirmenjian and Brunngraber. mit, mitochondria. Rat whole brain; negatively stained with PTA after overnight fixation in 10% formalin. $\times$ 33 800 (*From Lemkey-Johnston and Dekirmenjian, 1970*)

Plate 2.21 Glial fraction prepared from a clonal line of glial cells. Rat glial cells; OsO_4 fixation. $\times$ 30 400 (*From Cotman et al., 1971a*)

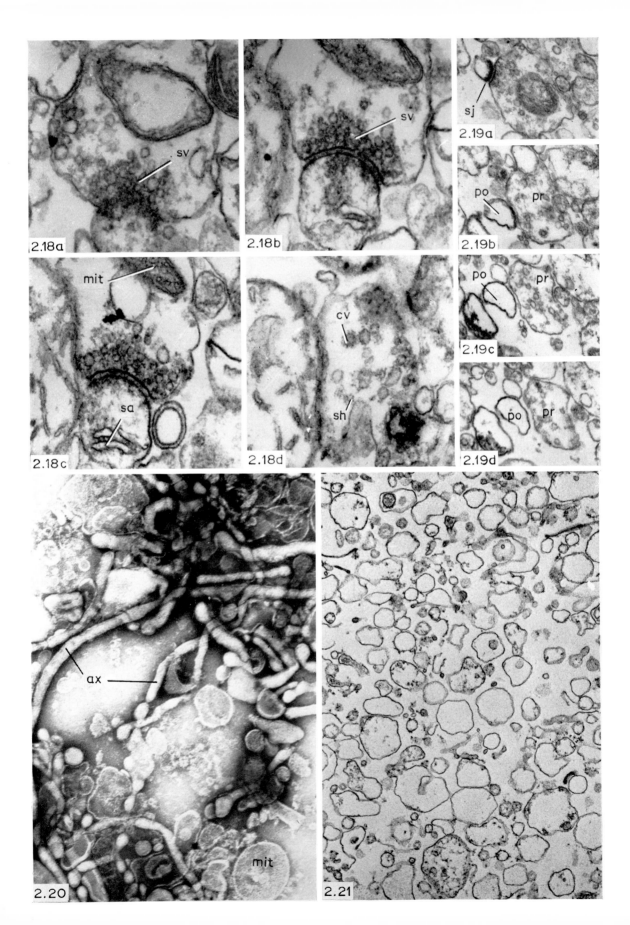

Plate 3.1 Synaptosome demonstrating a presynaptic component (pr), containing synaptic vesicles (sv) and a few vacuoles (v), a cleft region with cleft material (cm) and a postsynaptic membrane (pom). The postsynaptic thickening (pt) can be distinguished at one point from the postsynaptic membrane with its unit membrane (arrow). The enveloping membrane around the presynaptic component is intact. Rat cerebral cortex; OsO_4 fixation following resuspension in a Krebs-phosphate medium. $\times$ 114 000

Plate 3.2 This synaptosome resembles that shown in Plate 3.1. A mitochondrion (mit) is recognizable, while vacuoles (v) are prominent in the midst of the synaptic vesicles (sv). Details of preparation and material as for Plate 3.1. $\times$ 74 100

Plate 3.3 The postsynaptic component (po) of this synaptosome, of which a part is shown, is unusually large in comparison to the presynaptic component (pr). The cleft region is clearly demonstrated, and the asymmetrical arrangement of the membrane differentiations is readily discerned. cm, cleft material; pt, postsynaptic thickening. Details of preparation and material as for Plate 3.1. $\times$ 117 000

Plate 3.4 Synaptic vesicles (sv) of varying sizes and a mitochondrion (mit) dominate the presynaptic component of this synaptosome. cm, cleft material; pmm, paramitochondrial membrane; po, postsynaptic component. *Octopus vulgaris* supraoesophageal ganglia; potassium permanganate fixation. $\times$ 72 100

Plate 3.5 Two cleft regions, *cv* and *b*, are evident in this synaptosomal profile. Cleft material (cm) is present in both instances, while the respective pre- and postsynaptic membranes (prm and pom) are parallel. Synaptic vesicles (sv) are seen on both sides of cleft *a*. gm, granular material. Details as for Plate 3.4. $\times$ 71 250

Plate 3.6 A number of coated vesicles (cv) can just be recognized interspersed amongst synaptic vesicles (sv) in this synaptosome. Rat cerebal cortex; aldehyde–OsO_4 fixation. $\times$ 51 300

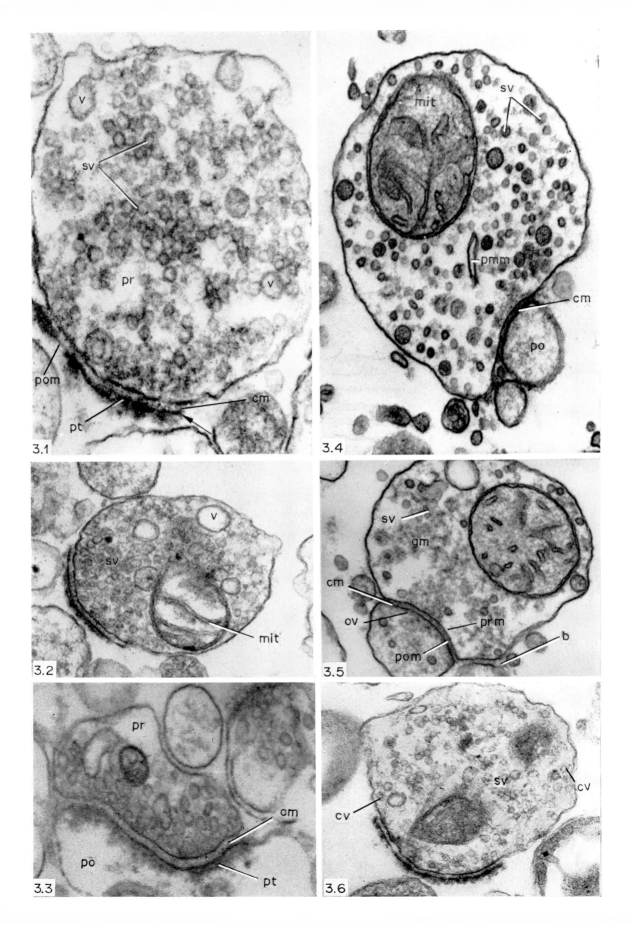

Plate 3.7 Negatively-stained synaptosome showing enclosed synaptic vesicles (sv) and a possible mitochondrial outline (mit). A number of the profiles are probably postsynaptic processes (po). Rat cerebral cortex; negatively-stained with ammonium molybdate. $\times$ 22 800

Plate 3.8 This negatively-stained synaptosome is surrounded by numerous white profiles (wp) which are the result of sucrose 'bubbling'. This is a typical manifestation of moderate sucrose contamination. po, postsynaptic process; sv, synaptic vesicles. Details as for Plate 3.7. $\times$ 28 000

Plate 3.9 Synaptic vesicles are not clearly defined in this synaptosome. Instead the external membrane of the synaptosome is obscuring the organelles present in the presynaptic component (pr). The cleft region (c) is well-defined. po, postsynaptic process. *Octopus vulgaris* optic lobe; negatively-stained with PTA. $\times$ 46 360

Plate 3.10 Large granular vesicles (lgv) are seen within this synaptosome, the background of which consists of a cytoplasmic framework (cf). Details as for Plate 3.9. $\times$ 43 700

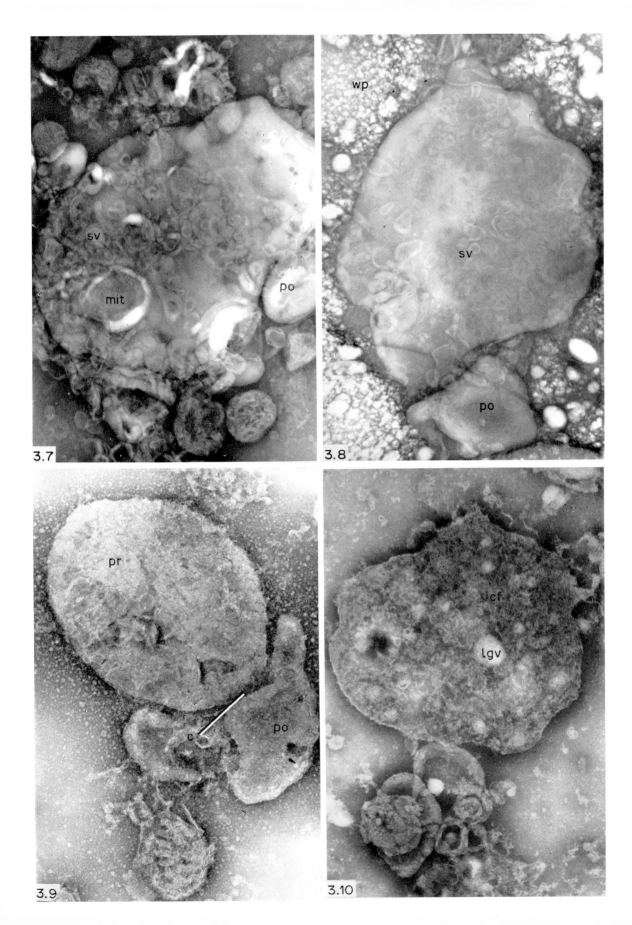

3.7

3.8

3.9

3.10

Plate 3.11 Synaptosomal fraction (P$_2$B) prepared under hypertonic conditions. The synaptosomes (s) are slightly shrunken with a dense cytoplasmic matrix. Vesicles (sv) are just recognizable against this dense background. The synaptosomes are variable in shape and size. Bat cerebral cortex; potassium permanganate fixation. × 34 390

Plate 3.12 A further example of a hypertonically prepared synaptosomal fraction. Synaptosomes (s) are more difficult to define, although mitochondria (mit) are readily recognizable. The profiles labelled *p* are difficult to categorize. Some (arrows) have mitochondrial characteristics and can be distinguished from definite postsynaptic membranes (pmm). Mouse cerebellum; potassium permanganate fixation. × 25 650

Plate 3.13 Synaptosome following incubation in phosphate buffered glucose-salines. Rat cerebral cortex; OsO$_4$ fixation. × 51 300

Plate 3.14 Synaptosome following incubation in phosphate buffered glucose—salines and electrical stimulation. Rat cerebral cortex; OsO$_4$ fixation. × 69 920

Plate 3.15 Synaptosome (type A) prepared using a non-osmicated technique. The presynaptic terminal (pr) is clearly delineated, the internal and external coats of the membrane being visible at certain points (arrows). cd, cleft densities; dp, dense projections; mit, mitochondria; pfd, postsynaptic focal densities; pn, presynaptic network. Rat cerebral cortex; glutaraldehyde fixation, PTA staining. × 74 100

Plate 3.16 Synaptosome (type B) prepared using a non-osmicated technique. The postsynaptic membrane is continuous along the length of the junction and is thickened (pt). The cleft material is composed of thickened, transversely orientated bars (tb). pn, presynaptic network. Rat cerebral cortex; glutaraldehyde fixation, PTA staining. × 145 920

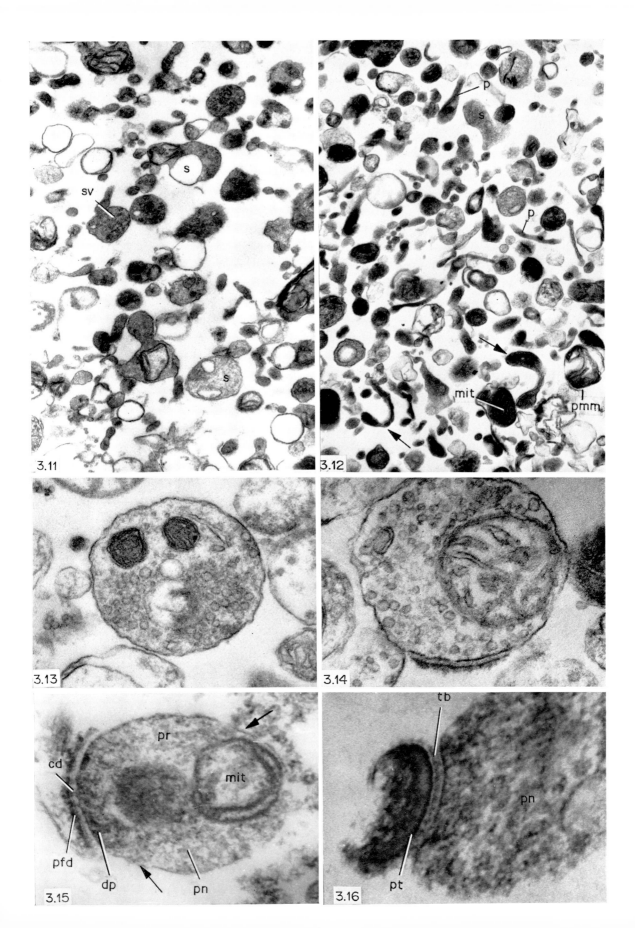

Plate 3.17 Synaptosomes separated from the P_1C fraction of a medulla/spinal cord homogenate. Vesicles (sv) are packed together in the dense cytoplasm. A few tubules (t) occur amidst the vesicles, together with vacuoles (v) of varying sizes. mit, mitochondria. Rat medulla/spinal cord; OsO_4 fixation. $\times$ 68 680

Plate 3.18 Synaptosome from the P_1D fraction of a medulla/spinal cord homogenate. The postsynaptic membrane with its postsynaptic focal densities (pfd) is evident. Rat medulla/spinal cord; OsO_4 fixation. $\times$ 72 675

Plate 3.19 This large synaptosome in a cerebellar P_1 fraction is probably derived from a mossy fibre synapse. A number of synaptic junctions are evident around its periphery (arrows). Serial sections through this synaptosome revealed that up to ten junctions could be seen. Rat cerebellum; OsO_4 fixation. $\times$ 34 200

Plate 3.20 A neurosecretosome derived from the posterior pituitary gland. The large neurosecretory granules (lng) are clearly seen. Bovine posterior pituitary gland; negatively stained with PTA. $\times$ 31 350 (*From LaBella and Sanwal, 1965*)

Plate 3.21 Synaptosomes from *Octopus* brain to demonstrate their appearance in non-osmicated material. The presynaptic spicules (ps) represent the dense projections of mammalian synaptosomes. pn, presynaptic network; sp, synaptic plate; vp, vesicular profiles. *Octopus vulgaris* supraoesophageal ganglia; glutaradehyde fixation, PTA staining. $\times$ 61 750 (*From Jones, 1970a*)

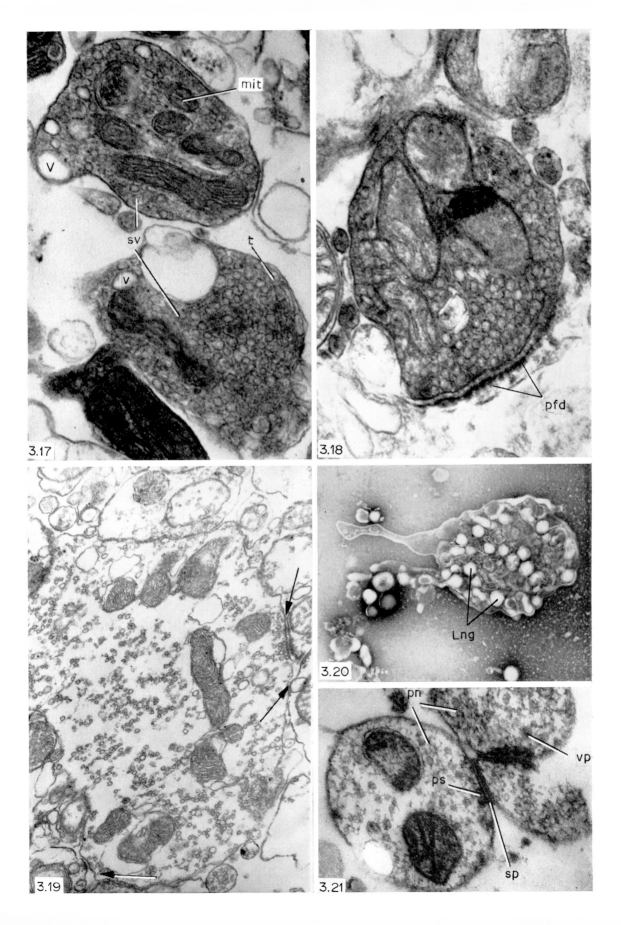

Plate 3.22 Negatively-stained synaptic vesicles. Arrows point to tail-like attachments to/of the vesicles. Mouse whole brain; negatively stained with sodium phosphotungstate. $\times$ 45 600 (*From Kuriyama et al., 1968a*)

Plate 3.23 Negatively-stained synaptic vesicles showing (1) connections between vesicles, (2) vesicles with 'tails', and (3) lengths of fibrillar material. Guinea-pig forebrain; negatively-stained with PTA. $\times$ 126 350 (*From Whittaker, 1966a*)

Plate 3.24 Synaptic junction from intact, non-fractionated, non-osmicated tissue. The dense projections (dp) are distinguishable from the presynaptic network (pn), the cleft densities (cd) are interconnected, while the postsynaptic thickening (pt) is essentially continuous. mit, mitochondrion. Rat cerebral cortex; glutaraldehyde fixation, PTA staining. $\times$ 114 000

Plate 3.25 This synaptosome, prepared in the same manner as the junction in Plate 3.24, should be compared with the intact junction. Dense projections are poorly demonstrated in the synaptosome due, in part, to the tight packing of the network (pn) close to the cleft. The cleft densities (cd) are more discrete, while relatively discrete postsynaptic focal densities (pfd) are visible in the postsynaptic component (po). Rat cerebral cortex; glutaraldehyde fixation, PTA staining. $\times$ 114 000

Plate 3.26 Low-power view of a synaptosomal fraction maintained in tissue cluture for 4h. The synaptosomes (s) are intact, synaptic vesicles (sv) are well preserved and cleft regions (c) are prominent. Rat cerebral cortex; synaptosomes incubated in a Krebs-phosphate medium and exposed to electrical pulses; OsO_4 fixation. $\times$ 16 150

Plate 3.27 Synaptosomes maintained in tissue culture for 24h. Most synaptosomes appear well preserved, although there is some loss and clumping of vesicles (sv). Details as for Plate 3.26. $\times$ 15 580

Plate 3.28 Synaptosomes maintained in tissue culture for 5 days. Severe autolysis is present by this stage. Although synaptosomes (s) and mitochondria (mit) are still recognizable, great loss of structure has occurred. Synaptic vesicles are represented within the synaptosomes by a poorly-defined, granular matrix. Details as for Plate 3.26. $\times$ 32 300

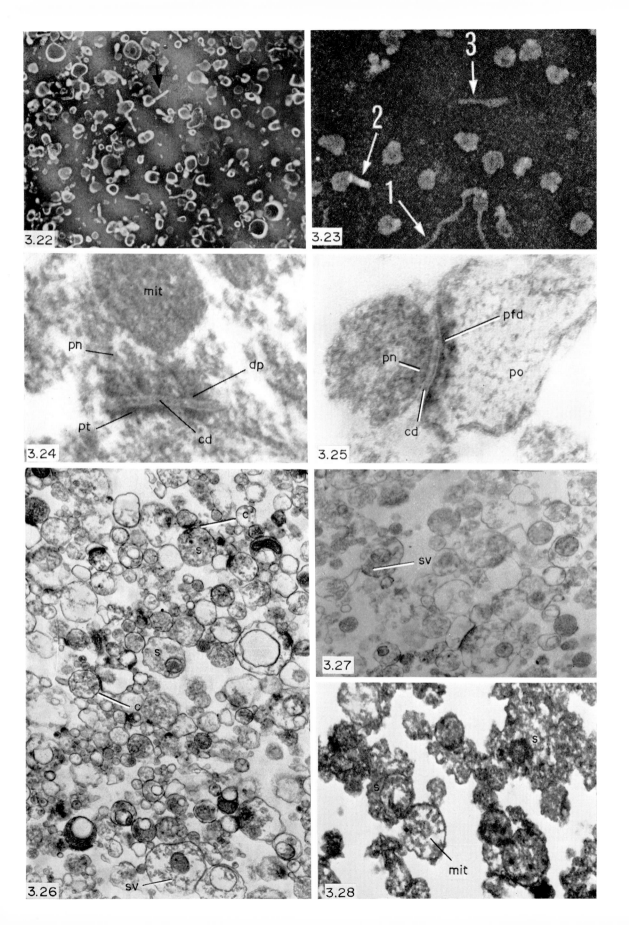

Plate 3.29 Synaptogenesis. A typical profile present in a 'synaptosomal' fraction early in post-natal development. The presence of ribosomes (r) and neurofilaments (nf) suggests a postsynaptic origin. The dense material (dm) localized close to its periphery, sometimes lies alongside a definite presynaptic process, with granular material (gm) intervening. Rat cerebral cortex; glutaraldehyde–OsO$_4$ fixation. $\times$ 49 970 (*From Jones and Revell. 1970a*)

Plates 3.30–3.32 Synaptogenesis. Typical synaptosomes from 5 (3.30), 7 (3.31) and 21 (3.32) day material. Granular material (gm) is conspicuous in the cytoplasm of the 5 day synaptosome, while there is an increase in the number of synaptic vesicles (sv) with development. Mitochondria (mit) are present in the 7 and 21 day material. Details as for Plate 3.29. Plate 3.30 $\times$ 30 875; Plate 3.31 $\times$ 25 500; Plate 3.32 $\times$ 34 200. (*From Jones and Revell, 1970a*)

Plate 3.33 Synaptogenesis. Part of the lightest fraction (1) obtained from 1 day old cerebral cortex. The profiles are characterized by amorphous granular material (gm), in addition to which a few vesicular structures (v) can be recognized. Rat cerebral cortex; glutaraldehyde–OsO$_4$. $\times$11 640 (*From Gonatas et al., 1971*)

Plate 3.34 Synaptogenesis. Some of the profiles in the heaviest fraction (3) obtained from 8 day old cerebral cortex. Vesicles are present in some of them, which are probably synaptosomes (arrows). Details as for Plate 3.33. $\times$ 18 050 (*From Gonatas et al., 1971*)

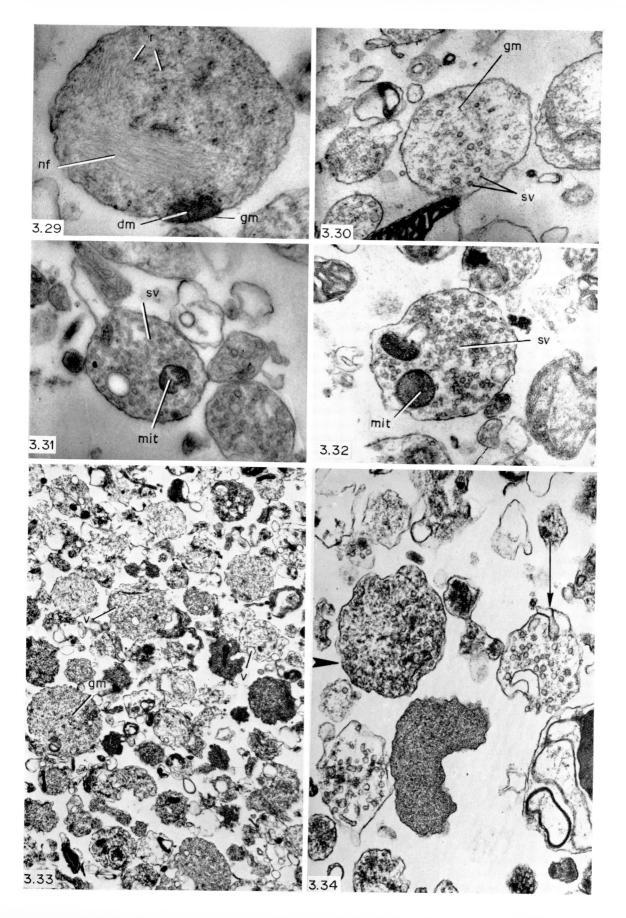

Plate 4.1 EM autoradiograph of rat area postrema. A neuronal perikaryon is illustrated, with labelling of the nucleus and ubiquitous labelling of the cytoplasm. ER, entoplasmic reticulum; n, nucleus. Intraventricular injection of ^{3}H-NE; aldehyde–OsO$_4$ fixation. $\times$ 23 750 (*From Sotelo, 1971b*)

Plate 4.2 EM autoradiograph of rat area postrema, showing an axon terminal synapsing on a dendrite. A few DCV are present (arrows) in the labelled terminal. Details of preparation of material as for Plate 4.1. $\times$ 34 200 (*From Sotelo, 1971b*)

Plate 4.3 EM autoradiograph of rat cerebral cortex slice incubated with ^{3}H-GABA. Clusters of silver grains are present over nerve terminals. Aldehyde–OsO$_4$ fixation. $\times$ 32 300 (*From Iversen and Bloom, 1972*)

Plate 4.4 EM autoradiograph of rat striatum homogenate pellet incubated with ^{3}H-GABA. Synaptosomes are evident, some of which (arrows) are labelled. Preparation as for Plate 4.3. $\times$ 31 350 (*From Iverson and Bloom, 1972*)

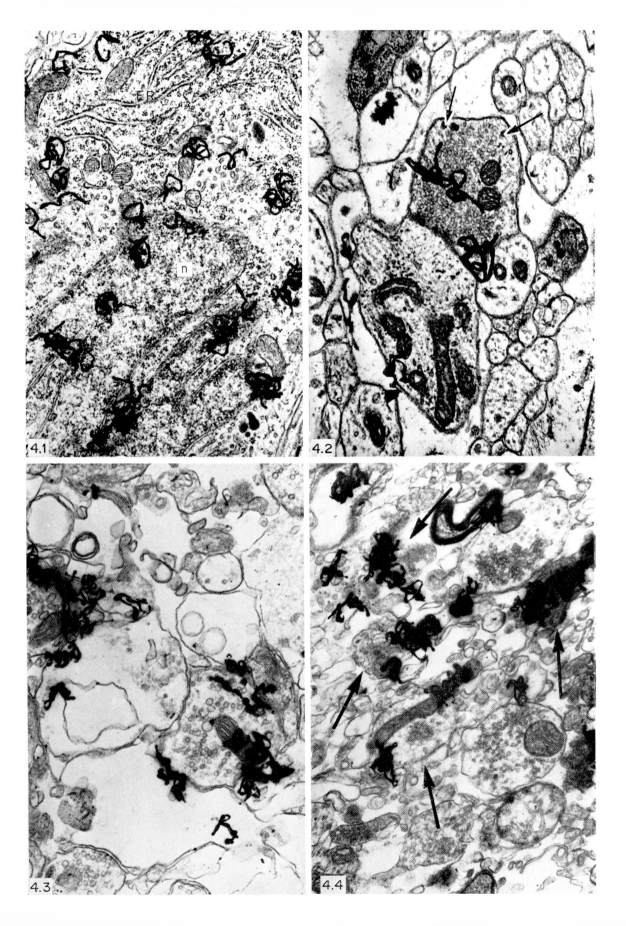

Plate 4.5 EM autoradiograph of rat spinal cord slice incubated with ^{3}H-glycine. Silver grains are present over a number of terminals (b_1–b_6). Aldehyde–OsO$_4$ fixation. $\times$ 11 400 (*From Hökfelt and Ljungdahl, 1971a*)

Plate 4.6 EM autoradiograph of rat spinal cord slice incubated with ^{3}H-glycine. The grains have accumulated over an oligodendroglial cell body, a nerve terminal and an axon (thick arrows indicate the latter two locations). The thin arrows point to two unlabelled terminals. Preparation as for Plate 4.5. $\times$ 11 875 (*From Hökfelt and Ljungdahl, 1971a*)

Plate 4.7 EM autoradiograph of rat spinal cord slice incubated with ^{3}H-glycine to show heavily labelled 'flattened-vesicle' axon terminal (f) and unlabelled 'round-vesicle' terminals (r). Aldehyde–OsO$_4$ fixation. $\times$ 57 000 (*From Matus and Dennison, 1972*)

Plate 4.8 EM autoradiograph of spinal cord homogenate pellet incubated with ^{3}H-glycine. Clusters of grains are seen over synaptosomal profiles (arrows). Preparation as for Plate 4.3. $\times$ 9 500 (*From Iversen and Bloom, 1972*)

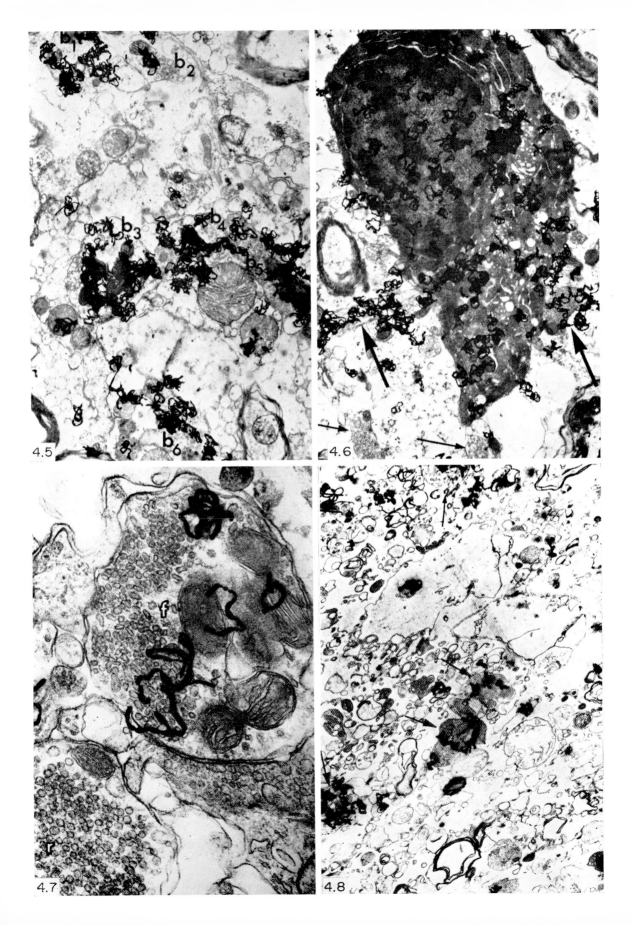

Plate 4.9 EM autoradiograph of chicken ciliary ganglion (GC) 1.5 h after the intracerebral injection of ^{3}H-lysine. Numerous grains are present over the presynaptic terminal (calyx, Ca), particularly over the plasma membranes (pm) and (as also shown in the inset) synaptic vesicles (sv). mit, mitochondria. Preganglionic axons (Ax) are not labelled. Aldehyde–OsO$_4$ fixation. × 17 100 (*From Droz et al., 1973*)

Plate 4.10 Preparation and material as for Plate 4.9; 18 h after injection of ^{3}H-lysine. The preterminal segment of the axon (PS) and the presynaptic terminal (Ca) are heavily labelled. The majority of the grains are located over presynaptic membranes (pm) and synaptic vesicles (sv) (see also inset), with a lesser number over mitochondria (mit) and axoplasm free of vesicles (ax). × 10 640 (*From Droz et al., 1973*)

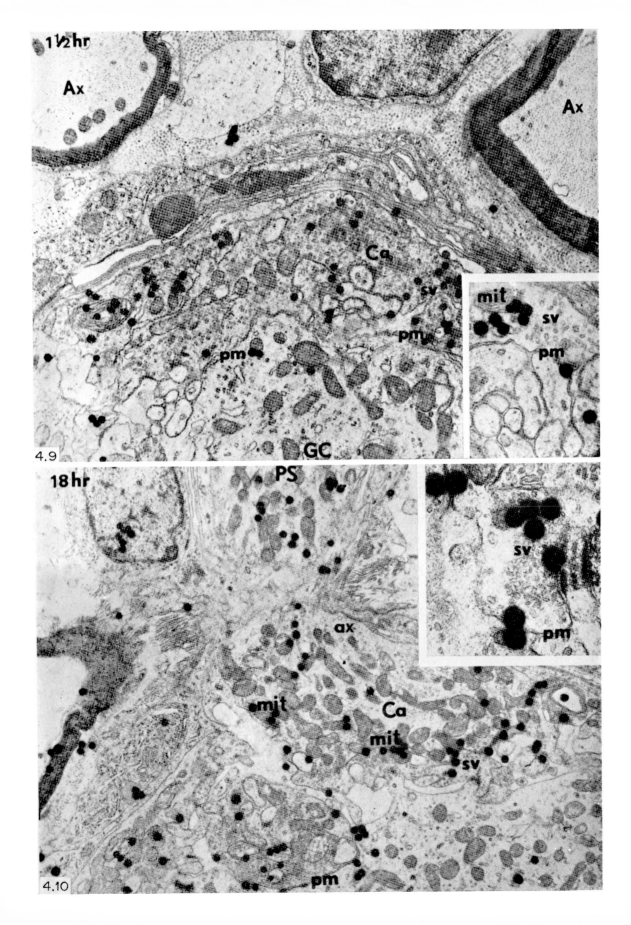

Plate 4.11 Comparison of the effects of amino acetylation and carboxy methylation on, in the left column, uranyl (U) and lead (L) treated synapses and, in the right column, BIUL treated synapses. C, controls; M, methylation; A, acetylation; A + M, acetylation followed by methylation. Cat subfornical organ; glutaraldehyde (G) fixation. × 66 500 (*From Pfenninger, 1971a*)

Plate 4.12 Ruthenium red staining of rat cerebral cortex. The ruthenium red reaction product is predominantly located extracellularly (arrows). Cytoplasmic ground substance and synaptic vesicles (sv) are essentially free of reaction product. Aldehyde–OsO$_4$ fixation. × 171 000 (*From Bondareff 1967*)

Plate 4.13 Ruthenium red staining of synaptosome derived from rat cerebral cortex. The reaction product is principally located in the cleft region and over the external aspect of the terminal membrane (arrows). Some intracellular penetration of the stain has occurred, in the region of the postsynaptic thickening (pt) and between the synaptic vesicles (sv). × 76 760

Plate 4.14 Test tube experiments and electrophoretic studies with bismuth iodide. In *a* the reactions of polyamino, hyaluronic and sialic acids with bismuth iodide have been tested using unfixed and glutaraldehyde-fixed substrates. With unfixed substrates the three basic polyamino acids react, and with glutaraldehyde-fixed substrates only polylysine and polyhistidine. The electrophoretic experiment depicted in *b* shows that after 10 (I) and 20 (II) minutes bismuth iodide moves towards the anode, resulting in its immobilization and precipitation with the basic polyamino acids. (*From Pfenninger, 1971a*)

Plate 4.15 Trypsin digestion for 1 h of sections of rat cerebral cortex. Only the postsynaptic membrane (arrow), the postsynaptic thickening and part of the cleft material are visible. Aldehyde-OsO$_4$ fixation. × 124 450 (*From Barrantes and Lunt, 1970*)

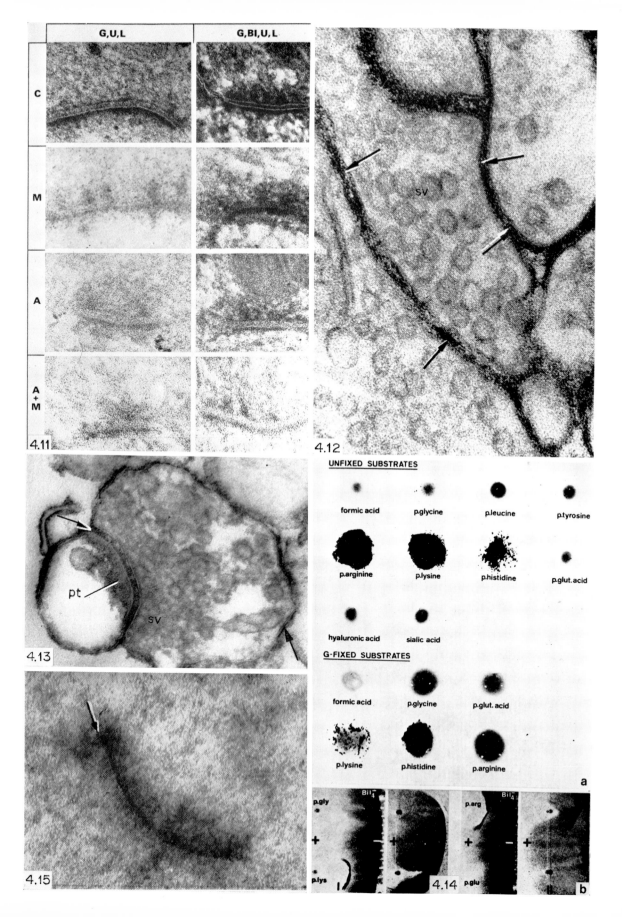

4.11

	G, U, L	G, Bi, U, L
C		
M		
A		
A + M		

4.12

sv

4.13

pt

sv

4.15

UNFIXED SUBSTRATES

formic acid   p.glycine   p.leucine   p.tyrosine

p.arginine   p.lysine   p.histidine   p.glut.acid

hyaluronic acid   sialic acid

G-FIXED SUBSTRATES

formic acid   p.glycine   p.glut. acid

p.lysine   p.histidine   p.arginine

a

p.gly   Bil⁻₄   p.arg   Bil⁻₄

+   +   +   −   +

p.lys   4.14   p.glu   b

Plate 4.16 Frozen section of rat hypothalamus stained with PTA, following exposure to soybean trypsin inhibitor and trypsin for 2 h. The stained material is present in all elements of the synaptic junction. The arrows point to dense projections. Aldehyde fixation. $\times$ 209 000 (*From Bloom and Aghajanian, 1968*)

Plate 4.17 Material similar to that in Plate 4.16 exposed to trypsin for 2 h. Dense projections (arrows) are barely visible. M, mitochondrian $\times$ 248 900 (*From Bloom and Aghajanian, 1968*)

Plate 4.18 A series of experiments to illustrate the opening of synaptic contacts in cat and rat subfornical organs, stained using the BIUL technique and incubated prior to glutaraldehyde fixation. a, control, no incubation; b and d, $0.1M$–$NaClO_4$; c, $3M$ sucrose; e, $0.1M$–EDTA; and f, $0.5M$–$NaClO_3$. dp, dense projections; po, postsynaptic opacity (thickening). $\times$ 92 625 (*From Pfenninger, 1971b*)

Plates 4.19 and 4.20 Rat spinal cord stained for AChE. The axosomatic terminal in Plate 4.19 is characterized by the lack of enzyme staining around the presynaptic process, unlike that in Plate 4.20 which is heavily stained (arrow points to cleft region). The rough endoplasmic reticulum (er) is heavily stained in both instances, whereas the synaptic vesicles (sv) and mitochondria (mit) are not. Aldehyde–OsO_4 fixation. Plate 4.19 $\times$ 24 985; Plate 4.20 $\times$ 51 585 (*From Lewis and Shute, 1966*)

Plates 4.21 and 4.22 Rat spinal cord stained for ChAc. Electrondense precipitate is present in terminals A and A_1 but not in A_2. It is also seen in the dendrite, D. *indicates an artifact. Aldehyde–OsO_4 fixation. Plate 4.21 $\times$ 74 765; Plate 4.22 $\times$ 56 050 (*From Kása, 1971*)

Plate 4.23 A synaptosome derived from rat cerebral cortex and stained for AChE. Precipitate is present over its limiting membrane and postsynaptically. Aldehyde–OsO_4 fixation. $\times$ 57 000 (*D. G. Jones; originally published in Whittaker, 1969b*)

Plates 4.24 and 4.25 Sections of chicken forebrain showing the distribution of immunofluorescence after incubation with anti-membrane-γ-globulin and fluoresceinisothiocyanate (FITC)-conjugated goat anti-rabbit-γ-globulin. Plate 4.24 $\times$ 171; Plate 4.25 $\times$ 713 (*From Livett et al., 1974*)

Plate 4.26 Immunofluorescence of a folium from chicken cerebellum after incubation with anti-membrane-γ-globulin. G, granular layer; M, molecular layer; P, Purkinje cells; W, white matter. $\times$143 (*From Livett et al., 1974*)

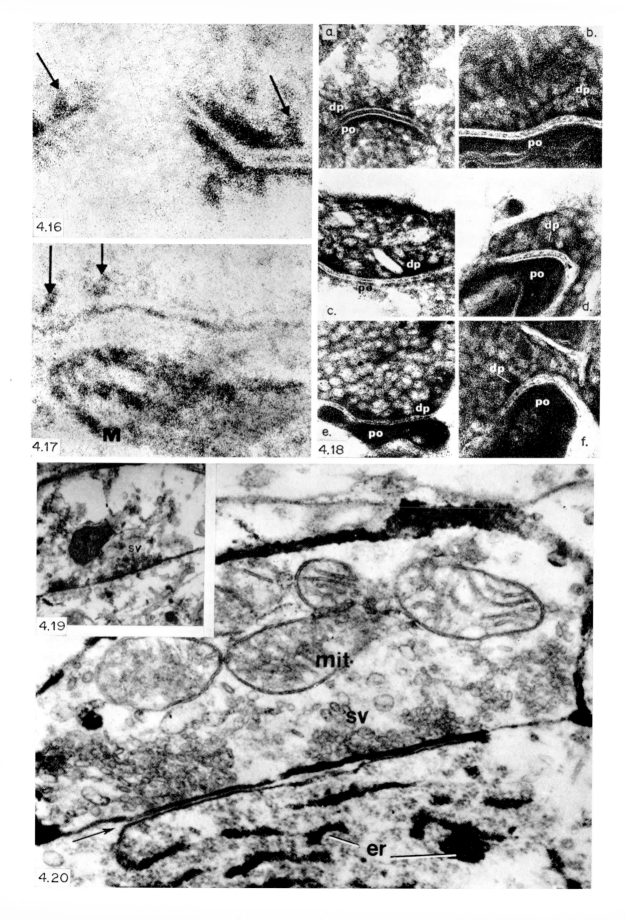

4.16

4.17 M

a. dp po

b. dp po

c. dp po

d. dp po

4.18 e. po dp

f. dp po

4.19 sv

4.20 mit sv er

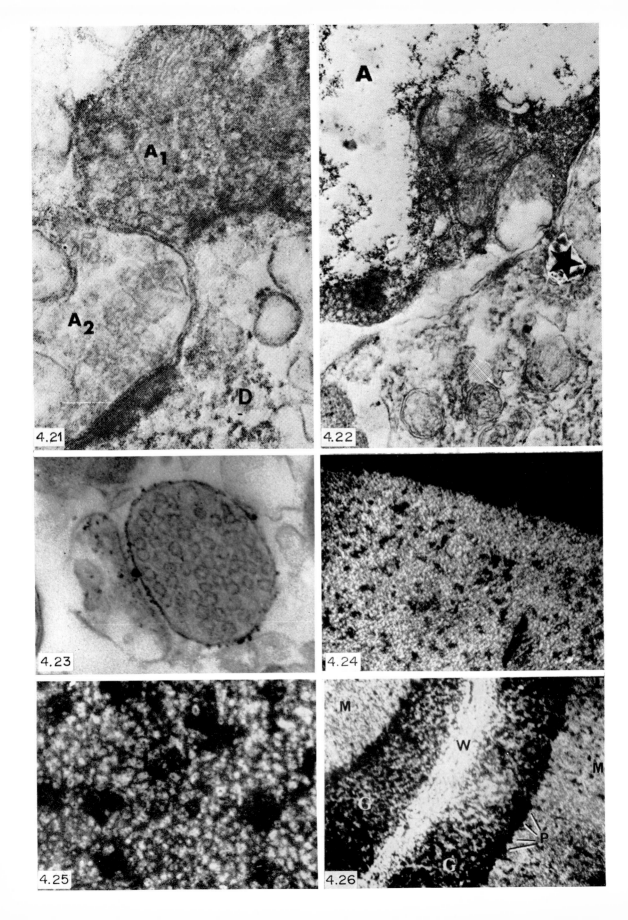

volume ratio, maintain their integrity given appropriate osmotic conditions. The 'stickiness' of the synaptic or contact region ensures the integrity of the synaptic junction during and subsequent to tissue disruption. Synaptosomes as a whole therefore, survive the liquid shear forces necessary to rupture many other tissue elements as well as sedimentation through the hypertonic sucrose density gradients necessary to separate them from other neuronal constituents.

In spite of the mode of formation of synaptosomes all available evidence suggests that the membrane enveloping them is continuous (Plates 3.1–3.6). This is true with respect to morphological criteria (e.g. Gray and Whittaker, 1962; Jones, 1969; Jones and Bradford, 1971a), their content of soluble cytoplasmic components and freely soluble metabolites (Whittaker, 1965; Mangan and Whittaker, 1966; Bradford and Thomas, 1969), and their osmotic properties whereby they swell and shrink in media of varying tonicity (Marchbanks, 1967; Keen and White, 1970). Furthermore, they are capable of performing like whole cells, with high linear respiration producing lactate and amino acids, generating ATP and phosphocreatine and accumulating K^+ and extruding Na^+ against a concentration gradient (Ling and Abdel-Latif, 1968; Bradford, 1969; Bradford and Thomas, 1969; see De Belleroche and Bradford, 1973b).

Whittaker's (1969b) designation of synaptosomes as 'miniature non-nucleated cells' is appropriate, and recent neurochemical investigations using synaptosomes to study oxygen and glucose utilization, putative neurotransmitters, the active transport of certain ions and molecules, and synaptosomal responses to depolarizing influences (for review see De Belleroche and Bradford, 1973) further justify it. The close correspondence between the junctional regions of synaptosomes and nerve endings *in situ* (Jones and Brearley, 1972a, b; Jones, 1973d) together with the obvious similarities of the presynaptic terminals in fractionated and intact situations help to substantiate the concept of the synaptosome as a *morphological* tool (Jones, 1972). It is to be hoped that with the extension of autoradiographic and immunological techniques to fractionation studies, the morphological usefulness of synaptosomes will be exploited.

3.1.2   Fixation techniques

Developments in understanding synaptosomal morphology have, not surprisingly, reflected corresponding developments in characterizing synaptic ultrastructure. The fixation and staining techniques current in the early 1960s were the ones employed by those involved in the initial synaptosomal studies. It is not surprising therefore, that Gray should have used OsO_4 fixation combined with PTA staining in his work with Whittaker (1960, 1962) on synaptosomal ultrastructure, in view of the proven value of this combination in classifying cerebral cortex synapses (Gray, 1959a; Fig. 3.1). Similarly De Robertis and his associates (1962a) looked to OsO_4 fixation and lead staining, as a consequence of their previous experience with these in intact synaptic tissue (De Robertis, 1956; De Robertis and Franchi, 1956).

In spite of this divergence between the two groups of workers, neither technique was utilized to its fullest degree, with the result that similar structural principles emerged.

Because the morphological studies were undertaken as controls for biochemical investigations, little interest was displayed in detailed ultrastructural features. Indeed, after the initial studies had been carried out, the majority of published EMs of synaptosomal fractions for the next few years were low-power ones, concerned only with demonstrating the enrichment of fractions. This trend was reflected in the work of Whittaker's group in the mid-1960s when permanganate was adopted as a fixative because of the readiness with which it delineated synaptosomal profiles (see Clementi *et al.*, 1966b; also Whittaker, 1965; Whittaker and Sheridan, 1965). Although permanganate was used for some higher-power investigations of synaptosomal ultrastructure (Israël and Whittaker, 1965; Whittaker, 1966b), it too was mainly confined to low-power studies (Plates 3.4 and 3.5).

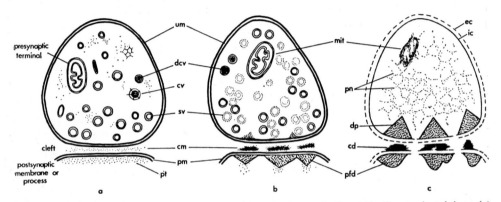

Figure 3.1 A comparison of synaptosomes after different methods of fixation and staining: (a) aldehyde–OsO$_4$, uranyl and lead; (b) OsO$_4$–PTA; (c) glutaraldehyde–PTA. cd, cleft densities; cm, cleft material; cv, coated vesicles; dcv, dense-cored vesicles; dp, dense projections; ec, external membrane coat; ic, internal membrane coat; mit, mitochondria; pfd, postsynaptic focal densities; pm, postsynaptic membrane; pn, presynaptic network; pt, postsynaptic thickening; sv, synaptic vesicles; um, unit membrane.

Combined aldehyde – OsO$_4$ fixation and double staining with uranyl and lead salts is now regularly employed in synaptosomal investigations (e.g. Kuriyama, Sisken, Ito, Simonsen, Haber and Roberts, 1968c; Del Cerro *et al.*, 1969; Ross, Andreoli and Marchbanks, 1971; Dowdall and Whittaker, 1973), although the greater rapidity associated with fixation in OsO$_4$ alone has ensured a continuing place for this procedure in these studies (De Robertis *et al.*, 1967a; Jones and Bradford, 1971a; Osborne, Bradford and Jones, 1973.). (Compare Plates 3.1–3.3 with Plate 3.6.).

With the advent of non-osmicated fixation techniques, primarily glutaraldehyde fixation and block PTA staining (Bloom and Aghajanian, 1966), for delineating the paramembranous densities at synaptic junctions, the way was opened for investigating the contact region between the pre- and postsynaptic components of synaptosomes (Jones, 1969; 1970a; Plates 3.15 and 3.25; Fig. 3.1). It provided a means of characterizing more accurately than had been previously possible different types of synaptosomes, and has also proved a ready way of assessing the synaptic complexes (Cotman *et el.*, 1971b; Cotman and Taylor, 1972) and postsynaptic membranes (Garey *et al.*, 1972).

Initially, fractionated pellets were treated as blocks of whole tissue (Gray and Whittaker, 1962), the pellets being fixed, stained and embedded under identical conditions (De Robertis *et al.*, 1962a, 1963). The results were reasonably satisfactory, although infiltration problems were present in much the same way as with whole tissue blocks. It was soon realized however, that as most of the fractions were obtained as suspensions and not pellets, it would be preferable to fix them in suspension thereby overcoming infiltration problems (Fig. 3.2).

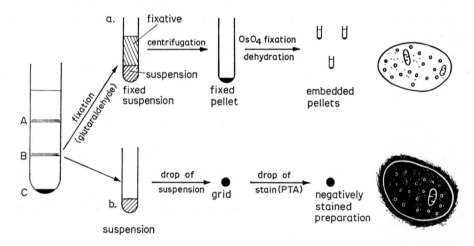

Figure 3.2 An outline of: (a) the method of fixation frequently employed in the preparation of positively stained, embedded fractions; and (b) the stages involved in the negative staining of fractions. Layer B, which is the starting-point of these procedures, is a synaptosomal fraction.

Fixation in suspension had been utilized early on by Palade and Siekevitz (1956a, b) and was employed in brain fractionation studies by Whittaker and Sheridan (1965). It has subsequently been used fairly extensively by other workers, including Jones, (1967, 1968, 1969), Gonatas, Autilio-Gambetti, Gambetti and Shafer (1971), Ross *et al.* (1971), Jones and Brearly (1972b, 1973) and Osborne *et al.* (1973).

Routinely, suspensions are fixed by the addition of approximately five volumes of ice-cold fixative, the time required for fixation being less than for the fixation of pellets. As a rough guide the time of fixation can be reduced to about 50% of that employed for whole tissue blocks, that is, 30–60 minutes for 0·6% potassium permanganate, 1% OsO_4 and 2–6% glutaraldehyde (Jones, 1967). The fixed suspensions are then sedimented to obtain a fixed pellet, by centrifuging at 5 000 *g* for 10–15 minutes at 0°–4°C (Whittaker and Sheridan, 1965; Jones, 1967, 1968, 1969). More vigorous centrifugation conditions are sometimes employed (e.g. 20 000 *g* for 30 minutes by Ross *et al.*, 1971), although the more gentle conditions are adequate under most circumstances.

Suspensions may be used for fixation even when dealing with a pelleted fraction (e.g. fraction C of Whittaker's schedule), by resuspending the pellet in a small quantity (2 ml) of the original homogenization medium (Jones, 1967). The resulting suspension is treated exactly as above. If further fixation is required, as in the case of the post-fixation of aldehyde-fixed material with OsO_4, the fixed pellet is treated as a whole tissue block, the period of OsO_4 fixation being of the order of 45–60 minutes (Jones and Revell, 1970a). Dehydration and embedding are carried out as desired.

The discussion so far has assumed that the fraction is isotonic. Frequently however, this is not so as when, for example, the fraction is formed as a band between 0·8M and 1·2M layers of sucrose. In these instances the hypertonic suspension is diluted with distilled water to restore isotonic conditions, before proceeding with fixation. When this stage is omitted the synaptosomes generally have a shrunken, dense appearance due to the hypertonic conditions under which they were fixed (Lemky-Johnston and Larramendi, 1968; Plates 3.11 and 3.12).

In spite of the advantages inherent in fixing fractionated material in suspension form, the fixation of pellets is nevertheless widespread. They may be treated in the same way as whole tissue blocks (e.g. De Robertis et al., 1967b; Rodriguez de Lores Arnaiz, Zieher and De Robertis, 1970), or the pellet may be left intact and fixed overnight, that is, for 16–18 h (Del Cerro et al., 1969). In the latter method the periphery of the pellet is usually well fixed and is suitable for EM, whereas the core of a pellet 1 cm or more in diameter is less satisfactory and may obviate detailed examination of this region. This is an important point to bear in mind when considering the distribution of organelles throughout a pellet.

All procedures up to the final fixation stage are routinely carried out at 0–5°C. The claim that slight warming of synaptosomal preparations (to 8°C) increases the frequency of tubular figures within the synaptosomes (Israël and Whittaker, 1965) is questionable. It is difficult to repeat these results (Jones, 1974), while the remarkably good preservation of synaptosomes after a period of incubation at 37°C in a physiological medium (Hökfelt, Jonsson and Lidbrink, 1970; Jones and Bradford, 1971a) throws further doubt on them. It is a matter of debate therefore whether, from a morphological standpoint, the cold conditions need be as rigorously preserved as at present.

3.1.3   Negative staining

Alongside the above techniques which are applicable only to embedded and sectioned material another means of viewing fractionated tissue, namely negative staining, was adapted for use with mammalian brain fractions by Horne and Whittaker (1962). They suggested the method should prove useful (a) for the rapid evaluation of subcellular fractions, (b) as a means of visualizing extremely small structures such as synaptic vesicles, (c) for visualizing complex structures, and (d) for providing information on the molecular structure of membranes and organelles. Experience has suggested that its principal value with regard to synaptosomes and synaptic vesicles is confined to (a) and (b), although on a broader front it has contributed significantly to (d). It is an effective, if sometimes inconsistent, means of rapidly demonstrating the structures present in a fraction, especially where the structures are of the dimensions of synaptic vesicles or smaller.

In spite of these useful attributes it does not occupy as prominent a place in fractionation work in the 1970s as might have been anticipated in the early 1960s. After repeated use by Whittaker and co-workers (Whittaker *et al.*, 1964; Whittaker and Sheridan, 1965; Sheridan *et al.*, 1966; Whittaker, 1966a) for demonstrating synaptosomes and synaptic vesicles, it is largely confined by other workers to investigations of axonal segments (Lemkey-Johnston and Larramendi, 1968, 1973; Lemkey-Johnston and Dekirmenjian, 1970), to surveys of vesicle fractions (De Robertis *et al.*, 1962 b, 1963; Israël *et al.*, 1970) or to studies of the morphological constituents of coated vesicles (Kanaseki and Kadota, 1969; Kadota and Kadota, 1973b, c) or receptor proteolipids (Vásquez, Barrantes, La Torré and De Robertis, 1970; De Robertis, 1971).

There are a number of reasons for this decline in the popularity of negative staining in synaptosomal studies. As already mentioned it gives inconsistent results, while perhaps more important, its delineation of ultrastructural detail is poor (Jones, 1971, 1972; Plates 3.7–3.10). These disadvantages are not compensated for by the rapidity of the procedure, as minor ultrastructural features are of considerable importance in view of the fact that an increasing number of studies now undertaken, particularly pharmacological and immunological ones, alter normal morphology.

Negative staining techniques for mammalian subcellular fractions do not differ significantly from those in general use (Brenner and Horne, 1959), and were adapted for this specific purpose by Horne and Whittaker (1962). Fixation prior to staining is generally employed, when a dilute suspension of particles is fixed by the addition of an equal volume of ice-cold 10 % (w/v) formaldehyde in 0·32M sucrose previously neutralized to pH 7·4 with 0·33N–NaOH (see Whittaker *et al.*, 1964). A drop of the fixed suspension is placed on a grid (which may have a collodion or formvar supporting membrane and be coated with carbon) and after a minute or so most of the liquid is withdrawn with a piece of filter paper lightly applied to the side of the grid (Fig. 3.2). A drop of 1 % (w/v) PTA previously neutralized to pH 7·4 with 2N–NaOH is placed on the grid and left for approximately a minute. It is then removed with filter paper in the same way as before (Fig. 3.2). With the exception of ammonium molybdate (see below), negative stains require prior fixation. Lemkey-Johnston and Dekirmenjian (1970) investigated the length of time required for optimal fixation with PTA staining and concluded that, while long (3–24 h) fixation with either formalin or aldehydes gave the best morphological preservation of synaptosomes, it prevented visualization of internal structures. The latter were best demonstrated after 1–1·5 h fixation.

More elaborate techniques for applying the solutions to the grid may be used. For example, the suspension and stain may be mixed beforehand and then sprayed onto the grid (see Horne, 1965). The results of such techniques are probably not superior to those of the simpler one already described, while the techniques themselves are more difficult to carry out.

The main barrier to the successful negative staining of brain fractions is sucrose contamination. When severe this gives rise to a 'bubbling' of the phosphotungstate under the electron beam. When less severe it may manifest itself as a pattern of small regular white circles similar in appearance to small membrane fragments or even vesicles (Plate 3.8). The presence of these circles is highly deceptive and they can all too easily be mistaken for synaptic vesicles. Their regularity and sharply outlined contours, plus the fact that they sometimes appear only after exposure to the electron beam, are useful criteria for recognizing them.

Sucrose contamination, while a factor to be reckoned with in mammalian fractions, becomes a major problem in situations where the tissue has been homogenized in 0·8M or 1M sucrose as opposed to 0·25M or 0·32M sucrose for mammalian fractions. Consequently fractionation studies of octopus brain were circumscribed for a number of years by the lack of a satisfactory negative staining technique. This was finally overcome by using either 0·8M sucrose as the homogenization medium plus ammonium molybdate as the stain, or 1·1M glucose for homogenization and negatively staining with PTA (Jones 1971). (See Plates 3.9 and 3.10).

Another barrier to successful staining is the comparatively large size of synaptosomes. Negative staining works best and is most consistent when applied to small organelles. Synaptic vesicles and mitochondria are therefore more conducive to successful negative staining than the larger synaptosomes. It is this factor which leads to the erratic and somewhat unpredictable results of the negative staining of synaptosomal fractions.

The discussion so far has considered only phosphotungstate negative staining, because most of the negative staining studies of brain fractions have employed this stain. Of the other stains commonly used in negative staining techniques, we will mention only ammonium molybdate. Muscatello and Horne (1968), in a study of the effect of the tonicity of negative staining solutions on the structure of membrane-bounded systems, concluded that membrane organization is well preserved in the presence of ammonium molybdate without prior fixation (see also Munn, 1968; Plates 3.7 and 3.8). By contrast other negative stains, including PTA and lithium tungstate, damage membrane systems by hypotonic disruption in the absence of previous fixation.

In their work Muscatello and Horne (1968) selected an ammonium molybdate concentration which would give a solution of osmolarity equal to that of the homogenizing medium, namely, 2·5% for 0·32M sucrose. Adapting this procedure for the 0·8M sucrose used for homogenization of octopus tissue, a 6% solution gave satisfactory results, delineating the synaptosomal membrane and contained synaptic vesicles very clearly (Jones, 1971). The vesicular limiting membrane is clearly demarcated due to the penetration of the stain, and resembles that of mammalian synaptic vesicles resuspended in sodium phosphate buffer prior to negative staining with PTA (Whittaker and Sheridan, 1965).

In general terms negatively-stained synaptosomes appear as thin-walled bags, in which synaptic vesicles can be distinguished to varying degrees (Plates 3.7 and 3.8). This is probably dependent on the extent to which the stain has been able to penetrate into the bag. When penetration is considerable the vesicles are clearly seen, whereas a lesser degree of penetration accentuates the synaptosomal limiting membrane at the expense of the vesicles (Horne and Whittaker, 1962). Fixation prior to staining is an important factor (Whittaker et al., 1964, Muscatello and Horne, 1968), although as we have just seen this does not apply to ammonium molybdate staining.

The postsynaptic membrane or process is sometimes visible (Horne and Whittaker,

1962; Jones, 1971). Unfortunately little definition of structures within the process is possible, and little detail can be made out of material within the cleft (Plate 3.9). Occasionally a band or plate parallel to the pre- and postsynaptic membranes is present (Jones, 1971). The definition of the synaptic contact region is however, poor compared with that possible in embedded, positively-stained synaptosomes.

The morphological characterization of isolated synaptic vesicles has proved a more congenial task for negative staining techniques. As outlined in Sections 2.4.2 and 2.4.5 it has played an important role in helping localize synaptic vesicles to certain fractions in vertebrate brain (De Robertis *et al.*, 1963; Whittaker *et al.*, 1964; Whittaker and Sheridan, 1965) and *Torpedo* electric organ (Israël, 1970; Soifer and Whittaker, 1972). Beyond this it has contributed to a fuller understanding of their detailed morphology (Whittaker, 1966a).

Whittaker and Sheridan (1965) noted that the limiting membranes of negatively-stained vesicles were not clearly seen in freshly prepared unfixed preparations, apparently due to failure of the stain (phosphotungstate in their case) to penetrate to the interior of the vesicle. On suspension in phosphate buffer the bilayered structure of the membrane reappeared, perhaps a result of phosphotungstate penetration. From these results they inferred that phosphate induces a change in the vesicle wall and/or disperses a solid or liquid core, thereby permitting phosphotungstate to penetrate to the interior of the vesicle.

Synaptic vesicles sometimes display 'tails' and lengths of fibrillar material (Whittaker, 1966a) in negatively-stained preparations. These are similar in some respects to positively-stained appearances associated with vesicles, and will be discussed in the appropriate section (3.2.5).

3.2 ADULT SYNAPTOSOMAL MORPHOLOGY

3.2.1 Species and brain regions studied

Since the first descriptions of synaptosomes in the early 1960s (Gray and Whittaker, 1960, 1962; De Robertis *et al.*, 1961a, b, 1962a) there has been a gradual extension of the range of species from which synaptosomes have been derived. By far the bulk of the work has been confined to rat and guinea-pig central nervous tissue, and no effort has been made to carry out a systematic survey of even a few groups of animals. Additionally, most of the studies have been primarily neurochemical in nature, and where ultrastructural investigations have been undertaken they have served as morphological controls. Very few studies have been chiefly concerned with morphology.

Table 3.1 shows the species from which synaptosomes have been isolated. Guinea-pig and rat studies have been excluded, as they are covered in Table 3.2. Although some of the studies shown in Table 3.1 do not include morphological controls, they are referred to for the sake of completeness.

Table 3.2 summarizes the principal regions used in synaptosomal investigations, and cites some of the main studies undertaken.

Table 3.1 Major species from which synaptosomes have been isolated (excluding rat and guinea-pig; see Table 3.2)

Species	Selected references
Bovine	LaBella and Sanwal, 1965
	Bindler *et al.*, 1967
	De Robertis, 1968
	Fahn *et al.*, 1969
	Andreoli *et al.*, 1970
	Wilson and Cooper, 1972
Cat	Lemkey-Johnston and Larramendi, 1968
	Fiszer and De Robertis, 1969
	Fonnum *et al.*, 1970
Cephalopod: Octopus	Jones, 1967, 1968, 1970a, b, 1971
	Florey and Winesdorfer, 1968
Loligo	Heilbronn *et al.*, 1971
	Welsch and Dettbarn, 1972
	Dowdall and Whittaker, 1973
Coypu	Whittaker and Sheridan, 1965
Dog	Laverty *et al.*, 1963
Fish: Teleost	Whittaker and Greengard, 1971
Torpedo	Sheridan *et al.*, 1966
	Israël and Gautron, 1969
	Israël *et al.*, 1968, 1970
	Heilbronn, 1972
	Soifer and Whittaker, 1972
	Whittaker *et al.*, 1972
	Morris, 1973
Frog	Abood *et al.*, 1967
Monkey	Metzger *et al.*, 1967
Mouse	Weinstein *et al.*, 1963
	Barondes, 1966, 1968
	Feit and Barondes, 1970
	Pilcher and Jones, 1970
Pigeon	McCaman *et al.*, 1965
Rabbit	Hebb and Whittaker, 1958
	McCaman *et al.*, 1965
	Fonnum, 1967
Sheep	Tuček, 1967
	De Belleroche *et al.*, 1975

The latter table does not include developmental studies, a number of which have been carried out during antenatal and postnatal development of the rat brain. Synaptosomes are recognizable from an early age, and their centrifugation characteristics during development as well as corresponding changes in their morphology and biochemistry have been investigated (Abdel-Latif and Abood, 1964; Abdel-Latif, Brody and Ramahi, 1967; Spence and Wolfe, 1967; Del Cerro *et al.*, 1969; Gonatas *et al.*, 1971; Kornguth *et al.*, 1972). These synaptosomes have been shown to be useful models for studying synaptic developmental sequences (Jones and Revell, 1970a, b). Synaptosomes have also been demonstrated in the developing chick embryo cerebellum (Kuriyama *et al.*, 1968c).

Table 3.2 Principal brain regions from which synaptosomes have been isolated

Region	Selected references
RAT	
Cerebral cortex	De Robertis *et al.*, 1962a, 1967b De Robertis, 1967 Whittaker, 1968a Jones, 1969 Barrantes and Lunt, 1970 Cotman and Flansburg, 1970 Gambetti *et al.*, 1972
Cerebellum	Rabié and Legrand, 1973 Hajós *et al.*, 1974 Tapia *et al.*, 1974
Hippocampus	Bondareff and Sjöstrand, 1969 Jones, 1969
Hypothalamus	Clementi *et al.*, 1970 Hökfelt *et al.*, 1970 Lagercrantz and Pertoft, 1972
Nucleus caudatus putamen	Hökfelt *et al.*, 1970
Striatum	Sattin, 1966 Kuhar *et al.*, 1970 Gfeller *et al.*, 1971 Lagercrantz and Pertoft, 1972
Spinal cord and medulla	Johnston and Iversen, 1971 Osborne *et al.*, 1973
GUINEA-PIG	
Forebrain	Gray and Whittaker, 1962 Horne and Whittaker, 1962
Cerebral cortex	Whittaker and Sheridan, 1965
Cerebellar cortex	Israël and Whittaker, 1965
Spinal cord	Ross *et al.*, 1971
OTHERS	
Basal ganglia	De Belleroche *et al.*, 1975
Caudate nucleus	Fahn *et al.*, 1969
Cerebellum	Lemkey-Johnston and Larramendi, 1968 Pilcher and Jones, 1970
Hypothalamus	Andreoli *et al.*, 1970
Lateral vestibular nucleus	Fonnum *et al.*, 1970
Pituitary stalk	Andreoli *et al.*, 1970
Posterior pituitary	LaBella and Sanwal, 1965 Bindler *et al.*, 1967
Subfornical organ	Akert and Pfenninger, 1969
Sympathetic ganglia	Giacobini *et al.*, 1971 Wilson and Cooper, 1972

The subcellular fractionation of peripheral nervous tissue and in particular autonomic nerves, while not strictly relevant to synaptosomal literature, is worthy of mention. De Potter, Smith and De Schaepdryver (1970) in a study of bovine splenic nerve distinguished five types of particle, including lysosomes, mitochondria, NE vesicles and microsomal particles. Using the same tissue, Klein and Thureson–Klein (1971) were able to obtain a homogeneous population of isolated NE storage vesicles, which they characterized by EM. A small yield of synaptosomes containing NE has been obtained from vas deferens by Bisby and Fillenz (1969), but perhaps one of the most successful attempts at separating cholinergic synaptosomes and vesicles from peripheral tissue is that of Wilson and co-workers using bovine superior cervical ganglia (Wilson and Cooper, 1972; Wilson, Schultz and Cooper, 1973; Section 2.3.6).

An encouraging start has been made in utilizing synaptosomes in paraclinical investigations, including thyroid deficiency and malnutrition (Gambetti et al., 1972; Rabié and Legrand, 1973).

3.2.2   Synaptosomal ultrastructure

The rationale behind the formation of synaptosomes from intact nerve endings has been considered in an earlier section (2.1.1). Once formed, synaptosomes consist of a limiting membrane enclosing the contents of the presynaptic terminal, namely synaptic vesicles and one or more mitochondria (e.g. Plates 3.2 and 3.4). Granular material, glycogen, DCV and coated vesicles, vacuoles and occasionally lysosomes and derivatives of endoplasmic reticulum may also be present (Plate 3.5). The junctional region, with its constituent cleft material, and a postsynaptic membrane or process are seen in a percentage of profiles (Section 3.1.1). The subsynaptic web, described by De Robertis et al., (1963) in some of their early work, shows up well in many synaptosomal preparations.

This description is an all-embracing one, resulting from study of the synaptosomes derived from mammalian cerebral cortex, or in more general terms, mammalian forebrain or even whole brain. Within these areas however, there is a striking variation in the appearance of synaptosomal profiles, particularly with regard to their outline and the density of the cytoplasmic background (e.g. Gray and Whittaker, 1962). In some situations, for example the hippocampus, the shape of certain synaptosomes (Jones, 1969) conforms to that of identifiable terminals such as the mossy endings which appear as large presynaptic bags (Hamlyn, 1961, 1962). Such variations however, are not considered sufficient grounds for distinguishing between different synaptosomal populations unless additional relevant criteria are also present (Section 3.5).

The above considerations refer to synaptosomes prepared for EM in one of the usual ways, e.g. aldehyde–OsO_4 fixation and double staining with uranyl and lead salts. Such general appearances are well known. Details of synaptosomes prepared from specific regions of the mammalian CNS are given in the following section (3.2.3).

Because synaptosomes are osmotically-sensitive, their appearance is dependent to a degree upon the tonicity of the fraction in which they sediment. This applies especially to sucrose gradients in which the typical synaptosomal fraction of Whittaker (B) sediments at the 0·32M–0·8M interface. Synaptosomes prepared for EM from this fraction frequently have a shrivelled, irregular appearance with dense cytoplasm and indistinct vesicles, these features being characteristic of a hypertonic environment (Plates 3.11 and 3.12). Better preservation of synaptosomes is claimed for Ficoll gradients, and these synaptosomes generally display a more regular, rounded outline, with an even distribution of vesicles and intact mitochondria (e.g. Autilio *et al.*, 1968; Garey *et al.*, 1972; Section 2.3.2). The latter synaptosomes are far more satisfactory for quantitative morphological investigations than those from sucrose gradients (see Plate 2.4).

When synaptosomes from sucrose gradients are subsequently incubated in a physiological medium, e.g. Krebs–phosphate medium at 37°C (Jones and Bradford, 1971a; Bradford, Bennett and Thomas, 1973), their morphological and biochemical characteristics are remarkably similar to synaptosomes from Ficoll gradients. They are rounded and possess clearly-defined features (Plates 3.13 and 3.14). The enclosed vesicles can be readily subdivided into agranular, coated and dense-cored, while when the junctional zone is in the plane of section, the aggregation of vesicles alongside it, the cleft material and the postsynaptic thickening are all evident (Jones and Bradford, 1971a). One further feature of both incubated/sucrose and Ficoll synaptosomes is the presence of vacuoles within their cytoplasm. Although not visible in all profiles, these vacuoles are a frequently observed feature of these synaptosomes in contrast to synaptosomes fixed immediately after removal from a sucrose gradient.

The contracted appearance of unincubated, sucrose synaptosomes is a result of their shrinkage during preparation, allowing sucrose to enter and interact with the fixative and stain. During incubation, sucrose diffuses out of the synaptosomes, which take up fluid and hence assume a more regular outline (De Belleroche and Bradford, 1973b).

The usual figure given for the diameter of synaptosomes derived from the P_2 fraction of rat or guinea-pig cerebral cortex is approximately 0·5 μm (Clementi *et al.*, 1966b). Examination of published micrographs suggests a figure of about 0.6 μm (e.g. Gray and Whittaker, 1962—guinea-pig brain; Whittaker, 1968a—rat forebrain) and so the range 0·5–0·6 μm serves as a useful guide to synaptosomal diameter for much mammalian brain work. This holds true for incubated/sucrose synaptosomes and those prepared on Ficoll gradients.

The junctional region of synaptosomes, intervening between their pre- and post-synaptic components, can be examined using the same techniques as employed on intact synapses (Section 1.3.1). Accurate estimates of the percentage of synaptosomal profiles with intact junctional regions are hard to come by, although postsynaptic membranes or processes are invariably visualized attached to presynaptic components in the majority of sections examined from synaptosomal preparations. A number of factors are relevant for any estimate: (a) the plane and thickness of the section and the likelihood of sectioning this region, (b) the volume of the presynaptic component of the synaptosome compared with the area of the junctional region, (c) possible variations in the percentage of synaptosomal profiles with intact junctional regions in different parts of the brain, and (d) variations in the size and number of junctional regions associated with different nerve endings.

The junctional region is highlighted in material prepared by the glutaraldehyde–PTA method (Jones, 1969; Jones and Bearley, 1972b). While these results parallel those of intact synaptic junctions (Section 3.3), they still merit consideration in their own right. Prepared in this way, the majority of cortical synaptosomes have the following features: (a) a presynaptic network in which a hexagonal arrangement of the constituent strands can sometimes be identified, (b) trilaminar pre- and postsynaptic membranes, (c) dense projections on the presynaptic side of the junction, (d) cleft densities within the cleft, and (e) postsynaptic focal densities on the postsynaptic side of the junction and corresponding in general position to the adjacent cleft densities (Plates 3.15 and 3.16). These features are depicted in diagrammatic form in Figs. 3.1, 3.3 and 3.4.

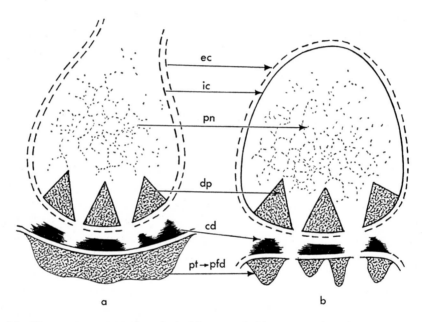

Figure 3.3 Diagram to compare the principal features of: (a) a synapse from intact cerebral cortex, and (b) the corresponding synaptosome. The features highlighted are those which would appear in non-osmicated material fixed in glutaraldehyde and block-stained with PTA. The synaptosome consists of pre-and postsynaptic components with the intervening cleft region. cd, cleft densities; dp, dense projections; ec, external membrane coat; ic, internal membrane coat; pfd, postsynaptic focal densities; pn, presynaptic network; pt, postsynaptic thickening.

In addition, the presynaptic component is enveloped by a membrane which is visible over the greater part of its circumference (Plate 3.15). This is an important distinction between fractionated and intact junctions, and renders synaptosomes easily identifiable in material prepared in this manner. The cleft densities and postsynaptic focal densities lie alongside one another and display a 1:1 correspondence in position along much of the length of the cleft. The dense projections are also adjacent to a cleft density and postsynaptic focal density in some instances, the three densities constituting a synaptic subunit (Jones, 1969).

110

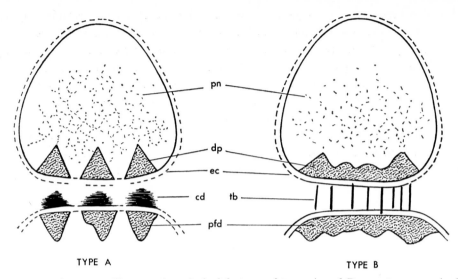

Figure 3.4 Diagram to illustrate the principal features of types A and B synaptosomes. cd, cleft densities; dp, dense projections; ec, external membrane coat; pfd, postsynaptic focal densities; pn, presynaptic network; tb, transverse bars. This diagram is based on the appearance of synaptosomes in glutaraldehyde–PTA material.

On closer examination of the dense projections they have a very irregular outline with their border forming spike-like extensions (Jones and Brearley, 1972b). The network in the vicinity of the dense projections is fairly opaque, and its strands are intimately related to the spikes of the dense projections (Jones, 1969; Jones and Brearley, 1972b; Plate 3.16, also Plate 1.10). While it is dangerous to be dogmatic about the nature of this association because of the overlapping of profiles within the thickness of sections, its constancy suggests a continuity between the dense projections and network strands. If this is the case it is likely that a functional connection exists between the two structures, a connection of potential importance in neurotransmission (Gray, 1966; Akert *et al.*, 1969; Jones, 1970b).

3.2.3 Specific examples of synaptosomes

While much early fractionation work concentrated on large heterogeneous brain areas, such as forebrain or even whole brain, the trend of more recent years has been to use specific, more highly specialized regions. The cerebral cortex with its well-recognized organization has perhaps been the most popular region with investigators, with the cerebellar cortex, spinal cord, hypothalamus and posterior pituitary coming into increasing prominence. Table 3.2 summarizes the many regions from which synaptosomes have been separated. In the present section we will consider those synaptosomes peculiar to spinal cord, cerebellum, hypothalamus and the posterior pituitary.

Ross *et al.* (1971) in their study of guinea-pig spinal cord found synaptosomes principally in their B_2 and B_3 fractions, that is, between the 1·0M and 1·2M layers of sucrose and at the lower limit of the 1·2M layer respectively. Those in the B$_2$ band are large (approximately 0·3 μm^2 in area—see Section 3.4.1) and are filled with agranular synaptic vesicles approximately 48 nm in diameter. Rarely, larger DCV are present. The synaptosomes coming down in the B$_3$ fraction differ in that they have a denser matrix and therefore appear much darker. They are also smaller, although the number of mitochondria and the vesicle size are similar. The authors suggest that the smaller size and more compact appearance of these synaptosomes is due to shrinkage caused by the higher osmotic pressure of this region of the gradient. It is significant that resuspension in 0·32M sucrose prior to fixation eradicates the gross discrepancies in size and appearance.

Osborne *et al.* (1973), in a study of the medulla and anterior two-thirds of rat spinal cord, obtained synaptosomes from the crude nuclear fraction ('heavy synaptosomes') and from the crude mitochondrial fraction. Both preparations consisted of well-preserved synaptosomes, with no obvious size differences between them. Many of the 'heavy' synaptosomes however, contained several large mitochondria (Plates 3.17 and 3.18). These 'heavy' synaptosomes were not dissimilar to those isolated from the crude mitochondrial fraction by Ross *et al.* (1971). Vacuoles and DCV were frequently observed, while the synaptic vesicles in many synaptosomes were packed together to give these synaptosomes a dark appearance (Plates 3.17 and 3.18). This effect may be due, as suggested by Ross *et al.* (1971), to hypertonic conditions (1·2M sucrose), although the fact that dark and light synaptosomes can generally be distinguished within the same fraction minimizes the significance of this possibility (Osborne *et al.*, 1973).

The synaptosomes with a light cytoplasmic matrix have unevenly distributed vesicles which vary more in size than those in dark synaptosomes (Plate 3.19). The synaptosomal fractions contain, in addition to synaptosomes, amorphous membrane fragments and occasional large profiles. The latter, which contain mitochondria and granular material, have a postsynaptic relationship to one or more synaptosomes and may be dendritic in origin (Jones, 1974). They underline the need for careful morphological identification of all profiles within reputedly synaptosomal fractions.

This point is forcibly brought out by Lemkey-Johnston and co-workers in their studies of fractions from cerebellum and whole brain (Lemkey-Johnston and Larramendi, 1968; Lemkey–Johnston and Dekirmenjian, 1970), in which they claim that synaptosome preparations are more heterogeneous than the studies of other workers would suggest. The major thesis of these papers has already been studied (Section 2.6.2), and our only concern here is to touch upon some of the findings of the cerebellum investigation (Lemkey–Johnston and Larramendi, 1968).

Synaptosomes were prominent in two of the fractions resulting from discontinuous density gradient centrifugation of their mitochondrial fraction, P$_2$. These were P$_2$B and P$_2$C, between the 0·8M and 1·0M layers and the 1·0M and 1·2M layers of sucrose respectively. The P$_2$B fraction demonstrated fields filled with tubular and oval profiles between 0·12 and 0·2 μm in diameter (Plate 2.20). They interpreted the tubular structures as non-myelinated axons, because neurotubules were occasionally seen in them and because they expected to find derivatives in this material of components of the granule cell axon from the molecular layer (the parallel fibre). The tubules however, were shrunken and had a dense axoplasm.

Fraction P_2C contained similar tubular structures, with in this instance recognizable synaptic bulbs, either along their length or as discrete synaptosomes. Unfortunately, they had undergone a considerable degree of shrinkage (estimated by the authors as 35%) due to their preparation under hypertonic conditions. Their dense, shrivelled appearance means that little information about their internal composition can be elicited from the published micrographs. Negative staining gave similar results, but did not add to the morphological information.

In a more synaptosome-oriented investigation of guinea-pig cerebellar cortex, Israël and Whittaker (1965) separated synaptosomes from the crude nuclear (P_1) and crude mitochondrial (P_2) fractions. Those from P_1 were large (2–5 μm diameter) and were thought to be derived from the mossy fibre endings of the granular layer (cf. Plate 3.19), while those from P_2 were much smaller (0·5 μm diameter) and may have originated from endings in the molecular layer. Large synaptosomes (3–5 μm diameter) have also been reported by Younoszai (1968) and Del Cerro *et al.* (1969) in cerebellar nuclear fractions, the latter workers also isolating a routine synaptosomal subfraction from their crude mitochondrial fraction.

Further attempts at separating these mossy fibre terminals by Hajós *et al.* (1974) and Tapia, Hajós, Wilkin, Johnson and Balázs (1974) revealed that conventional means of tissue disruption failed to provide 'naked' mossy fibre terminals in sufficient numbers. To overcome this drawback these workers used manual fragmentation with a modified Dounce homogenizer, the sucrose homogenization medium containing 1mM–$MgSO_4$. Due to the lack of any generally accepted biochemical markers for the mossy fibre terminals, the isolation procedure was guided by EM controls.

Rate centrifugation* yielded a nuclear fraction characterized by glomerulus particles (intact portions of the mossy fibre terminals with their contained synaptic vesicles and mitochondria, plus dendritic extensions of the synapsing granule cells), non-glomerular neuropil fragments (originating probably from the molecular layer), myelinated axons and nuclei. Typical synaptosomes sedimented in the mitochondrial fraction. Approximately 60% of the total protein was sedimented in the nuclear fraction, and 10% in the mitochondrial, this high level in the nuclear fraction pointing to the integrity of the glomerulus particles. These particles are about 20 times larger than conventional synaptosomes and usually display numerous synaptic membrane specializations (Hajós *et al.*, 1974).

Isopycnic centrifugation* of the nuclear fraction using a discontinuous sucrose gradient produced a fraction containing glomerulus particles and non-glomerular neuropil fragments, the glomerulus particles constituting half of the total tissue volume (Tapia *et al.*, 1974). Of the area of the glomerulus particles themselves, 60% was accounted for by intact mossy fibre terminals. The mossy fibre terminals contributed 95% of the presynaptic area in this fraction. The remaining fractions were composed of myelin fragments and nuclei.

* For definitions of these terms refer to Section 2.2.1.

On subfractionation of the mitochondrial fraction derived from hypothalamus or pituitary stalk, Andreoli, Ceccarelli, Cerati, Demonte and Clementi (1970) obtained three synaptosomal fractions. Of these, the two lightest fractions contained various membranes, myelin fragments and dense core granules in addition to the synaptosomes. Of the synaptosomes, about 15% of them contain DCV (100 nm across) the remaining ones being filled with agranular synaptic vesicles (45 nm in diameter). The third and densest fraction, particularly in the pituitary stalk, was characterized by an increased percentage of synaptosomes with very large DCV (200 nm diameter).

Parallel biochemical studies by these workers demonstrated that in the subfractions, 5-HT and NE distribute chiefly in the synaptosome-rich fractions, with a preponderance of 5-HT in the lightest synaptosomal fraction and of NE in the heaviest. A large amount of 5-HT was also recovered in the high speed supernatant, possibly a result of release of bound 5-HT during the fractionation procedure. In this regard the distribution of 5-HT differs from that of other brain areas (e.g. Michaelson and Whittaker, 1963; Zieher and De Robertis, 1963; Levi and Maynert, 1964).

While the morphological results allow for the possibility of two or even three synaptosomal populations, and while the slightly different distributions of 5-HT and NE tend to support the reality of this subdivision, no firm conclusions can be drawn. This is principally because of the overlapping of the synaptosomal types within each fraction and because of the overall heterogeneity of the fractions.

Subcellular fractionation of the median eminence of the hypothalamus by Clementi, Ceccarelli, Cerati, Demonte, Felici, Motta and Pecile (1970) demonstrated that dopamine, NE and 5-HT were present in higher concentrations in the synaptosomal subfractions, with NE concentrated in the lightest synaptosomal fraction and 5-HT in the heaviest. This is at variance with the results of Andreoli *et al.* (1970) in whole hypothalamus, although as the synaptosomes from the three synaptosomal fractions of median eminence did not reveal any clear differences the significance of this is difficult to assess. Dopamine was concentrated in the middle synaptosomal band, suggesting that the three neurotransmitters are stored in different populations of nerve endings. This conclusion however, is rendered tentative by the lack of convincing morphological evidence.

Synaptosomes containing neurosecretory granules have been separated from the posterior pituitary and characterized morphologically, hormonally and enzymically by LaBella and co-workers (LaBella and Sanwal, 1965; Bindler, LaBella and Sanwal, 1967). These synaptosomes have been termed *neurosecretosomes* by Bindler *et al.* (1967) and are best visualized by negative staining (Plate 3.20). Neurosecretory granules, appearing with or without electron-dense centres, and smaller rounded or flattened microvesicles ('synaptic vesicles') characterize the neurosecretosomes, which can be separated in highly purified fractions.

Three almost homogeneous populations of neurosecretosomes were obtained on subfractionation, the vasopressin/oxytocin ratio increasing from the lightest to the densest fraction (Bindler *et al.*, 1967). Although the neurosecretosomes in these fractions appear identical, and although complete separation of vasopressin and oxytocin was not achieved, vasopressin and oxytocin may well be stored in different types of nerve ending.

3.2.4 Non-mammalian synaptosomes

Although the literature on non-mammalian synaptosomes is sparse it merits attention because of its interest on morphological and biochemical grounds. As we have seen previously, the majority of studies have used squid brain or *Torpedo* electric organ as the sources
of synaptosomes. The principal reason for this is the high level of ACh within these tissues
and hence their potential usefulness to an understanding of cholinergic mechanisms of
neurotransmission (Section 2.3.7). A source of synaptosomes with high 5-HT, dopamine
and NE levels is the fresh water mussel, *Anodonta cygnea* (Hiripi *et al.*, 1973). These
synaptosomes will also be considered in this section.

Synaptosomes separated from the supraoesophageal ganglia of *Octopus vulgaris*
(Jones, 1967), the optic ganglia of *Octopus dofleini* (Florey and Winesdorfer, 1968) and
the head ganglion of *Loligo pealii* (Dowdall and Whittaker, 1973) have been fixed in a
variety of ways using potassium permanganate, OsO_4 and glutaraldehyde–OsO_4 respectively. The resulting synaptosomes have much in common and are similar in general
appearance with mammalian synaptosomes isolated on Ficoll gradients or on sucrose
gradients with subsequent physiological incubation. They are well-preserved and have
regular, rounded perimeters (Plates 3.4 and 3.5). Agranular synaptic vesicles and mitochondria are their usual distinguishing features, with DCV and vacuoles often present.
Some synaptosomes contain only DCV, or large vesicles with diffuse dense contents.
Occasionally, flattened vesicles may predominate in some synaptosomes following
aldehyde fixation (Jones, 1967). Postsynaptic processes are sometimes recognizable
alongside presynaptic components (Plates 3.4 and 3.5), although postsynaptic membranes
are rarely encountered. In conventionally-prepared preparations postsynaptic components
appear to be less frequent than in the bulk of mammalian preparations.

The mean diameter of the synaptosome profiles in the supraoesophageal lobes was
found by Jones (1967) to be 0·93 μm, and in the optic lobes 0·62 μm, synaptosomal
profiles varying from 0·1–3·2 μm in diameter. The agranular synaptic vesicles exhibit a
wide range of diameters, 15–120 nm, far greater than in most mammalian brain regions
(Jones, 1967). They are in accordance however, with studies on intact *Octopus* nervous
tissue (Barber, 1966; Barber and Graziadei, 1966). Furthermore 70% of the vesicles are
between 25–50 nm in diameter, a figure agreeing quite well with those given by Gray and
Young (1964) for the intact vertical lobe, and Dilly *et al.* (1963) on the intact optic lobe.
More recent studies by Gray (1970b, c) in the vertical and optic ganglia have identified
vesicles in two groups, 30–50 nm and 90–100 nm.

Florey and Winesdorfer (1968) described three types of synaptosomes in terms of their
vesicular content: (a) those packed with vesicles, 55–75 nm in diameter, and of medium
density, (b) those with vesicles, 25–70 nm across, and of low density, and (c) those
containing DCV, 70–100 nm across, in addition to their population of agranular vesicles.
Jones (1967) estimated that 4% of all vesicles in synaptosomal fractions were dense-cored,
having a mean diameter of 72 nm.

Further studies of octopus synaptosomes have concentrated on the structure of the
synaptic contact region between the pre- and postsynaptic components (Jones, 1968,

115

1970a, b). Using the glutaraldehyde–PTA method, notable differences have been detected between the arrangement in octopus and that described for mammalian junctions (Plate 3.21). The octopus presynaptic densities have an irregular appearance, are closely associated with elements of the presynaptic network and are often continuous with each other at their base on the internal coat of the presynaptic membrane. They are termed presynaptic spicules and probably correspond to the dense projections in mammals. An electron-density within the cleft and extending the length of the junction is not subdivided into the relatively discrete cleft densities typical of many mammalian junctions (Jones, 1969). This is the synaptic plate (Jones, 1970a). Many of the spaces of the presynaptic network have densely-staining vesicular profiles within them, rather than the clear profiles found in mammalian terminals (Jones, 1970b). Their number and size suggest they represent a range of synaptic vesicles.

In spite of interest recently shown in fractionating *Torpedo* electric organ, very limited emphasis has been placed on the resulting synaptosomes, particularly their morphology. Micrographs of only a few different synaptosomes are shown in the publications of Israël's group (e.g. Israël and Gautron, 1969), and these are surrounded by a variety of vesicular profiles and membrane-bound bodies. The synaptosomes themselves frequently have an incomplete limiting membrane, are about 1·3 μm across and contain a moderate number of vesicles and perhaps a single mitochondrion.

Synaptosomes filled with DCV are obtained by osmotically shocking the mitochondrial fraction of *Anodonta cygnea* (Hiripi *et al.*, 1973). They are variable in size, rounded and invariably occupied only by DCV. When osmotic shock is excluded, the synaptosomes are shrunken and very dense, the DCV appearing either as naked granules or merging with the dark background.

3.2.5   Synaptic vesicles

While ultrastructural analysis of synaptic vesicles is not confined to vesicular or even synaptosomal fractions, being equally well carried out on intact tissues, the advent of fractionation procedures proved a stimulus to their study. This was a result of the successful application of negative staining techniques for the visualization of vesicles (Section 3.1.3). The latter technique has opened the way for the study of vesicular interrelationships, as well as of coated vesicles and their association with cytoplasmic figures. The negative staining of vesicles has prompted questions concerning basic structural principles, and has driven investigators to look more critically at positively-stained vesicles and their characteristics.

The full range of synaptic vesicle types is present in synaptosomal and vesicular fractions, including typical spherical agranular vesicles, flattened agranular vesicles, DCV, vesicles with diffuse dense contents, ZIO-positive and negative vesicles, and coated vesicles. Of these, flattened vesicles have not been frequently reported even in aldehyde-fixed material, although De Robertis, Pellegrino de Iraldi, Rodriguez de Lores Arnaiz and Zieher (1965) have described them in aldehyde-fixed synaptosomes prepared from rat anterior hypothalamus while De Robertis (1968) has demonstrated them in similarly prepared synaptosomes from cat cerebral cortex. In this latter investigation De Robertis also described flattened and 'tubular' vesicles in a vesicular fraction from cat cerebral cortex, and noted that they are far more abundant here than in the corresponding situation of rat brain. As previously mentioned, synaptosomes containing a preponderance of flattened vesicles have been described in *Octopus* tissue (Jones, 1967), although these synaptosomes are relatively infrequent.

Agranular synaptic vesicles vary in both size and number within the synaptosomes from a given brain or brain region. Whittaker (1968a), in synaptosomes from rat fore-brain, noted that many of the synaptosomes contain a few vesicles with a diameter of approximately 70 nm, and the remainder a diameter of approximately 45 nm. The number of vesicles counted however, was small, and some of the profiles regarded as large vesicles may have been vacuoles. More significant was the observation that of the small vesicles, 87% of the variance was within individual synaptosome profiles, 9% between synaptosomes in the same field and 4% between different fields of the same block. These figures underline the necessity of careful scrutiny of as wide a range of samples as possible before coming to firm conclusions regarding the significance of apparent differences in vesicle sizes.

In a detailed quantitative study of vesicle diameters in synaptosomes from the supra-oesophageal lobes of *Octopus* brain, Jones (1967) noted a range of 15–120 nm, with 70% of the profiles between 25–50 nm (Section 3.2.4). This was in close agreement with the figures given (in less detailed studies) for intact tissues of *Octopus* brain (Gray and Young, 1964). The size distribution in each of the individual primary fractions was similar. It should be noted that vesicle diameters are more variable in octopus brain than in most regions of the mammalian CNS.

A parallel study by Jones (1970c) on the size distribution of vesicles in vesicular fractions from octopus brain produced a range of 10–140 nm with 70% between 30–80 nm in diameter. In this case 20% of the vesicle profiles were between 40–50 nm, and 15% between 60–70 nm in diameter. No significant differences were detected between the size distribution of vesicles in the three fractions containing them. This was taken to imply that because vesicles of the same appearance and size have different sedimentation properties, they may represent different populations.

A difficulty encountered in analysing synaptic vesicle sizes is the presence of large vesicular profiles in certain synaptosomes. These have been interpreted as vacuoles (Jones and Bradford, 1971a). They are a feature of some synaptosomes but are not usually found in intact terminals. They are of the order of 110–160 nm in diameter, are commonly present in synaptosomes which have been incubated during preparation (Jones and Bradford, 1971a) and are also found in synaptosomes prepared on Ficoll gradients (Autilio *et al.*, 1968; Garey *et al.*, 1972) as well as in synaptosomes from some CNS regions (e.g. spinal cord; Osborne *et al.*, 1973). Little is known at present about the origin or nature of these vacuoles, although a possible relationship between them and the cisternae of neuromuscular junctions is commented on in Section 5.4.3.

Detailed investigations of the ultrastructure of isolated synaptic vesicles have confirmed their remarkable resemblance to those seen *in situ* (Whittaker and Sheridan,

1965; Plates 2.7 and 2.8). The positively-stained vesicles appear as hollow structures bounded by a unit membrane, which has the typical trilaminar arrangement and dimensions originally described for permanganate-fixed unit membranes (Robertson, 1959). Whittaker and Sheridan did note however, that the profiles of isolated vesicles varied more than those *in situ* and they sought to account for this diversity in terms of the effect of the plane of section and the overlapping of profiles in closely packed clumps.

Negatively-stained, isolated vesicles differ in a number of characteristics from positively-stained, sectioned ones, although they closely resemble the vesicles seen in negatively-stained synaptosomes. In negative staining, occasional vesicles have a clear limiting membrane although it is poorly defined in the majority of profiles. In these latter instances there is a central area of electron-density in the vesicle, apparently caused by the pooling of the stain on top of a collapsed spherical structure (Whittaker and Sheridan, 1965). Varying degrees of stain penetration into vesicles, accompanied sometimes by 'lipping' of the vesicles, serve to produce a wide range of vesicle appearances in negative staining (Section 3.1.3).

High power EM investigations of isolated vesicles, both positively- and negatively-stained, have been used to comment upon concepts of membrane organization (Whittaker and Sheridan, 1965; Whittaker, 1966a; Jones, 1973b). The validity of the proposed schemes depends upon the extent to which they conform to concepts issuing from physical and biochemical approaches to membrane structure (e.g. Robertson, 1966; Stoeckenius and Engelman, 1969; Hendler, 1971).

Vesicular fractions provide a good opportunity for study of connections between vesicles (Plates 3.22 and 3.23). While filaments or tubules associated with vesicles may well be identifiable in intact nerve terminals, the increased distance between vesicles plus the relatively small number of vesicles in a given volume of suspension render the vesicular preparation a particularly good one for this type of investigation.

Whittaker (1966a), using a mammalian vesicle fraction, demonstrated the existence of a number of profiles in negatively-stained preparations. These fell into three categories, (a) connections between vesicles, (b) vesicles with 'tails', and (c) lengths of fibrillar material (Plate 3.23). In the light of these observations Whittaker (1966a) postulated that the fibrillar material connected to synaptic vesicles represents collapsed sections of a system which opens during stimulation to release the transmitter. The ultrastructural evidence on which this idea is based is meagre, the validity of the connections between vesicles and filaments requiring substantiation using a range of techniques. Further observations of connections between vesicles have been made by Jones (1970c) on positively-stained, isolated vesicles from *Octopus* brain, the linking strands appearing to have a tubular structure in many instances. While similar, even though less distinct, interconnections have been reported in octopus synaptosomes (Jones, 1967, 1968), their functional significance remains difficult to define. They may represent a response to excessive metabolic demands, being involved in the production and turnover of vesicles within the terminal. Alternatively, or perhaps additionally, they may take some part in the movement of vesicles and hence transmitter towards the synaptic cleft. In regard to the former possibility, the observations of Smith on the relationship between vesicles and microtubules in lamprey CNS are interesting and perhaps relevant (Järlfors and Smith, 1969; Smith, 1971).

Much of the ultrastructural work on coated vesicles by Kanaseki and the Kadotas (Kanaseki and Kadota, 1969; Kadota and Kadota, 1973b, c) has employed fractions of the vesicles, positively- and negatively-stained (Section 2.4.4; Plate 2.10). Kanaseki and Kadota (1969) described four vesicle types. The first is a vesicle with a diameter of 50–100 nm and with 1–8 subparticles attached to its surface. These subparticles are demonstrated best by uranyl acetate negative staining and appear as hollow cylinders 10 nm across (see also Kanaseki, 1973). The second type of vesicle has a 50 nm diameter and is contained in a 'basket' 100 nm across and composed of a network of regular pentagons and hexagons (with sides 24 nm in length). The third vesicle type may be a modification or derivative of the second type, being only partially enclosed by a basket arrangement, while the fourth type consists of a basketwork but no central vesicle. The significance of these various appearances has already been discussed in Section 1.3.3, while they are illustrated in Plates 1.16 and 1.17.

The flocculent material isolated along with plain synaptic vesicles and coated vesicles by Kadota and Kadota (1973c) has been classified by them into (a) fine particles, (b) short tubelike structures and (c) meshwork-like structures (Plate 2.11). The fine particles are interpreted by the Kadotas as consisting of 4 globules, 3·5 nm in diameter, arranged in an open square. The short tube-like structures have a linear array in the majority of instances, with a few spiral or helical arrangements.

3.3 COMPARING SYNAPTOSOMES AND *IN SITU* SYNAPSES

The discussion in Chapter 2 and thus far in the present chapter has been based on the underlying assumption that the features displayed by synaptosomes are representative of those of *in situ* synapses. The biochemical basis for this assumption will be considered in the next chapter (4.2). In this section we will concentrate on the morphological evidence for this assumption, the evidence falling into two principal categories. The first examines the ultrastructural correspondence between the junctional region of synaptosomes and intact synaptic junctions, while the second consists of a study of the survival of synaptosomes in tissue culture.

Detailed morphological studies of synaptosomes are of limited value if it is not known whether they accurately reflect the morphology of intact synaptic junctions. It is important to know therefore if fractionation procedures distort the ultrastructure of the synaptic region to an appreciable degree. If they do, synaptosomes cannot be used as indicators of the morphological integrity of synaptic junctions (Jones, 1972). This would be true in spite of the remarkable way in which the pre- and postsynaptic terminals of synapses are held together during tissue fragmentation. The existence of synaptosomes as discrete entities does not ensure the accurate morphological reproducibility of the cleft and paramembranous regions.

In order to investigate this problem Jones and Brearley (1972a, b) examined synaptic junctions from rat cerebral cortex and then compared them with cortical synaptosomes, placing particular emphasis on the paramembranous densities and presynaptic network. By employing a non-osmicated fixation technique and block PTA staining these structures were clearly delineated, allowing a quantitative comparison to be carried out (Section 1.3.1).

The essential features of the junctional regions in the fractionated and intact material correspond, in that each displays a presynaptic network, trilaminar pre- and postsynaptic membranes, presynaptic dense projections, cleft densities and some form of postsynaptic thickening (compare Plates 3.24 and 3.25; Fig. 3.3). There are however, a number of differences which in qualitative terms can be reduced to the general principle that continuities in intact synaptic junctions are broken up and appear as discontinuities in synaptosomes. The cleft densities and postsynaptic thickening show a greater degree of focalization in synaptosomes, so much so that the continuous postsynaptic thickening of intact junctions is represented by more-or-less discrete focal densities in synaptosomes. While the dense projections are similar in both situations they are more difficult to distinguish clearly in synaptosomes on account of the close packing of the presynaptic network around their apices. Finally, at low magnification synaptosomes are more readily identified than intact junctions because the limiting membrane of their presynaptic terminal is visible, in contrast to its counterpart in intact junctions (Plates 3.24 and 3.25).

On comparing the preparations quantitatively, the overall similarity already noted is reinforced. Jones and Brearley (1972a, b) measured nine indices on intact and fractionated synaptic junctions and subsequently compared them. The indices used were: (a) height of dense projections; (b) width of dense projections at their base along the presynaptic membrane; (c) distance between the central points of adjacent dense projections; (d) gap between the nearest points of adjacent dense projections at their bases; (e) distance between the internal electron-opaque coats of the pre- and postsynaptic membranes; (f) width of the intracleft electronopacity; (g) width of the intermediate, electron-translucent coat of the postsynaptic membrane; (h) height of the postsynaptic thickening; and (i) length of the postsynaptic thickening (Fig. 1.5).

In terms of these indices, (a), (c), (d) and (h) are significantly smaller in synaptosomes than intact junctions, suggesting there is some shrinkage of the dense projections and postsynaptic thickening during fractionation procedures. By contrast (h), the width of the dense projections at their bases, is significantly larger in synaptosomes. A possible explanation to account for these differences is that the presynaptic terminal is compressed during fractionation, decreasing the height and separation of the dense projections but increasing their width. This explanation is rendered more likely by the crowding of the network strands around the apices of the dense projections in synaptosome profiles (Fig. 3.3). Differences may also be expected in vesicular diameter and number, although these have not as yet been investigated.

The remaining indices are strikingly similar before and after fractionation. The cleft region is unaffected by the procedures, as is the length of the postsynaptic thickening. This is important as most EM controls of fractionation studies use conventional preparative techniques which highlight the overall shape of the presynaptic terminal and the length of the postsynaptic membrane. There is no reason to suppose that synaptosomes are not accurate representations of *in situ* synapses, as long as the minimal shrinkage factor is taken into account. The studies of Jones and Brearley (1972a, b) in which the emphasis was placed on the junctional region are searching comparative investigations in view of the critical part played by the junctional region in synaptosomal formation. These results point therefore to the usefulness of the synaptosome for reproducing the essential features of the intact synaptic junction. Consequently the synaptosome may be considered a morphological tool (Jones, 1972), a valid model of the synaptic junction for morphological investigations.

Further evidence pointing to the same conclusion was provided by Adinolfi (1972a, b). Working on *in situ* synapses he demonstrated that the sequence of changes in the structural maturation of synaptic junctions does not differ significantly from the results of Jones and Revell (1970a, b) using isolated synaptosomes.

An alternative method of testing whether synaptosomes accurately reflect the events and morphology of intact synapses is to delineate the period in which they can survive as a useful, metabolically active preparation. Synaptosomes can be followed over periods of even a few days in tissue culture (Bradford, Jones and Booher, 1975). During 8 h in culture the basal level of synaptosomal respiration shows a marked reduction compared with the respiratory rates of samples previously incubated in tissue culture fluid for varying periods of time. Nevertheless stimulated respiratory levels remain high (Table 3.3). This is also true after 24 h, when basal respiration had fallen to low levels. A res-

Table 3.3 Basal and electrically stimulated respiration of synaptosome suspensions (from Bradford et al., 1975)

O_2 uptake (μ mol O_2/100mg protein/h)

Incubation period (h)	Krebs-Phosphate medium	Tissue culture medium	
	Basal respiration	Basal respiration	Stimulated respiration
0	62 ± 4	55 ± 7	78 ± 8
2	62 ± 4	53 ± 6	75 ± 9
3	58 ± 5	—	—
3·5	50 ± 3	—	—
4	40 ± 5	41 ± 6	58 ± 8
6	20 ± 6	35 ± 7	58 ± 14
8	—	23 ± 7	52 ± 16
10	13 ± 8	—	—
24	—	12 ± 8	46 ± 16
2 days	—	13 ± 9	16 ± 9
5 days	—	6 ± 8	10 ± 6

Synaptosomes were incubated at 37°C in Krebs-phosphate medium in Warburg flasks or in tissue culture fluid in glass bottles without stirring for the period indicated. After incubation, suspensions in tissue culture fluid were centrifuged at 5000 g/20 min to deposit synaptosomes which were then resuspended in Krebs-phosphate medium and incubated again at 37°C in Warburg respirometer flasks containing gold ring electrodes. Pulses were passed for 20 min after a preincubation period of 30 min. Values are mean $\pm$ S.D. for five preparations in each case.

piratory response could still be evoked by electrical pulses after 2 days, although even this was minimal after 5 days.

Morphologically, synaptosomes maintained in culture for 24h show remarkably good preservation of structure, having a continuous terminal membrane and containing

121

recognizable synaptic vesicles, vacuoles and mitochondria (compare Plates 3.26 and 3.27). Pre- and postsynaptic membranes are visible in some instances and intact junctional regions in others (Bradford *et al.*, 1974). They compare well with routinely incubated synaptosomes (Jones and Bradford, 1971a) and with *in situ* nerve-endings (e.g. Adinolfi, 1972a; Jones and Brearley, 1972a). After 2 days in culture synaptosomes can still be identified although obvious deterioration is evident, the limiting membrane being deficient in places and the vesicles appearing as an indistinct granular network. More severe damage is present after 5 days (Bradford *et al.* 1975; Plate 3.28).

When these results are compared with those of degeneration studies of rat cerebral cortex (Colonnier, 1964), the only indication of degeneration after 24 h in culture is a decrease in the number of synaptic vesicles. After 2 days in culture the granular appearance of the vesicles resembles that of vesicles in degenerating synaptic knobs of the cerebral cortex 1–3 days after undercutting (Colonnier, 1964). This comparison underlines (a) the survival of synaptosomes in tissue culture for periods of up to 24h, a conclusion supported by metabolic and stimulation studies, and (b) the similarity of the ultrastructural processes inherent in the degeneration of synaptosomes and of *in situ* synapses. Each conclusion lends support to the contention that synaptosomes are reliable indicators of intact synaptic morphology.

Another means of assessing the survival of synaptosomes in tissue culture is to compare their morphology with that of synaptosomes derived from brain tissue stored at room temperature for periods of up to 20h prior to fractionation (Swanson, Harvey and Stahl, 1973). After 20h at room temperature the proportion of identifiable synaptosomes had dropped from 45–60% (control) to 12–25%, while the percentage of dense unidentified bodies had increased from approximately 10% to 31–40% The synaptosomes themselves display obvious autolytic changes, with membrane breakage, swelling and a loss of distinct vesicles. The principal changes after 3h at room temperature were an increase in the granularity and density of synaptosomes, and a decrease in the percentage of synaptosomal profiles.

While the distinction between the control and 3h conditions may be less clear-cut than the authors suggest, it is evident that autolysis is proceeding far more rapidly in this instance than in the culture synaptosomes. Furthermore, after 20h at room temperature there is a moderate shift in SDH activity from the mitochondrial to the synaptosomal fraction. Synaptosomes maintained in tissue culture for 24h therefore show little in the way of autolytic changes, these changes becoming prominent only after 2 days in culture.

3.4 DISTINGUISHING SYNAPTOSOMAL POPULATIONS

In spite of the potential value of knowing whether different populations of synaptosomes can be distinguished on morphological grounds, the present state of our knowledge is fragmentary and all too uncertain. This in part stems from difficulties encountered in equating the different types of synaptic junctions described in intact tissue (Gray's types 1 and 2, Colonnier's asymmetric and symmetric, Uchizono's round and flat vesicle-containing endings) with the range of appearances found in synaptosomal fractions.

Allied to this is the fact that the commonly-used gradients for separating brain fragments do not distinguish between synaptosomal populations; hence the importance of morphological differences for their potential characterization. More recent attempts at labelling brain slices and subsequently separating synaptosomes on a continuous density gradient have yielded more hopeful results, but even so the morphological side of these studies is not entirely satisfactory.

Routine morphological examinations of synaptosomes have shown that synaptosomal profiles vary on a number of counts. This variation includes differences in size, synaptic vesicle content, shape and packing, mitochondrial population, characteristics of the cleft (or contact) region, length of the postsynaptic membrane, and nature of the postsynaptic thickening and process.

Mere tabulation of observed differences is not sufficient to demonstrate distinct populations, especially as many of the differences noted apply to synaptosomes from more than one brain region or even species. Nevertheless it has some merit in drawing attention to the *kind* of differences capable of morphological description and elucidation, and hence the sort of differences to be looked for in future investigations designed to characterize synaptosomal populations.

3.4.1. Synaptosomal size

As discussed previously (Section 3.2.2) synaptosomes are generally considered to have a diameter of the order of 0·5–0·6 μm. While there is considerable variation in their size in certain brain regions, and while it is often difficult to identify with certainty what are commonly regarded as grazing sections through synaptosomes, this figure is a useful one for most purposes. It must not however, obscure the possibility that different populations of synaptosomes may be distinguishable in terms of size. In some situations, e.g. spinal cord, this is obvious. In other areas, e.g. cerebral cortex, this is not as obvious, and it is in these latter areas that critical investigations are taking place.

In an attempt to separate synaptosomes into different morphological types on a continuous sucrose gradient, Whittaker (1968a) analysed synaptosomal profiles from different fractions of rat forebrain using a number of criteria, including synaptosomal size. Each fraction examined contained two populations, the main one with synaptosomal profiles of less than about 0·3 μm^2 in area and a smaller one with areas of up to 0·7 μm^2. Those profiles with an area less than 0·3 μm^2 had a mean area of around 0·16 μm^2. In the absence of recognizable qualitative differences between synaptosomes in adjacent fractions, Whittaker was forced to investigate the existence of quantitative differences. A preliminary analysis indicated that the mean areas of synaptosomal profiles from the middle of the gradient were 12% greater than those from the top or bottom. In addition, within any one fraction there were small differences in profile areas from one block to another, and between different regions of the same block. Although these data are not sufficiently precise to separate different populations of synaptosomes with confidence, the approach is an important one highlighting its possibilities as well as suggesting pitfalls for interpretation, e.g. stratification within pellets.

Iversen and Bloom (1972) in an autoradiographic study of homogenates of hippo-campus and hypothalamus were unable to detect any size differences between GABA labelled synaptosomes and unlabelled profiles. By contrast in cerebral cortex the labelled synaptosomes were larger than the unlabelled ones (0·61 μm compared with 0·35 μm).

A number of reports have been published on other regions of the mammalian CNS and these include much larger synaptosomes than those mentioned above. In the cerebellar cortex synaptosomes ranging in diameter from 2–5 μm and derived from large mossy fibre endings have been reported in the P_1 fraction (Israël and Whittaker, 1965; Whittaker, 1966b), although the published micrographs show synaptosomes with a diameter of only 1·2–1·4 μm. Synaptosomes reportedly up to 5 μm in diameter have also been reported by Younoszai (1968) and Hajós et al. (1974) in cerebellar cortex. Of greater significance than the mere size of these particles is the fact that they are predominantly located in a nuclear fraction whereas conventional synaptosomes sediment in the mitochondrial fraction. Synaptosomes derived therefore from one set of endings (mossy fibre terminals of the cerebellar granular layer) can be separated from those representing another set of endings (from the cerebellar molecular layer).

Spinal cord studies similarly reveal the presence of large synaptosomes admixed with ones of more usual dimensions. For instance, Ross et al. (1971) have described synapto-somes in three subfractions of the mitochondrial fraction from guinea-pig spinal cord. Those in B_1 (junction of 0·8M and 1·0M sucrose) have a diameter around 0·2 μm, and are accompanied by numerous other membranous elements. Those in B_2 (1·0–1·2M) constitute 20% of the profiles in this fraction, vary from 0·1–2·0 μm in their longest dimension and have a mean profile area of 0·3 μm^2 (compared with 0·18 μm^2 for forebrain synaptosomes in Whittaker's 1968a paper). Many of these synaptosomes have a diameter of the order of 1·5 μm, larger than that of the synaptosomes in B_3 (lower limit of 1·2M) which have a mean profile area of 0·18 μm^2.

This study raises a number of interesting points which are inevitably encountered when attempting to distinguish between synaptosomal populations. The first is that neither size differences alone, nor even size differences accompanied by ultrastructural differences, are sufficient to distinguish between populations. The synaptosomes of fractions B_2 and B_3 differ on both counts, and yet these differences may well reflect the osmotic conditions under which they sediment and are resuspended (see Section 3.2.3). The fractions themselves are too heterogeneous to allow meaningful biochemical charac-teristics to emerge. Secondly, for ultrastructural differences to be significant they must involve differences in at least one of the following: the number, size, shape or type of vesicles, the number, size or type of mitochondria, or the type of junctional region. In the study of Ross et al. (1971) the only difference, apart from size, between the synaptosomes of B_2 and B_3 lay in the density of the cytoplasm—a feature all too susceptible to osmotic conditions. Lastly, similar-sized synaptosomes may belong to different synaptosomal populations. This may be true even in the absence of observable ultrastructural differences.

3.4.2   Vesicular ultrastructure

In spite of the potential value afforded by differences in synaptic vesicle morphology as a basis for distinguishing between synaptosomes, only limited progress has been made in this direction.

Perhaps the most readily-recognizable difference between synaptosomes occurs between those containing DCV and those containing agranular vesicles. So obvious is this distinction however, that its value for distinguishing between synaptosomal populations is limited, reflecting as it does readily observed differences in *in situ* nerve endings. Synaptosomes containing DCV have been separated in large numbers and sometimes in enriched fractions from a variety of sources including hypothalamus (Hökfelt *et al.*, 1970; Andreoli *et al.*, 1970), hypophysis (LaBella and Sanwal, 1965; Bindler *et al.*, 1967; Plate 3.20), nucleus caudatus putamen (Hökfelt *et al.*, 1970), pituitary stalk (Andreoli *et al.*, 1970), median eminence (Clementi *et al.*, 1970), basal ganglia (De Belleroche, Bradford and Jones, 1975) and from an invertebrate such as *Anodonta* (Hiripi *et al.*, 1973).

Synaptosomes containing round vesicles can be distinguished from those containing flattened ones (De Robertis *et al.*, 1965; Jones, 1967; De Robertis, 1968) although they have not as yet been obtained in isolation from each other. Even hippocampal synaptosomes labelled with either GABA or glycine could not be distinguished in terms of their vesicle characteristics (Iversen and Bloom, 1972). This is disappointing in view of the association of labelled glycine with flattened vesicles reported in spinal cord slices (Matus and Dennison, 1971).

Distinguishing between synaptosomes on the basis of variation in the size or number of the contained vesicles has proved even more elusive. Major differences in the size of vesicles within synaptosomes can be detected even in mammalian central nervous tissue. However, as demonstrated by Whittaker (1968a; Section 3.2.5) far greater variation occurs within individual synaptosomal profiles than between synaptosomes.

3.4.3   Mitochondrial content

The number of intraterminal mitochondria has been noted to vary between synaptosomes located in different fractions of sucrose density gradients (Gfeller *et al.*, 1971). As these fractions also vary in their content of neurotransmitter – specific synaptosomes, the ultrastructural variations assume an important role in identifying particular synaptosomes, and hence synapses, with particular neurotransmitters. Following on from this, Iversen and Bloom (1972) noted that in homogenates of various brain regions the only consistent difference between unlabelled synaptosomes and those labelled with ^3H – GABA was the higher density of mitochondria within the cytoplasm of the latter. A considerably higher proportion of the labelled terminals had one or more mitochondria than did the unlabelled terminals.

Cotman *et al.* (1970), in a study of the sedimentation of brain subcellular particles using an analytical differential centrifugation procedure, claimed to distinguish between a fraction in which all the synaptosomes contained at least one mitochondrion and another in which there was a greater preponderance of synaptosomes without any mitochondria. The fractions in question sedimented at 24–67 $\times$ 10^7 w^2t and 85–102 $\times$ 10^7 w^2t respectively, and also differed in synaptosomal size—0·75–1 μm in diameter compared with 0·5 μm respectively. The micrographs illustrating the respective fractions are far from convincing however, in that few synaptosomes are shown and those that are, are difficult to interpret. Further, the fractions also contain numerous isolated mitochondria and other contaminants such as postsynaptic membranes.

Weinstein, Roberts and Kakefuda (1963) suggested that synaptosomes rich in mitochondrial inclusions are concentrated in slightly higher densities of sucrose than those containing few or no inclusions. It is difficult to substantiate this idea in terms of their published micrographs, and no quantitative findings were reported. Whittaker (1968a) however, attempted to investigate this conclusion by evaluating the mean areas of the profiles of mitochondria contained within synaptosomes, and also the proportion of the total synaptosome profile areas occupied by mitochondrial profiles. His statistical analysis failed to demonstrate that a higher proportion of the total synaptosome volume is occupied by mitochondria in the denser fractions. By counting the percentage of profiles containing mitochondria he obtained results which implied the presence in the lighter fractions of a population of synaptosomes lacking mitochondria. His results suggest therefore that the size of the mitochondria and/or synaptosomes may vary between fractions. Further quantitative studies of this possible relationship are required before it can be used as a criterion to distinguish synaptosomes of varying morphological type.

3.4.4 Junctional (cleft) region

As discussed in Section 3.1.1 the term *synaptosome* is sometimes used to denote the presynaptic component alone, as opposed to a more satisfactory morphological definition which also takes account of the cleft region and postsynaptic component. This distinction becomes important when attempting to distinguish between synaptosomal fractions in terms of size differences.

For instance, Gfeller *et al.* (1971) in their attempt to distinguish between populations of synaptosomes, found that synaptosomes with intact clefts occurred more frequently in the denser fractions. Of the synaptosomes sedimenting in the denser fractions 40% had clefts compared with only 10% in the lighter fractions. These percentages may be compared with figures obtained by Jones (1974) in synaptosomal fractions of rat cerebral cortex, where approximately 30% of synaptosomal profiles had definite cleft and postsynaptic components and 60% possible cleft and postsynaptic components.

Unable to find any difference between the circumference of the presynaptic components of synaptosomes in their fractions, Gfeller *et al.* (1971) took account of this differential incidence of cleft and postsynaptic components in order to postulate an overall size difference. This is a valid and useful procedure when dealing with separate fractions. Unfortunately, it provides no means of recognizing different synaptosomes, and hence different synaptosomal populations, within a single fraction. Neither does it throw light on possible morphological differences between synapses functioning with different neurotransmitters.

Answers to this latter point are more likely to come from an examination of the ultrastructure of the junctional region itself, either in synaptosomes which will be considered here, or intact synapses. Detailed features of the junctional region were considered earlier in this chapter (Section 3.2.2); our present concern is with the possibility of identifying more than one type of synaptosome on the basis of the morphology of this region. Conventional preparative techniques for EM investigations have thrown little light on this problem as the junctional region is not sufficiently well characterized using these methods. By contrast, use of the glutaraldehyde–PTA technique has suggested possible differences which may constitute the basis needed for formulating population characteristics.

In a study of synaptosomes derived from adult rat cerebral cortex, Jones (1969) described two typical appearances of synaptosome profiles, and these he termed types A and B. These are represented in Fig. 3.4, as well as in Plates 3.15 and 3.16. Type A is distinguished by discontinuous pre- and postsynaptic paramembranous densities along the length of the cleft, and constitutes what may be described as a *discontinuous–discontinuous* junction (Plate 3.15). Dense projections, cleft densities and postsynaptic focal densities are all prominent. Type B profile by contrast is characterized by paramembranous densities which have a continuous appearance along their length of apposition and which give rise to the so-called *continuous–continuous* junction (Plate 3.16). In this, pre- and postsynaptic regions are continuous, the external coats of both having transversely-orientated bars between them rather than cleft densities.

The separation of two synaptosomal types on qualitative grounds alone is open to criticism, as it may simply reflect a sectioning artefact. Jones (1969) found that of 100 synaptosomes counted 45 fell readily into the type A and 32 into the type B bracket. This left 23 which were either intermediate in appearance or possessed junctional regions which were too indistinct to be classified. Type B therefore could represent obliquely-sectioned type A profiles, type B representing the 'continuous' extreme of a continuum and type A the 'discontinuous' opposite extreme. In spite of this possibility the concept of two distinct types is not unexpected in view of the findings of Gray (1959a, 1969a), Colonnier (1968), Akert (1971) and others, and their subdivision of synapses into two or more populations (Section 1.2.1).

A more direct attack on the question of two synaptosomal populations had to await quantitative studies on glutaraldehyde–PTA prepared material (Jones and Brearley, 1972b). As outlined in a previous section (3.3) nine junctional indices were measured. On plotting their size distribution in histogram form six of the histograms display two peaks, suggesting the existence of two synaptosomal populations. The most conspicuous peaks are displayed by the indices for dense projection height, width and separation, the height and length of the postsynaptic thickening and the width of the cleft.

It is tempting to conclude from these indices that two synaptosomal types can be distinguished. Unfortunately at present, this distinction can be applied only to synaptosomes *en masse* and not to individual synaptosomes. Hence it is difficult to correlate these quantitative findings with the qualitative concepts of discontinuity and continuity. In spite of this drawback these findings support the postulate that different types of synaptosomes can be distinguished using morphological criteria. What is required is an extension of these quantitative findings to ones which can be used on individual synaptosomes.

Study of the postnatal development of synaptosomes also points to the existence of two types of synaptosome (Jones and Revell, 1970a). The stages through which synaptosomes and their junctional regions pass is dealt with in some detail in the following section (3.5) Suffice it to say at this juncture that the junctional region, while relatively symmetrical and undifferentiated for the first 4 postnatal days, begins to take on characteristics of either type A or B synaptosomes from day 5 onwards.

3.5 DEVELOPMENTAL STUDIES

These have proved of value in monitoring pre- and postnatal changes in the activities of ACh, AChE, ATPase, phospholipids, phosphoproteins (Abdel-Latif and Abood, 1964, 1965; Abdel-Latif et al., 1967; Abdel-Latif, Yamaguchi, Yamaguchi and Chang, 1968; Abdel-Latif, Smith and Ellington, 1970), lecithin (Abdel-Latif and Smith, 1970), ChAc, SDH, LDH (Gonatas et al., 1971), aspartate amino-transferase (Piras, Szijan and Gómez, 1970), components of the GABA system (Kuriyama et al., 1968c), gangliosides (Spence and Wolfe, 1967) as well as proteins, lipids and nucleic acids (Cuzner and Davison, 1968; Banik and Davison, 1969). Because developmental studies have principally been conducted with biochemical correlates most of the early studies regarded the morphological aspects of development as secondary. Nevertheless it was soon realized that the distribution of organelles in density gradients is markedly different in developing and adult animals, rendering accurate morphological identification of fractions throughout development an essential prerequisite for biochemical studies.

3.5.1. Distribution of fractions during development

While the exact details of organelle localization depend upon the fractionation techniques employed, there is one overriding principle governing the localization of synaptosomes during early development. This is that around the time of birth synaptosomes occupy the highest fraction in a typical density gradient as opposed to their more usual denser fraction position in the adult (e.g. Abdel-Latif and Abood, 1964; Spence and Wolfe, 1967). As the majority of developmental studies have been carried out on rat brain, in which synaptic maturation takes place principally after birth (Jones et al., 1974), most developmental studies have concentrated on postnatal changes.

Fig. 3.5 summarizes the relative movements of organelles within density gradients throughout the postnatal period. Gonatas et al. (1971), working with rat cerebral cortex, placed the crude mitochondrial fraction on a discontinuous Ficoll gradient consisting of 5%, 7·5%, 13% and 20% solutions of Ficoll. Five fractions resulted, although in terms of their organelle content the work can be summarized by reference to only three fractions.

The lightest fraction in *day 1* material consisted principally of intact processes lacking synaptic vesicles (Plate 3.33). These measured 0·5–3 μm in diameter, were densely packed throughout the thickness of the pellet and contained amorphous granular material, possibly vacuoles, ribosomes and/or fibrils (cf. Plate 3.29). They accounted for 94% of the processes in this material and probably represent immature dendrites or axons. The remaining 6% were processes containing synaptic vesicles, and were interpreted as 'presynaptic terminals' (synaptosomes). Free mitochondria, membranous debris and a few additional synaptosomes occupied the denser fractions.

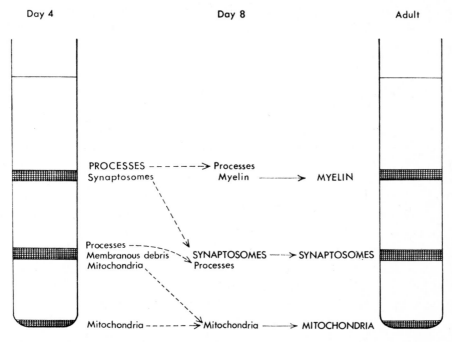

Figure 3.5 Diagram summarizing the distribution of subcellular brain constituents within discontinuous density gradients at representative ages during the postnatal developmental period in rats. Only principal fractions are depicted. The constituents in capital letters are the major components of fractions.

A similar overall distribution was observed in *day 4* material, except that the percentage of synaptosomes in the lightest fraction had increased to 22%. By *day* 8, myelin had made its appearance in small amounts in the lightest fraction, more empty processes were present, well-differentiated synaptosomes were increasingly common (40%) in the intermediate fraction and vesicles were sometimes observed in processes containing granular material (Plate 3.34). Appearances increasingly resembling the adult condition were found at *days* 12 *and* 18, with myelin occupying the lightest fraction, an increasing percentage of synaptosomes (55–75%) and a decreasing percentage of processes containing ribosomes and fibrils in the intermediate fraction, and an increasing preponderance of free mitochondria in the densest fraction.

Abdel-Latif and Abood (1964) working with foetal (14–16 days gestation) and 10 day rat whole brains and using a discontinuous Ficoll–sucrose–ethylenediaminetetraacetate (EDTA) gradient, obtained three or four fractions of differing distributions in the two age groups. Synaptosomes, unmyelinated axons and microsomal-like particulates occupied the lightest fraction in the embryonic material, while myelinated axons were present in the lightest fraction and synaptosomes in the intermediate fraction in the 10 day material. Mitochondria occupied the densest fractions in both cases. A modified procedure (Abdel-Latif et al., 1967) substantiated these findings.

Similar results were reported by Spence and Wolfe (1967) using discontinuous sucrose density gradients and working with rat whole brains. Much smaller morphological changes were recorded by Piras et al. (1970) who compared 5 and 30 day rat cerebral cortex. However, synaptosomes were present in three out of the five fractions obtained by them in both age groups, making accurate comparison a difficult procedure. Furthermore, their EMs are not sufficiently clear to enable satisfactory interpretation of comparable fractions by an observer.

The increase in the buoyant density of synaptosomes with maturation noted by Gonatas et al. (1971) may not be a general phenomenon. Oberjat and Howard (1973) examined this buoyant density shift for two classes of synaptosomes, and found that while catecholamine-storing synaptosomes exhibit it GABA-storing synaptosomes do not (Section 4.3).

3.5.2 Synaptosomal ultrastructure

The majority of studies have concentrated on the morphology of *postnatal* synaptosomes, and there is only limited information on their *prenatal* appearance. Much of what is known about the morphology of *prenatal* synaptosomes stems from the studies of Abdel-Latif and co-workers (Abdel-Latif and Abood, 1964; Abdel-Latif et al., 1967) on rat whole brain homogenates. They noted that embryonic synaptosomes appear more fragile than postnatal ones as many of them lack a limiting membrane, while their synaptic vesicles are clumped together (see also Kuriyama et al., 1968c). The vesicles are not well-defined although they are readily recognizable, and many of the synaptosomes lack a mitochondrion. By contrast *postnatal* synaptosomes, even from 1-day-old animals, contain well-defined synaptic vesicles and some mitochondria. In fact, as Abdel-Latif et al. (1967) point out, the synaptosomes of 1-day-old animals are more or less comparable to those of 25-day-old ones but are distinct from those of the embryo.

While this may be a somewhat subjective judgement and is certainly a qualitative one, their published EMs bear it out. A cautionary note is called for however, as the preservation of embryonic material may be inferior to postnatal material. Difficulty is commonly experienced in fixing very young material, and poor fixation may account for the lack of membranes and clumping of vesicles experienced by Abdel-Latif et al. (1967) in their embryonic synaptosomal fractions. Perhaps the most important point to bear in mind when considering synaptosomes during early development, whether pre- or postnatal, is the immense morphological variation at any one age. In view of this it is hazardous to draw too sharp a distinction between late prenatal and early postnatal synaptosomes, just as it is to draw far-reaching conclusions from one or two synaptosomal appearances.

In early development, whether pre- or postnatal, profiles can only be positively identified as synaptosomes by the presence of vesicles. As was intimated in the previous section (3.5.1) a highly-enriched synaptosomal fraction is not obtainable until around day 18 of postnatal life, before which time synaptosomes are associated with processes probably representing immature nerve endings, dendrites and axons (Gonatas *et al.*, 1971). In order to distinguish between neuronal and non-neuronal profiles, resort to serial sectioning may be required (Jones and Brearley, 1973; Section 2.6.1).

The number of synaptic vesicles within immature synaptosomes is small, sometimes as few as one or two, and an additional characteristic of these synaptosomes is the presence of diffusely distributed, amorphous granular material (Fig. 3.6A). The vesicles themselves

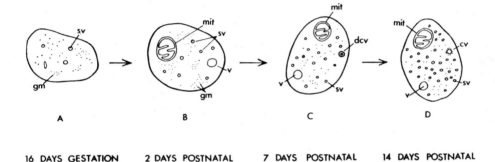

A   B   C   D

16 DAYS GESTATION   2 DAYS POSTNATAL   7 DAYS POSTNATAL   14 DAYS POSTNATAL

Figure 3.6 This diagram represents typical synaptosomal appearances at various stages in the development of rat cerebral cortex. The increase in vesicle numbers with maturation and the predominance of granular material in early development are features of general applicability. cv, coated vesicles; dcv, dense-cored vesicles; gm, granular material; mit, mitochondria; sv, synaptic vesicles; v, vacuoles.

may be ill-defined, particularly against the granular background, while their size is variable. The nature of this amorphous granular material is unclear, but as Gonatas *et al.* (1971) suggest, it could represent poorly preserved synaptic vesicles or microtubules, and may well have an artefactual basis.

As maturation proceeds there is an increase in the number of synaptic vesicles and a corresponding decrease in granular material (Plates 3.30–3.32). Mitochondria, which are infrequent in the earliest synaptosomes, become a regular feature, while other varieties of vesicles such as DCV and coated vesicles are frequently observed from the seventh postnatal day onwards. Vacuoles are also recognizable in postnatal synaptosomes (Fig. 3.6 B–D).

An increase in the number of synaptic vesicles is one of the most striking features of synaptic development. It has been repeatedly noted in synaptosomal studies (e.g. Del Cerro *et al.*, 1969; Jones and Revell, 1970a; Gonatas *et al.*, 1971), in which a sharp increase in the number of vesicles per synaptosome occurs around day 7 in rat studies (Jones and Revell, 1970a). Although no detailed quantitative estimations have been

131

made, this trend corresponds with that noted in intact cerebral cortex in which the rate of increase per unit area of presynaptic bags is most marked between 4 and 7 days, while the numbers more than double from the fourteenth day to adult life (Armstrong-James and Johnson, 1970; see Section 1.4.1).

Alongside the increase in vesicle numbers per synaptosome there is an overall increase in synaptosome numbers during development. This is reflected in the relative difficulty which is experienced in finding synaptosomes during early development, as well as in the changing proportions of synaptosomes and non-specific processes in the lighter fractions as development proceeds (Gonatas *et al.*, 1971). Once again this trend is present in intact tissue where attempts have been made to quantify it (Aghajanian and Bloom, 1967c; Armstrong-James and Johnson, 1970).

As mentioned previously (Section 3.5.1), processes with ribosomes amongst their constituents are frequently seen in the lighter fractions during early development (Plate 3.29). Some of these can be positively identified as postsynaptic, linked as they are to presynaptic terminals by paramembranous thickenings (Jones and Revell, 1970a). This finding is confined to the first 4 to 6 postnatal days, during which time the postsynaptic component is larger than its presynaptic counterpart. This is the reverse of the adult picture and the reason may be that up to the seventh postnatal day dendritic spines have not formed with the result that synaptic contact is made with the relatively large dendritic trunk (Jones and Revell, 1970a; Section 1.4.2). If this is the case, some at least of the ribosomes observed in fractions are present in immature dendrites.

3.5.3   Junctional region

The discussion so far has concentrated on general features of synaptosomal development. Attention in this section will be directed to one specific area of the synaptosome, that is, the junctional region between its pre- and postsynaptic components.

Using conventional methods of preparation (glutaraldehyde and OsO_4 fixation; uranyl and lead staining) Jones and Revell (1970a) reported that the synaptosomal junctional region in rat cerebral cortex was characterized by desmosome-like symmetrical thickenings until the fourth postnatal day, after which it became increasingly asymmetrical (Fig. 3.7). Up to day 4 therefore, pre- and postsynaptic components could only be distinguished by the presence of synaptic vesicles and possibly ribosomes in the respective terminals. From days 5 and 6 onwards the postsynaptic thickening increased in width relative to the presynaptic one and the cleft material took on a more organized appearance. Further development involved the focalization of the postsynaptic thickening to form discrete postsynaptic focal densities. The majority of junctions on day 7 and later were distinctly asymmetrical.

With the glutaraldehyde–PTA method (Section 3.2.2) Jones and Revell (1970b) noted that the internal coats of pre- and postsynaptic membranes initially appeared as undifferentiated plaque-like thickenings (Fig. 3.7). These were gradually replaced over the 5–7 day postnatal period by dense projections and postsynaptic focal densities respectively. Similarly, the external coats of the synaptic membranes, after initial fusion forming a plate-like structure, focalized by day 5 to form the cleft densities or transverse bars of the adult junctional region.

The emergence of the adult forms of the paramembranous densities is therefore a gradual process, the initial continuous densities along the length of the junction breaking down in stages until the typical adult form is attained (type A in Fig. 3.7). In the majority

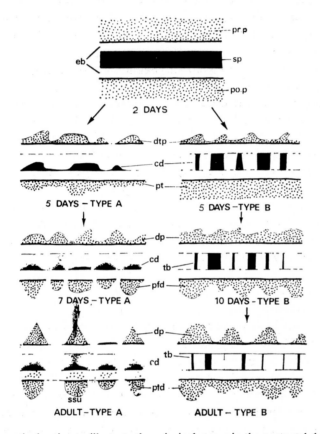

Figure 3.7 Schematic drawing to illustrate the principal stages in the postnatal development of the junctional region in rat synaptosomes. This scheme is based on the study of glutaraldehyde–PTA material and emphasizes the divergence of the two synaptosomal types. cd, cleft densities; dp, dense projections; dtp, dense triangular profiles; eb, electrontranslucent bands; pfd, postsynaptic focal densities; po.p, postsynaptic plaque; pr.p, presynaptic plaque; pt, postsynaptic thickening; sp, synaptic plate; ssu, synaptic subunit; tb, transverse bars. (Modified from Jones, 1972).

of junctions this is completed by day 21. Until the commencement of differentiation of the paramembranous densities at day 5, all junctions are basically similar in appearance, only one type of synaptosome being recognizable. From day 5 onwards two types, corresponding to types A and B of adult life, can be identified (Section 3.4.4; Fig. 3.7).

The similarity of synaptosomal morphology to that of intact synaptic junctions (Section 3.3) means that studies of this nature can be used to further fundamental concepts of neurotransmission mechanisms. The investigations outlined in this section have, as was discussed in the first chapter (1.4.3), contributed substantially to ideas concerning the role of synaptic vesicles in the maturation of dense projections.

3.5.4   Biochemical correlates

The shift of synaptosomes from the lighter to the heavier fractions during development is paralleled by an altered distribution of ChAc and AChE (Gonatas *et al.*, 1971). For instance, in 1-day-old rats 40% of these enzyme activities are localized in the lightest fraction compared with 20% in the 'future-synaptosome' fraction, whereas in adult animals the corresponding figures are 10% and 40% respectively. As these enzymes are localized in high concentrations in synaptosomes (Aldridge and Johnson, 1969; De Robertis *et al.*, 1962a), this is the sort of movement anticipated with maturation. In similar fashion LDH, a cytoplasmic marker, shows comparable changes with age, while the percentage of protein recovered in the 'future-synaptosome' fraction doubles from day 1 to the adult (Gonatas *et al.*, 1971).

The rate of increase of specific activity of ChAc in the 'future-synaptosome' fraction corresponds fairly closely with the rate of increase of the percentage of synaptosomal profiles in this fraction from day 8 onwards. The rate of increase of specific activity of AChE parallels the ChAc increase from day 12 (Gonatas *et al.*, 1971). Both enzymes however, have much slower rises in the early postnatal period than that of the synaptosomes. This discrepancy between biochemical and morphological observations during the first 8 postnatal days may reflect the relatively small number of synaptic vesicles in immature synaptosomes (cf. Bodian, 1966a), although the tardiness of the AChE rise points to immaturity of the receptor mechanism of the synaptic membranes.

The rise in specific activity of AChE during maturation of rat brain is gradual, levelling off after 18 days (Gonatas *et al.*, 1971) or even falling slightly (Abdel-Latif *et al.*, 1970). A similar trend appears to hold in the developing chick embryo brain (Burdick and Strittmatter, 1965; Iqbal and Talwar, 1971), while the concentration of ACh also increases evenly with age in both situations (Abdel-Latif *et al.*, 1970). The absence of abrupt changes in the development of AChE could indicate that it is not directly related to the appearance of electrical activity in the brain. By contrast, $(Na^+–K^+)$–ATPase specific activity increases abruptly on the 21st day of gestation in rat, the period during which electroencephalographic (EEG) activity is first detectable (Abdel-Latif *et al.*, 1967, 1970).

The gradual increase in the ACh specific activity with age correlates with the apparently gradual increase in vesicle numbers. This observation in itself however, provides no direct information about the origin of neurotransmitter substances during maturation. Abdel-Latif *et al.* (1970) also noted that AChE activity was much lower in the synaptosomal than the microsomal fraction. While both fractions may be decidedly heterogeneous, the gradual increase in the synaptosomal AChE and minimal decrease in the microsomal AChE in the first 10–12 postnatal days may indicate some movement of this enzyme from the cell body to the synaptic terminal over this period.

Chapter 4: Synapses and Synaptosomes as Functional Units

4.1 SUBCELLULAR LOCALIZATION OF PUTATIVE TRANSMITTERS

Studies into the chemical and enzymic composition of synaptosomes constitute the fundamental *raison d'etre* of synaptosomal investigations, enabling as they do analysis of the presynaptic terminal plus a small portion of the postsynaptic process in isolation from the remaining elements of the CNS. Synaptosomal preparations have, not surprisingly, proved excellent model systems for the study of central chemical transmitters, especially ACh, NE and the physiologically active amino acids. Furthermore, they have proved useful in localizing the constituent enzymes of the cholinergic system, namely ChAc and AChE, and hence have contributed to the establishment of a coordinated picture of the organization of the cholinergic terminal. A similar claim may be made for the monoaminergic terminal.

In assessing analytical studies of synaptosomes Whittaker (1969c) has drawn attention to a number of cautions which need to be borne in mind. These are: (a) the degree of contamination of synaptosomal preparations (Section 2.6); (b) the chemical heterogeneity of the preparations; (c) the possibility of soluble substances diffusing out of synaptosomes

Table 4.1 Markers for subcellular fractions of brain tissue (Modified from Whittaker, 1972)

Organelle	Marker	Investigations
Nuclei	deoxyribonucleic acid	Aldridge and Johnson, 1959
Myelin	cerebrosides	Eichberg *et al.*, 1964
Synaptosomes	ACh (bound), ChAc, glutamate decarboxylase, NE, 5–HT	e.g. Whittaker, 1959 Gray and Whittaker, 1962 Michaelson and Whittaker, 1963 Fonnum, 1965
Mitochondria	SDH, fumarase etc.	Aldridge and Johnson, 1959
Soluble cytoplasm	LDH, K^+	Johnson and Whittaker, 1963 Stahl *et al.*, 1963 Mangan and Whittaker, 1966
Microsomes	AChE, $(Na^+–K^+)$–ATPase, $5'$–nucleotidase	Aldridge and Johnson, 1959 Skou, 1960
External synaptosome membranes	AChE, $(Na^+–K^+)$–ATPase, $5'$–nucleotidase	Hosie, 1965 Harwood and Hawthorne, 1969
Glial fragments	butyrylcholinesterase	Cavanagh *et al.*, 1954
Lysosomes	acid hydrolases	Koenig *et al.*, 1964

during preparation; (d) fractionation of tissue at low ionic strengths may modify subcellular distribution patterns; (e) cell constituents may be destroyed during fractionation; and (f) the presence of a particular substance in a fraction is no guarantee that this is the dominant substance in that fraction.

The emphasis placed upon ACh in synaptosomal investigations stems from the observation that it is a useful *chemical marker* for synaptosomes. Besides this, it is readily bioassayed in picomolar quantities using a thin slip of the dorsal muscle of the leech (Szerb, 1961; Gaddum, 1965). This concept of chemical markers is a fundamental one for fractionation procedures, because if it can be established that a particular substance has a specific subcellular localization this substance can be regarded as a marker for the organelle in which it is located (Whittaker, 1965). Examples of markers routinely used in brain tissue are given in Table 4.1.

The development of subcellular fractionation techniques and associated concepts has been discussed previously (Sections 2.1.1–2.1.3), and has been extensively reviewed with especial emphasis on the cholinergic system by Whittaker (e.g. 1965, 1969a, b, c, 1971b, 1972) and De Robertis (1967) amongst others.

4.1.1   The cholinergic system

The fractionation schemes employed by Whittaker, De Robertis and their respective co-workers for the separation of synaptosomes and synaptic vesicles have been outlined in Chapter 2 (Schemes 2.1, 2.2, 2.4 and 2.5). The distribution of the principal chemical markers in the primary fractions and also in the subfractions resulting from synaptosomal rupture are depicted in Figs. 4.1 and 4.2.

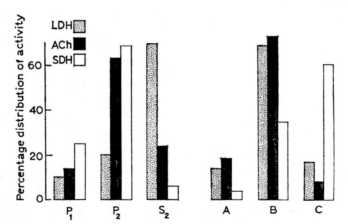

Figure 4.1   Distribution of LDH, bound ACh and SDH in the primary fractions of guinea-pig brain. (Modified from Whittaker, 1965).

(i) *Distribution of ACh.* The early work of Whittaker (1959), and the yet earlier study of Brodkin and Elliott (1953) had demonstrated the existence of more than one form of 'bound' ACh within synaptosomes (Section 2.1.2). This followed from the observation

136

that mild disruptive treatments which would be expected to break down lipoprotein membranes released only about 50% of the bound ACh (the 'labile-bound' fraction). By contrast all of it is released by more vigorous treatments (the 'stable-bound' fraction). Further work by Johnson and Whittaker (1963) and Whittaker *et al.*, (1964) helped localize these two categories of bound ACh.

The *labile-bound* fraction of ACh is not only ruptured by suspension of synaptosomes in water but is destroyed in the absence of a ChE inhibitor. This fraction (synaptosomal

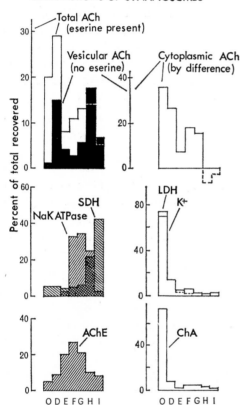

Figure 4.2 Distribution of the components of the cholinergic terminal and of marker substances in the fractions obtained by hypotonic rupture of synaptosomes. (From Whittaker, 1971b).

cytoplasmic ACh) behaves much like any soluble cytoplasmic constituent and exchanges with 14C-ACh added to the suspension medium (Marchbanks, 1968a).

The *stable-bound* fraction survives hypotonic treatment of synaptosomes, analysis of the disrupted organelles demonstrating its presence in synaptic vesicles (Whittaker *et al.*, 1964; Fig. 4.2). Fig. 4.2 shows that the vesicles have a bimodal distribution in this gradient, band D consisting principally of monodisperse vesicles and band H of vesicles intermingled with damaged synaptosomes. The stable-bound ACh (vesicular ACh) has a corresponding distribution, with its highest specific concentration in the isolated vesicle fraction, D. Added radioactive ACh does not exchange with this vesicular ACh under a variety of conditions (Marchbanks, 1968a).

137

In addition to these forms of bound ACh a proportion of the total tissue ACh is in the *free* state, and is recovered in the high speed supernatant (chiefly S_3; also S_2 as in Fig. 4.1). The proportion of ACh which is in the free form varies from approximately 20% in the cerebral cortex and caudate nucleus where cholinergic neurons are mainly represented by their terminals, to about 90% in ventral roots and nerve trunks containing cholinergic axons (Whittaker, 1971b). It is quite possible that free ACh represents cytoplasmic ACh present in axons and cell bodies, and is released when these structures are broken down during homogenization. This distinguishes it from both forms of bound ACh which appear to be limited to nerve terminals.

The pertinent question in the light of these results is whether these three fractions of neuronal ACh are distinct, or whether they are derived from a pre-existing pool which is redistributed during subcellular fractionation (Whittaker, 1971b). In an attempt to answer this question Chakrin and Whittaker (1969) set out to determine the specific activities of the various pools after prior administration of radioactive choline *in vivo*. After 1 h they noted that of the three pools the free ACh was the least labelled, with the vesicular ACh coming next and the synaptosomal cytoplasmic ACh the most intensely labelled. From this, they concluded that the three pools of ACh turn over at different rates, and probably therefore represent distinct pools in intact tissue.

Assuming the reality of three ACh pools, from which pool is ACh released into the cleft in response to nerve stimulation? Considerable experimental effort has been devoted to answering this question, and while strides have been made in our understanding of the dynamic mechanisms at play, a clear-cut answer has not as yet been forthcoming.

Richter and Marchbanks (1971a), using cerebral cortical slices incubated with ^{3}H-choline with or without the addition of potassium chloride, demonstrated that the ACh had not become radioactively labelled to the full extent theoretically possible. In addition, the specific activity of the ACh released by K^+ was greater than that released in control incubations, suggesting it may come from a newly synthesized, more radioactive store. Nevertheless, the specific activity of the ACh released was less than that of the ACh remaining in the tissue, implying the existence of a pool of ACh in the tissue which is either turning over very slowly or is being synthesized from a less radioactive pool of choline. When synaptosomes were prepared from slices incubated with potassium chloride their vesicles contained ACh of a lower specific activity than the cytoplasmic ACh (Richter and Marchbanks, 1971b). It appears therefore that the more radioactively labelled ACh is lost preferentially during the preparation of synaptosomes from K^+ stimulated tissue. The slowly turning over pool of ACh predicted by Richter and Marchbanks (1971a) from their studies on cortical slices may well be represented by the synaptic vesicles by hypotonic disruption of synaptosomes.

This in turn implies that the vesicle population in nerve terminals is heterogeneous, a postulate supported by evidence from a variety of sources. Marchbanks and Israël (1971) have shown that when the ACh of synaptic vesicles is labelled by incubation with ^{3}H-choline, the radioactive and bioassayable ACh are heterogeneous and behave differently when the vesicles are submitted to isotonic gel filtration. The more radioactively labelled ACh is washed off the vesicles, while the bulk of the bioassayable ACh passes through in the void of the column. This suggests there is in the vesicle fraction from incubated slices a pool of ACh which is more highly labelled and less firmly bound, and which may represent the most recently synthesized ACh. Barker, Dowdall and Whittaker (1972), investigating the turnover of synaptosomal and stable-bound ACh isolated from cortical tissue, demonstrated that the ACh in fraction H differs from that in fraction D. They found, in contradistinction to the results of Chakrin and Whittaker (1969), that at short time intervals after the injection of radioactive choline (10–20 min) the ACh of fraction H is considerably more labelled than that of D. The labelled ACh in H is also heterogeneous and is inversely related to the yield of ACh in the fraction. Barker *et al.* (1972) explained these findings by assuming that H contains two pools of ACh, a small rapidly turning-over pool and a larger one similar in specific activity to that in D.

The significance of these and similar results for the vesicle hypothesis is discussed in Sections 5.3.1. and 5.3.2, in which the possible localization of these different ACh pools is considered. The important contribution of squid synaptosomal studies to issues such as choline uptake mechanisms is discussed in Section 2.3.7 and has been reviewed by Whittaker, Dowdall and Boyne (1972).

(ii) *Distribution of ChAc.* The isolation of synaptic vesicles by the Whittaker and De Robertis techniques gives diverging localizations for ChAc (Section 2.4.2). Both groups agree that it is present in relatively high concentration within the presynaptic terminals of cholinergic neurons. In this it corresponds to the distribution of ACh. It remains sequestered there when the terminals are detached by fractionation procedures to form synaptosomes (Hebb and Whittaker, 1958; Gray and Whittaker, 1962; De Robertis *et al.*, 1962a). On subfractionation of synaptosomes it is bound to synaptic vesicles according to De Robertis *et al.* (1963), while according to Whittaker *et al.* (1964) it is localized in the soluble cytoplasm of the synaptosome (fraction O—Fig. 4.2). In spite of this divergence of opinion both groups agree that bound ACh is present in the vesicle fraction. As highlighted by Schemes 2.4 and 2.5, the synaptosomal constituents were separated by differential centrifugation in De Robertis's laboratory and by density gradient centrifugation in Whittaker's.

In order to clarify the situation both Whittaker and De Robertis used the techniques of the other and repeated the other's experiments (Whittaker *et al.*, 1964; McCaman, Rodriguez de Lores Arnaiz and De Robertis, 1965). The limitations of this approach are obvious, although these studies highlight a number of features. Whittaker *et al.* (1964) found that the levels of ChAc and ACh in M_1, M_2 and M_3 corresponded to those they had previously obtained with their own techniques. The most striking difference between their results and those of De Robertis was the low level of ChAc in their vesicular (M_2) fraction in contrast to the high level in De Robertis's M_2 fraction. Negative staining of this fraction in Whittaker's hands revealed an extremely heterogeneous fraction, quite unlike that of De Robertis. A reason proposed by Whittaker for this difference was De Robertis's use of OsO_4 as a fixative prior to negative staining, a procedure likely to cause disintegration of the fragile synaptosomes on resuspension (Horne and Whittaker, 1962). While this may be a valid factor, it is unlikely to be as significant as suggested by Whittaker *et al.*, (1964).

This is because their micrographs of the negatively-stained M_2 fraction are not comparable to those of De Robertis *et al.*, (1963), in addition to which De Robertis's contentions are supported by a micrograph of positively-stained embedded tissue. It should also be noted that Whittaker's reconstruction of De Robertis's techniques employed guinea-pig brain, whereas De Robertis's own experiments were on rat brain. Further evidence presented by Whittaker for the heterogeneity of De Robertis's vesicular fraction are the presence in it of markers for external membranes, such as ChE (De Robertis *et al.*, 1963), $(Na^+–K^+)$-activated ATPase (Germain and Proulx, 1965) and ganglioside (Burton, Howard and Gibbons, 1964). These markers are absent from vesicle preparations isolated according to Whittaker's technique (see Whittaker, 1969c).

McCaman *et al.*, (1965) in De Robertis's laboratory laid the chief blame for the differences on Whittaker's failure to wash the nuclear fraction, claiming that this resulted in the loss of appreciable mitochondrial enzymes to this fraction. This by itself however, does not bear on the respective quality of the vesicle fractions and is therefore of limited relevance to the present discussion.

Another aspect of McCaman *et al*'s (1965) explanation for the differences in ChAc distribution is species variability. They concluded that ChAc is synaptic vesicle-bound in rat and rabbit cerebral cortex, partly vesicle-bound and partly soluble in guinea-pig, and soluble in pigeon. Saelens and Potter (1966) using rat forebrain synaptosomes and Tuček (1966) using whole rat brain and sheep caudate nucleus also claimed the enzyme behaved as though particle-bound.

In an investigation into the compartmentation of ChAc in synaptosomes Fonnum (1967) found it may be isolated in either a bound or soluble form depending on the final pH and ionic strength of the suspension after hypotonic rupture of the synaptosomes (Fig. 4.3). He found that the bound form is favoured by the fall in ionic strength and pH accompanying hypotonic treatment, whereas the soluble form is predominant under more physiological conditions of pH and ionic strength. Two further points of interest noted by Fonnum (1967) were: (a) the occluded form of the enzyme may not be bound to synaptic vesicles but to larger membrane fragments such as those derived from external synaptosomal membranes (1968); and (b) the species differences in the distribution of the enzyme may be due to species differences in its solubility (Fig. 4.3) and not, as suggested by McCaman *et al.* (1965), to variations in its compartmentation in the cholinergic neurons of different species.

In terms of the postulated localization of ChAc by Whittaker and co-workers, the main site of ACh synthesis in synaptosomes is in the cytoplasm where it is transported to synaptic vesicles by an uptake mechanism.

(iii) *Distribution of AChE.* The subcellular distribution of this enzyme is consonant with membrane localizations. Consequently its highest specific activity occurs in the microsomal fraction which is derived from endoplasmic reticulum, although it is also associated with the myelin and synaptosomal fractions. Fig. 4.2 shows that on rupture of the synaptosomes it is chiefly found in subfractions E, F and G which are derived mainly from fragmented external synaptosomal membranes. Compared with the distribution of another external membrane marker, (Na^+-K^+)-ATPase, AChE is relatively rich in fraction E. This is probably the result of microsomal contamination (Whittaker, 1971b). The relationship between the distribution of these two membrane markers in the synaptic plasma membrane fractions of different investigators is considered in Section 2.5.1.

Histochemical studies of intact cholinergic neurons confirm this distribution of the enzyme. It is confined to the rough endoplasmic reticulum and occasionally to tubules and areas of the nuclear envelope in cell bodies, to the axonal membrane and around much of of the presynaptic terminal (Lewis and Shute, 1966; Section 4.4.5). Synaptosomal investigations suggest its presence over the external membrane.

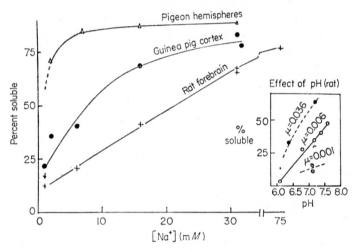

Figure 4.3 Effect of ionic strength on the binding of ChAc to membrane fragments. Data from Fonnum (1967). (From Marchbanks, 1969).

The coexistence of AChE and cytoplasmic ACh in neurons and their presynaptic terminals can be explained by assuming that the enzyme is *functionally* on the outside of the neuron (Whittaker, 1971b). This implies it is sequestered *within* the lumen of the endoplasmic reticulum and tubules, while it is attached to the *external* aspect of the axonal and terminal membranes.

4.1.2   Subcellular distribution of other biogenic amines

Although the bulk of subcellular fractionation studies of neurotransmitters have concentrated on ACh and its associated enzymes in cholinergic neurons, the distribution of other biogenic amines has been followed. Masuoka (1965) and Fuxe, Grobecker, Hökfelt and Jonsson (1967) were the first to demonstrate that the terminal varicosities of monoamine-containing neurons form synaptosomes during homogenization. They were able to show that fluorescent particles similar to terminal varicosities are present in synaptosomal fractions examined by fluorescence microscopy.

Amine analyses of subcellular fractions have been predominantly on whole brain preparations (e.g. Kataoka. 1962; Michaelson and Whittaker, 1962, 1963; Carlini and

Green, 1963; Zieher and De Robertis, 1963). More specifically, amine distribution in the brain stem (Levi and Maynert, 1964), hypothalamus (Andreoli *et al.*, 1970) and spinal cord (Ross *et al.*, 1971) has been studied. In these studies the specificity of the synaptosomal preparations for the binding of NE and 5-HT has been demonstrated. In the spinal cord study of Ross *et al.* NE and 5-HT were prominent in the two synaptosomal fractions, B_2 and B_3 (Section 3.2.3), with a concentration of 5-HT in B_2 and NE in B_3. A similar distinction was obtained by Andreoli *et al.* (1970) in hypothalamus and pituitary stalk, although Clementi *et al.* (1970) obtained the reverse (Section 3.2.3).

The association of NE with synaptic vesicles has been suggested by a number of workers, although the evidence is not as strong as for ACh. Michaelson, Whittaker, Laverty and Sharman (1963) for example observed a marked loss of NE from the particulate material of synaptosomes when the latter were osmotically shocked, although there was no sharp concentration of it in the vesicular fractions. One difficulty is the low level of amines in brain tissue.

5-HT, although present in the synaptosomal fraction, also appears in high concentration relative to protein in the P_3 fraction (Zieher and De Robertis, 1963). Dopamine closely resembles the distribution of LDH (Laverty, Michaelson, Sharman and Whittaker, 1963), and is less specifically concentrated in synaptosomes (from caudate nucleus and putamen) than ACh. In subfractions of synaptosomes approximately 80% of it is recovered in the supernatant.

4.1.3 Subcellular distribution of amino acids

Amino acids have been described as constituting a dominant compositional feature of synaptosomes (De Belleroche and Bradford, 1973b), in line with their importance in whole brain where glutamate, GABA, taurine (Agrawal, Davison and Kaczmarek, 1971) and *N*-acetyl glutamate (Reichett and Fonnum, 1969) occur in the largest amounts. Although only about 10% of the total amino acids are recovered in synaptosomes (Mangan and Whittaker, 1965; Whittaker, 1968b), biochemical and autoradiographic studies strongly suggest that GABA uptake is specifically associated with at least certain categories of nerve terminal, for example, the basket cells of the cerebellum (Hökfelt and Ljungdahl, 1972) and the amacrine cells of the retina (Ehinger and Falck, 1971; Graham, 1972). Likewise, glycine uptake is associated with the nerve terminals of the spinal cord (Hökfelt and Ljungdahl, 1971a; Matus and Dennison, 1971, 1972; Sections 4.3.2 and 4.3.3).

Early subcellular distribution studies on the compartmentation of GABA (Weinstein *et al.*, 1963), glutamate (Ryall, 1964) and amino acids in general (Mangan and Whittaker, 1965) failed to show a specific localization of amino acids in the synaptosomal fraction. This conclusion was reached in view of the small percentage of amino acids recovered in this fraction, their distribution resembling soluble cytoplasmic constituents and the similarity in distribution between pharmacologically active and inactive amino acids (Whittaker, 1968b).

More recently, in addition to the considerable body of evidence suggesting an inhibitory transmitter role for GABA, its subcellular localization in synaptic structures has been demonstrated autoradiographically (Section 4.3.2). Mechanisms for the specific binding and transport of GABA have been demonstrated for synaptosomal fractions isolated from adult (Kuriyama, Weinstein and Roberts, 1969; Martin and Smith, 1972; Snodgrass, Hedley-Whyte and Lorenzo, 1973) and developing (Kelly, Luttges, Johnson and Grove, 1974) brain. High affinity uptake systems for GABA have been described in brain fractions enriched in synaptosomes (Iversen and Johnston, 1971; Logan and Snyder, 1971).

Because amino acids are major candidates as transmitters in the CNS and as some of them are taken up by synaptosomes, their relationship to synaptic vesicles becomes an important issue. A number of investigations have been made into the recovery of amino acids in synaptic vesicle fractions, with conflicting results. On the one hand Agrawal *et al.* (1971) and Rassin (1972) were unable to detect a significant vesicle content of amino acids, whereas others including Kuriyama *et al.* (1968a, b), Farrow and O'Brien (1972) and De Belleroche and Bradford (1973a) have reported the presence of a number of amino acids notably glutamate, taurine and GABA in vesicle fractions. Furthermore, some members of this latter group of workers have also suggested that vesicle fractions may have a capacity for the uptake of such amino acids.

The reasons for the conflicting results are probably technical ones (see De Belleroche and Bradford, 1973a), the main weight of evidence appearing to indicate that a small but well-defined pool of physiologically active amino acids is associated with mammalian cortical synaptic vesicles. There are differences however, between the amino acid and ACh pools. While vesicular ACh isolated by gel filtration is released by passage of the vesicles through Sephadex equilibrated in water (Marchbanks, 1968a), amino acids are not. Although the amount of amino acids remaining associated with vesicles after passage through Sephadex columns is small (Table 4.2), it is still many times greater than

Table 4.2   Amino acid content of a purified cerebral cortex synaptic vesicle fraction (From De Belleroche and Bradford, 1973a)

Amino acid	nmol/g *original tissue*
Aspartate	3.97 ± 0.96
Glutamine	3.41 ± 0.63
Serine	2.20 ± 0.33
Glutamate	15.69 ± 2.33
Glycine	1.87 ± 0.32
Alanine	1.69 ± 0.45
GABA	3.74 ± 0.97

Synaptic vesicles were applied to Sephadex columns equilibrated in 0·4M sucrose. The amino acid contents of the void volume were determined after perchloric acid extraction and are shown as means ± S.E.M. from eight experiments.

comparable ACh levels (0·6–0·79 nmol ACh/g tissue—Whittaker and Sheridan, 1965; Marchbanks, 1968a). Finally, the significance of an amino acid presence in vesicles is not clear, especially with one such as taurine which could be the most enriched amino acid in them (De Belleroche and Bradford, 1973a). Among possible functions are an inhibitory transmitter role, a binding to ACh and the maintenance of ion gradients in vesicles.

4.2 METABOLIC PROPERTIES AND RESPONSES OF SYNAPTOSOMES

The morphological integrity of synaptosomes was discussed in a previous chapter (Section 3.3) while their biochemical complexity has been touched upon from a number of angles (Sections 2.3.1 and 4.1). The aim of the present section is to investigate the extent to which they display the metabolic properties and responses of *in situ* synapses. The result of this investigation will determine the validity of concepts which regard synaptosomes as small whole cells.

4.2.1 Respiratory properties

A number of workers have demonstrated that when suspensions of cortical synaptosomes maintained in a Krebs-Ringer medium buffered with Tris-HC1, glycylglycine or phosphate, are incubated at 37°C, they absorb oxygen in a linear fashion (Bradford, 1967, 1969; Whittaker 1969c; Balfour and Gilbert, 1970). The rate of absorption in the presence of 10mM glucose is of the order of 60–67 μmol. O_2/100 mg protein/h (Fig. 4.4), which is

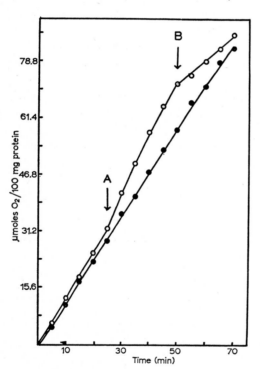

Figure 4.4 Repiratory response of synaptosomes to electrical stimulation. A, current on; B, current off; O, stimulated sample; ●, control sample incubated in parallel. (From Bradford, 1970)

comparable to that of cortical slices (McIlwain and Batchelard, 1971). Synaptosomes from other brain regions, such as hypothalamus and medulla/spinal cord, respire with similar rates under equivalent conditions (Edwardson, Bennett and Bradford, 1972; Osborne *et al.*, 1973).

Synaptosomes from mammalian brain are capable of high respiration in the presence

144

of a range of substrates, such as glucose, pyruvate and glutamate (Bradford, 1969). With glucose as substrate considerable amounts of ATP and phosphocreatine are synthesized, while these synaptosomes also have the capacity for the active accumulation of potassium ions (Bradford, 1967, 1969) and the extrusion of sodium ions (Ling and Abdel-Latif, 1968).

These metabolic activities imply, as Bradford and Thomas (1969) have pointed out, the presence within synaptosomes of the enzymes and co-factors involved in these processes. A number of enzymes involved in, for example, the glutamate cycle and the mitochondrial oxidation pathways, had previously been reported (Salganicoff and De Robertis, 1965; Balázs *et al.*, 1966; Abdel-Latif, 1966) in synaptosomal preparations. It was however, of considerable interest to find that synaptosomes incubated under conditions in which they display high respiration were able to transform substrates into intermediary metabolites (Bradford and Thomas, 1969). In particular, glucose may be converted into lactate, aspartate, glutamate, glutamine, alanine and GABA during 1h incubation periods with [U–^{14}C]-glucose. Furthermore, the incorporation of the radio-activity principally into CO_2, lactate, aspartate, glutamate, glutamine, alanine and GABA corresponded fairly closely to the incorporation characteristic of cortex slices (Beloff-Chain, Cantanzaro, Chain, Masi and Pocchiari, 1955). In contrast to cortex slices, very little glutamine was produced either from glucose or glutamate in synaptosomal preparations. Table 4.3 compares the incorporation of [U–^{14}C]-glucose into metabolites

Table 4.3 Incorporation of [U–^{14}C]glucose into metabolites by synaptosomes and cortex slices (From Bradford and Thomas, 1969)

Metabolite	Synaptosomes Dis./min $\times 10^{-3}$/100 mg protein	Cortex slices Dis./min $\times 10^{-3}$/g wet wt tissue
Aspartate	746 ± 90	479 ± 36
Glutamate	1887 ± 202	2425 ± 72
Alanine	315 ± 41	489 ± 29
GABA	307 ± 40	607 ± 9
Glutamine	traces	1136 ± 80
Lactate	10 326 ± 749	16 275 ± 483
Malate	not detected	115 ± 37
CO_2	4950 ± 421	6306 ± 191
Ethanol insoluble residue	59 ± 4	8 ± 2
Total counts in metabolites	18 590 ± 1065	27 840 ± 1709
No. of samples	12	9

Incubation was for 1 h at 37°C in 2 ml Krebs–tris medium containing 10mM glucose and 10 μc of [U–^{14}C] glucose. Values are means ± S.E.M.

by synaptosomes and cortex slices. The greater incorporation in slices results from their higher lactate production.

In spite of this discrepancy and of the differences in the pool sizes of the amino acids between cortex slices (Shaw and Heine, 1965) and synaptosomes (Bradford and Thomas, 1969), the considerable lactate production (16 μmol/100 mg protein/h; Bradford and Thomas, 1969) as well as the formation of ATP and phosphocreatine (Bradford, 1969; De Belleroche and Bradford, 1972a) demonstrate the usefulness of synaptosomes as metabolic models. Synaptosomal respiration is considerable for 20 minutes even in the absence of glucose. Linear respiration continues for 3–4 h in the presence of glucose, following which it slowly declines along with the amino acid pool sizes and potassium content (Table 4.4). By contrast, respiratory rates decline rapidly after 20 minutes when glucose is lacking. Refurbishing the glucose levels at 3 h or resuspending in fresh incubation medium has no effect on the pattern of declining O_2 uptake (Bradford et al., 1975). From this and similar work it has been estimated that the useful life of synaptosomal preparations may not exceed about 5 h (De Belleroche and Bradford, 1973b). In spite of this, tissue culture studies by the same workers demonstrate the remarkable morphological integrity of synaptosomes maintained for 24 h in culture (Section 3.3).

4.2.2 Membrane potentials

If, as demonstrated in the preceding section, synaptosomes are cell-like entities, it becomes important to demonstrate their intactness. A good index of this in functional terms is the existence of a trans-membrane potential (Bradford, 1971). Unfortunately, the small size of synaptosomes (0·5 μm) makes direct measurement of such potentials difficult. Evidence for them must therefore be established by inference, and this has been sought in terms of either the ion gradients across the membrane or the displacement of a membrane potential.

Electrical pulses and elevated extracellular potassium are two agents which depolarize in vivo (Bunešová and Bures, 1969) and in vitro (McIlwain, 1955). When applied to synaptosomes incubated at 37°C in physiological media, both produce effects similar to those observed in brain slices (see Hertz, 1969; Quastel, 1969) and indicative of membrane depolarization. Consequently, application to cortical synaptosomes of alternating rectangular pulses (sufficient to give a maximal respiratory response in slices (McIlwain and Joanny, 1963)) causes a large increase in respiratory and glycolytic rates as shown in Fig. 4.4 (Bradford, 1970). In parallel with these changes, there is a substantial loss of potassium and gain in sodium (Bradford, 1970, 1971), while certain amino acids—glutamate, aspartate and GABA—are preferentially released into the medium. These responses have been interpreted by Bradford (1970, 1971) as occurring as a result of depolarization of a trans-membrane potential generated by the synaptosomes.

The value of this potential has been put at −27 mV (Bradford, 1971). This is about half the value expected in nerve endings in situ. However, if account is taken of the membranous contamination of synaptosomal preparations and of the large proportion of the synaptosomal volume occupied by mitochondria and synaptic vesicles, this is a minimal value. Bradford has also estimated that a change from −27 mV to −7 mV may occur when pulses are applied for 30 minutes.

The above results on synaptosomes derived from cerebral cortex have also been obtained on synaptosomes from various other central brain regions, including cerebellum (De Belleroche and Bradford, 1973b), hypothalamus (Bradford et al., 1972, 1973), medulla and spinal cord (Osborne et al., 1973) and basal ganglia (De Belleroche et al., 1975).

The evidence presented here, plus that on the calcium uptake of synaptosomes

Table 4.4 Respiration, amino acid content and potassium content of incubated suspensions of synaptosomes (From Bradford et al., 1975)

Incubation time (min)	0	20	45	60	180	360
Respiration (μmol O_2/100 mg protein/h)	—	62 ± 4 (8)	61 ± 5 (8)	63 ± 4 (8)	57 ± 5 (8)	20 ± 4 (8)
Potassium Content (μeq/100 mg protein/h)	19·7 ± 0·71 (8)	17·0 ± 0·25 (4)	16·3 ± 0·45 (2)	17·9 ± 1·49 (8)	14·8 ± 0·45 (6)	11·2 ± 1·7 (4)
Amino Acid content (nmol/100 mg protein)						
Aspartate	3889 ± 202(8)	4770 ± 457(4)	4297 ± 68(2)	4487 ± 283(8)	1404 ± 348(4)	477 ± 73(4)
Glutamine	950 ± 34(6)	520 ± 24(2)	—	412 ± 21(6)	267 ± 70(4)	146 ± 22(4)
Serine	1231 ± 96(8)	748 ± 79(4)	767 ± 24(2)	659 ± 27(8)	467 ± 74(4)	302 ± 46(4)
Glutamate	7129 ± 189(8)	6386 ± 492(4)	5442 ± 100(2)	4587 ± 152(8)	1993 ± 168(4)	1614 ± 184(4)
Glycine	913 ± 156(8)	876 ± 175(4)	639 ± 119(2)	897 ± 80(8)	1007 ± 78(4)	549 ± 62(4)
Alanine	853 ± 100(8)	874 ± 115(4)	778 ± 61(2)	838 ± 25(8)	744 ± 95(4)	702 ± 135(4)
GABA	2517 ± 117(8)	1898 ± 218(4)	1315 ± 15(2)	1158 ± 76(8)	370 ± 27(4)	333 ± 20(4)

Synaptosomes were suspended in Krebs-phosphate medium and incubated at 37° C in Warburg respirometer vessels for the period indicated. Values of amino acids and potassium are for the synaptosomes deposited by centrifugation at the end of incubation. Amino acids in the incubation medium were also measured. Values are mean ± S.E.M. for number of experiments in parentheses.

(Blaustein and Wiesman, 1970), suggests that the synaptosome membrane is polarized and that, in the presence of adequate sources of energy, many small molecular weight electrolytes can be concentrated within synaptosomes (Bradford *et al.*, 1973).

4.2.3 Active transport

An important reason for postulating the existence of a synaptosomal trans-membrane potential and hence of an intact limiting membrane is the observation that various ions and molecules are actively transported either into or out of synaptosomes. Chief amongst these is the active extrusion of Na^+ (Ling and Abdel-Latif, 1968), and accumulation of K^+ (Bradford, 1969; Escueta and Appel, 1969) and Ca^{2+} (Lust and Robinson, 1968).

A number of factors are involved in each of these processes, while the Na^+ and K^+ transport systems appear to be closely interrelated. For instance, K^+ stimulates the efflux of Na^+ from synaptosomes whereas ouabain inhibits it (Ling and Abdel-Latif, 1968). Conversely, increasing the Na^+ concentration stimulates K^+ uptake, indicating the involvement of (Na^+-K^+)-activated ATPase (see Abdel-Latif, 1972). Further aspects of these uptake systems are that K^+ uptake occurs against a concentration gradient, while Na^+ uptake is an Mg^{2+}, energy and temperature-dependent process. The uptake of Ca^{2+} is stimulated by K^+ and appears to be an Mg^{2+} and ATP-dependent process (Yoshida, Kadota and Fujisawa, 1966; Lust and Robinson, 1968, 1970a, b; Stahl and Swanson, 1969).

The active transport of these ions indicates the presence of an Na^+ permeability barrier and of a system allowing the extrusion of Na^+ from the synaptosome. This, together with the pattern of Ca^{2+} entry, points to the occurrence of depolarization (see De Belleroche and Bradford, 1973b).

Synaptosomes also demonstrate amino acid accumulating properties, a characteristic of brain tissue. They probably possess high affinity uptake mechanisms for amino acids which may be implicated as transmitter substances (Logan and Snyder, 1971). Other transport systems in synaptosomes are those for biogenic amines, such as NE and 5-HT. These systems respond to high sodium and low potassium levels, are sensitive to ouabain and are inhibited by the presence in the medium of calcium (Bogdanski, Tissari and Brodie, 1968; Colburn, Goodwin, Murphy, Bunney and Davis, 1968; Tissari, Schönhöfer, Bogdanski and Brodie, 1969).

4.2.4 Synaptosome beds

The work outlined in the preceding three sections (4.2.1–4.2.3) has demonstrated the respiratory properties of synaptosomes, as well as their ability to accumulate a variety of ions against a concentration gradient. The increased metabolic rates, loss of K^+ and differential loss of physiologically active amino acids in response to the application of electrical pulses or increased medium potassium, have been interpreted as evidence for the existence of a trans-membrane potential. A drawback of these studies is their dependence upon suspensions of synaptosomes which have a very high fluid : tissue ratio. In an attempt to overcome this, De Belleroche and Bradford (1972a) devised a preparation having a low fluid: tissue ratio, and termed by them a 'synaptosome bed'.

In essence, the synaptosome bed preparation consists of a deposit of synaptosomes between nylon gauzes. De Belleroche and Bradford (1972a) found that these preparations respire, produce lactate, ATP and phosphocreatine, and metabolize [U–^{14}C]-glucose to glutamate, aspartate, alanine and GABA at similar rates to synaptosomes. On electrical stimulation, a significant increase (40%) in the rates of oxygen uptake and lactate production was noted. Electrical and potassium stimulation caused differential release of glutamate, aspartate and GABA, although the maximal amounts released (12–26%) were small compared to the values for suspensions (58–62%).

Cortex slices positioned between gauzes showed many similarities to the synaptosome beds, in terms of the glycolytic response to electrical stimulation. Of the amino acids measured however, only the release of GABA was significantly increased in response to electrical and potassium stimulation.

The advantages claimed by De Belleroche and Bradford (1972a) for synaptosome beds over synaptosomal suspensions in metabolic studies are: (a) the ease of manipulation and fixation of the beds, (b) direct contact between the synaptosomes and electrodes is prevented by the gauze. and (c) the low fluid: tissue ratio approximates more closely to the *in vivo* environment of nerve endings.

4.2.5   Release of putative transmitters

Electrical stimulation and elevated medium potassium levels (6mM rising to 56mM) are responsible for the differential loss to the medium of ACh (Marchbanks, 1969; Haga, 1971; De Belleroche and Bradford, 1972b), NE (Blaustein, Johnson and Needleman, 1972) and a number of amino acids. Those involved are the physiologically active glutamate, GABA and aspartate (Bradford, 1970; De Belleroche and Bradford, 1972a), their release occurring under conditions favourable to depolarization. The release of these substances is however, reduced when Ca^{2+} is omitted from the medium and prevented by the inclusion of EGTA which complexes with any endogenous Ca^{2+} (Table 4.5). Release of these amino acids has been recorded not only from cerebral cortical synaptosomes (Bradford, 1970) but also from hypothalamic (Bradford *et al.*, 1973) and medulla/spinal cord (Osborne *et al.*, 1973) ones. Glycine is additionally released in the latter situation. ACh is released by potassium from the crude mitochondrial fraction (Haga, 1972) and slices (Richter and Marchbanks, 1971a, b) of cerebral cortex.

The fact that physiologically active amino acids and ACh are released from *in vivo* preparations (Jasper and Koyama, 1969; Iversen, Mitchell and Srinivasan, 1971), supports the possibility that the synaptosomal response is typical of the *in situ* nerve ending.

Underlying this discussion is a desire to investigate the possible transmitter functions of these physiologically active amino acids (Curtis and Johnston, 1970, Krnjević, 1970; Johnson, 1972). Unfortunately, not only are the amino acids widely dispersed throughout tissues with a variety of metabolic and biosynthetic functions, but many synaptosomal preparations are probably heterogeneous, containing synaptosomes from neurons employing a variety of transmitters. In an attempt to overcome the heterogeneity problem Osborne et al. (1973) investigated the release of glycine from medulla/spinal cord synaptosomes, limiting the amino acids therefore to those functions most intimately involved in transmission. Glycine is likely to be an inhibitory transmitter in the spinal cord (Werman, Davidoff and Aprison, 1968; Curtis and De Groat, 1968), a contention supported by autoradiographic (Hökfelt and Ljungdahl, 1971a; Matus and Dennison, 1971, 1972) and electrical stimulation (Hopkin and Neal, 1970; Hammerstadt, Murray and Cutler, 1971; Roberts and Mitchell, 1972) studies. Osborne et al. (1973) detected glycine

Table 4.5 The effect of omission of calcium from the incubation medium on the amino acids accumulation in the medium (From De Belleroche and Bradford, 1973b)

	Amino acid content of supernatant (nmoles/100 mg *protein*)					
	Calcium-containing medium		*Medium without calcium*			
			Containing EGTA			*Without EGTA*
	Control	*Potassium-stimulation*	*Control*	*Potassium-stimulation*	*Electrical-stimulation*	*Potassium-stimulation*
Aspartate	146	333	134	103	195	245
Glutamine	211	294	118	118	145	186
Serine	530	660	287	329	230	484
Glutamate	249	635	256	259	346	484
Glycine	310	359	255	281	210	288
Alanine	410	535	261	244	249	386
GABA	47	133	41	45	50	79
No. of samples	6	6	5	6	6	4

Synaptosome beds were incubated in Krebs–bicarbonate medium in the presence of 10mM glucose at 37° C for 40 min. Medium with calcium contained 0·75mM calcium. EGTA was present at 0·5mM where indicated. After the first 30 min of incubation, potassium or electrical stimulation was started as indicated and continued for the remaining 10 min of incubation. Values given are mean values, standard errors were about 10% of the mean. Potassium stimulation was by elevation of medium potassium by 50mM and an equivalent volume of medium was added to the controls.

in high concentration in medulla/spinal cord synaptosomes, and noted both its stimulus-induced and calcium dependent release from the preparations. The suppression of glycine release by tetanus toxin (Osborne and Bradford, 1973; Osborne et al., 1973) points both to a presynaptic site of action of the toxin and to its *in vivo* action by preventing or diminishing the release of the inhibitory transmitters (see also Curtis, Felix, Game and McCulloch, 1973).

Synaptosomes from the nuclear fraction (Section 3.2.3; Plates 3.17 and 3.18) had similar metabolic properties to those from the mitochondrial fraction, although they did demonstrate an enrichment in their glycine content relative to other amino acids. This may suggest that the nuclear fraction contains a relatively higher proportion of synaptosomes derived from inhibitory nerve endings.

The electrical and potassium stimulation of synaptosomes is not confined to investigating putative transmitters. For instance, Edwardson et al. (1972) working with the knowledge that corticotrophin-releasing factor (CRF) and other trophic hormone releasing factors are concentrated in the synaptosome fraction of the hypothalamus (Mulder, Gueze and De Wied, 1970) have demonstrated that synaptosome preparations of this type can be used as model systems for studying the release of neurosecretory substances. Electrical and potassium stimulation causes the release of CRF, vasopressin and prolactin inhibitory factor into the incubating medium, this release being Ca^{2+} dependent. In subsequent work Bennett and Edwardson (1973) demonstrated inhibition of CRF release by corticosteroids applied *in vitro* and *in vivo*. ACh stimulates CRF release *in vitro*, a process blocked by atropine and dopamine.

4.3 AUTORADIOGRAPHY OF NEUROTRANSMITTERS

The technique of autoradiography serves to bridge the gap between biochemistry and morphology, allowing both the detection and location of radioactive atoms in biological structures (Droz, 1969). When used in conjunction with data derived from cytochemical techniques (Section 4.4), it helps reveal structures with particular chemical compositions, making them susceptible to quantitative analysis. Nowhere are these approaches more relevant than in the area of neurotransmitters.

EM autoradiography is being used to a considerable extent to localize neurotransmitters, principally monoamines (e.g. Aghajanian and Bloom, 1966, 1967a, b; Lenn, 1967; Descarries and Droz, 1970; Sotelo, 1971b; Bloom, 1972a; Sotelo and Taxi, 1973) and amino acids (e.g. Ehinger, 1970; Hökfelt and Ljungdahl, 1970; Bloom and Iversen, 1971; Ehinger and Falck, 1971; Matus and Dennison, 1971; Sotelo, Privat and Drian, 1972; Frontali and Pierantoni, 1973). The principle underlying these localization attempts is that transport systems with high specificity and high affinity for their substrates exist for virtually all the known transmitters (see Snyder *et al.*, 1973). In addition, the application of autoradiographic analysis of protein synthesis in synaptosomal fractions has made an important contribution to the debate on the sites of protein synthesis (Autilio *et al.*, 1968; Droz and Barondes, 1969; Bosman and Hemsworth, 1970; Cotman and Taylor, 1971), while attempts at separating synaptosomes into two or more populations on the basis of their neurotransmitter content have been significantly advanced by autoradiography (e.g. Iversen and Snyder, 1968; Green *et al.*, 1969).

4.3.1 Monoamine localization

This extensive field is introduced at this juncture because of the light it throws on the autoradiographic localization of amino acids, an area far less adequately worked through at present.

In peripheral tissues monoaminergic neurons have been identified using a range of techniques, namely, fluorescence microscopy, EM identification of DCV and EM autoradiography, the latter procedure both strengthening evidence already obtained using the other techniques and itself being validated by them (e.g. Hökfelt and Ljungdahl, 1971b). While the same principle applies in the CNS, EM identification of monoaminergic nerve terminals is more difficult (see Hökfelt, 1965), with the result that EM autoradiography assumes greater importance. In the CNS, labelled NE can be localized in nerve terminals and cell bodies of adrenergic neurons either when the labelled catecholamine is injected into the cerebrospinal fluid *in vivo* or when brain slices are incubated with labelled NE (Aghajanian and Bloom, 1966, 1967a; Ishii and Friede, 1967, 1968; Lenn, 1967; Fuxe, Hökfelt, Ritzen and Ungerstedt, 1968; Descarries and Droz, 1970; Hökfelt and Ljungdahl, 1971b). Examples of these localizations are shown in Plates 4.1 and 4.2. In these studies the uptake of labelled NE is not confined to adrenergic neurons but includes certain dopaminergic neurons in some situations.

The uptake of labelled 5-HT is primarily by 5-HT-containing neurons when studied by EM autoradiography (Aghajanian and Bloom, 1967b; Kuhar and Aghajanian, 1973). However, as Shaskan and Snyder (1970) have demonstrated, 5-HT is also taken up by adrenergic neurons, casting doubt on the specificity of the procedure in the absence of prior destruction of adrenergic terminals.

Synaptosomal studies undertaken by Coyle and Snyder (1969) suggest that in various regions of rat brain, labelled NE is taken up predominantly by synaptosomes. Quantitative EM autoradiographic studies in Iversen's laboratory (see Iversen and Schon, 1973), confirmed these results and carried them further, demonstrating that ^{3}H-NE is taken up in an 'all or none' fashion by certain synaptosomes and not others. More specifically, their results indicated that about 5% of all synaptosomes from rat cerebral cortex are noradrenergic, and about 16% of those from rat neostriatum dopaminergic.

An alternative to the above procedures in which the labelled amines themselves were applied exogenously is to administer the labelled precursor L-DOPA (3, 4-dihydroxyphenylalanine). Using this method, Descarries and Havrankova (1970) described autoradiographic labelling in neurons in the locus coeruleus and hypothalamus. An allied procedure is the localization of labelled drugs such as 6-hydroxydopamine, found by Ljungdahl, Hökfelt, Jonsson and Sachs (1971) in adrenergic nerve terminals.

4.3.2 Amino acids – GABA localization

The evidence favouring GABA as an inhibitory transmitter has been briefly considered previously (Section 4.1.4). Its transmitter role is assumed in the present discussion.

EM autoradiographic studies of labelled GABA uptake can be categorized according to whether carried out on (a) brain slices incubated *in vitro*, (b) homogenates incubated *in vitro*, or (c) labelled *in vivo*.

Slices and synaptosomes from rat cerebral cortex were found by Iversen and Neal (1968) to actively accumulate ^{3}H–GABA when incubated *in vitro*. This was in line with evidence previously obtained by a number of other workers (Elliott and Van Gelder, 1958; Weinstein, Varon, Muhlemann and Roberts, 1965). Furthermore, it was noted by Iversen and Neal that, following brief incubations with ^{3}H–GABA, the unchanged amino acid accumulated in the tissue without any significant accumulation of labelled metabolites. Also of relevance is the observation that electrical stimulation of cortical slices releases labelled GABA (Srinivasan, Neal and Mitchell, 1969), which has a subcellular distribution similar to that of endogenous GABA (Neal and Iversen, 1969). Against this background, Bloom, and Iversen (1971) adapted LM autoradiography for the localization of GABA-containing structures in the CNS (Ehinger, 1970) for an equivalent EM investigation.

Using cortical slices incubated *in vitro* with ^{3}H–GABA, Bloom and Iversen (1971) and later Iversen and Bloom (1972) found it localized over small nerve terminals and axons (Table 4.6; Plate 4.3). The labelling of nerve terminals occurred in an 'all or none'

Table 4.6 Localization of ^{3}H-GABA in rat cortical slices (From Iversen and Bloom, 1972)

	(Average % ± S.E.M. (n = 5)) Surface area	Silver grains
Glial cells	13 ± 1	2 ± 0·1
Neurone Perikarya + Dendrites	39 ± 3	11 ± 2
Myelinated Axons	5 ± 2	1 ± 0·1
Unmyelinated Axons	14 ± 1	11 ± 1
Nerve Terminals	23 ± 4	71 ± 2
Space	5 ± 1	3 ± 1

Values are means ± S.E. for five randomly selected low power electron micrographs. The area of tissue in each micrograph was 275 μm^2.

manner, the proportion of labelled terminals being constant at approximately 30% whatever the exposure times (Table 4.7). Further work on slices of cerebellum and substantia nigra confirmed these results, the percentage of labelled terminals rising to approximately 50% in the granular layer of cerebellum and the substantia nigra (Iversen and Schon, 1973).

In cortical slices Iversen and Bloom (1972) demonstrated that whereas ^{3}H–GABA accounted for 71% of all autoradiographic activity over nerve terminals, these terminals constituted only 23% of the total cellular surface area (Table 4.6). A similar analysis of the

Table 4.7 Proportion of labelled terminals after different exposure times (From Iversen and Bloom, 1972)

Sample	Proportion of labelled terminals as % 10 days exposure	20 days exposure	30 days exposure
Cerebral cortex slices—GABA	27·0 ± 2·4 (12)	27·2 ± 3·0 (5)	
Cerebral cortex homogenate—GABA	30·7 ± 2·38 (8)	33·7 ± 2·47 (12)	34·5 ± 2·52 (5)
Striatum homogenate—GABA	35·4 ± 2·36 (5)	30·8 ± 3·23 (4)	34·0 ± 1·45 (5)
Hippocampus homogenate—GABA	38·3 ± 2·84 (6)	45·4 ± 2·59 (6)	
Spinal cord homogenate—GABA	25·1 ± 2·00 (6)	24·0 ± 1·46 (5)	
Spinal cord homogenate—glycine	25·2 ± 2·32 (7)	29·4 ± 2·14 (7)	

distribution of silver grains over the various particulate bodies in homogenate samples of hypothalamus yielded a comparable result, 72% of the autoradiographic activity being located over synaptosomes (cf. Iversen and Johnston, 1971; Plate 4.4). The percentage of synaptosomes labelled varied considerably from 13% in cerebellar homogenates to 42% in hippocampus homogenates, with intermediate values being recorded by homogenates of medulla/pons, cerebral cortex, striatum and hypothalamus (Iversen and Bloom, 1972).

153

In spinal cord homogenates approximately 25% of synaptosomes are labelled by ^{3}H–GABA (Section 4.3.3).

Synaptosomal studies have a number of advantages over those using cortical slices. Firstly, as glial cells and nerve cell bodies are presumably either removed or at least present only as minor contaminants in synaptosomal preparations, alternative sites of ^{3}H–GABA uptake are removed (Iversen and Schon, 1973). Secondly, statistical analysis of the proportion of labelled terminals present in a population is far more readily and reliably accomplished using synaptosomes than intact slices. Lastly, the good preservation of tissue which is feasible using synaptosomal preparations opens the way for distinguishing synaptosomal populations on the basis of their transmitter content. However, as already discussed (Sections 3.4.1 and 3.4.2), synaptosomes labelled with ^{3}H–GABA in Iversen and Bloom's study had little in the way of obvious morphological features to distinguish them from unlabelled synaptosomes.

These results indicate that nerve terminals are the principal sites of uptake of ^{3}H–GABA in certain nerve terminals in the CNS, these terminals representing perhaps 30% of all synaptic terminals in many CNS regions (Iversen and Schon, 1973).

Labelled GABA uptake has also been studied in retinae (Lam and Steinman, 1971; Neal and Iversen, 1972), sympathetic ganglia (Bowery and Brown, 1972; Iversen and Schon, 1973), and crustacean nerve muscle preparations (Orkand and Kravitz, 1971). While these investigations are far more preliminary than those already discussed, they point to a diversified localization in these situations with a marked glial localization in retina and sympathetic ganglion.

In order to circumvent difficulties associated with the poor preservation of fine structure in tissue slices incubated *in vitro*, labelling with ^{3}H–GABA *in vivo* has been investigated (Schon and Iversen, 1972; Iversen and Schon, 1973). The pattern of neuronal labelling after *in vivo* experiments confirms that seen after *in vitro* studies, although labelling of neuronal perikarya was seen far more clearly in the *in vivo* situations. In addition to these neuronal sites of ^{3}H–GABA uptake after injection of the labelled amino acid *in vivo*, there are a number of non-neuronal sites—ependymal cells, pial membranes and cerebral blood vessels—regions with high GABA–Glu transaminase activity (Van Gelder, 1967). In a number of brain regions uptake over various glial elements, particularly oligodendroglia, is prominent in *in vivo* studies (Iversen and Schon, 1973).

4.3.3 Amino acids – glycine localization

A number of studies have demonstrated a specific, high affinity uptake system for glycine in spinal cord and brain stem (Neal and Pickles, 1969; Johnston and Iversen, 1971; Logan and Snyder, 1971, 1972; Neal, 1971). In EM autoradiographic studies Hökfelt and Ljungdahl (1971a) and Matus and Dennison (1971, 1972) reported labelling of ^{3}H–glycine over some nerve terminals, small myelinated axons and oligodendroglia (Plates 4.5 and 4.6). According to Hökfelt and Ljungdahl approximately 50% of boutons are labelled, while 30% of the total number of silver grains overlie boutons. Matus and Dennison, in their spinal cord material, were able to distinguish between terminals containing round vesicles and those characterized by flattened ones (Section 1.2.2), and they made the striking observation that silver grains were only found over those containing flattened vesicles (1971; Plate 4.7). Although only approximately 60% of these flattened vesicle terminals are labelled (1972), the association such as it is tends to confirm the postulated relationship between flattened vesicles and inhibition (see Gray, 1969a).

A drawback recognized by Matus and Dennison (1972) is that incubation with exogenous glycine *in vitro* results in tissue preservation which is far from optimal. This has so far curtailed any detailed analysis of the terminals labelled by ^{3}H–glycine, and is undoubtedly responsible for some of the discrepancies between the results of Hökfelt and Ljungdahl, and Matus and Dennison.

Iversen and Bloom (1972), in the study discussed previously (Section 4.3.2), analysed the uptake of ^{3}H–glycine by synaptosomes. Using EM autoradiography, a similar pattern of labelling was seen compared with ^{3}H–GABA, 25–30% of the synaptosomes being labelled (Plate 4.8). When a spinal cord homogenate was labelled by simultaneous exposure to a mixture of ^{3}H-glycine and ^{3}H–GABA, about 50% of the synaptosomes were labelled. As approximately 25% of synaptosomes were labelled when the amino acids were used separately, this result was interpreted by Iversen and Bloom as indicating that the two amino acids are accumulated by distinct subpopulations of the nerve terminals in spinal cord (Section 4.3.4).

No EM autoradiographic studies have so far been conducted on glutamate or other putative transmitter amino acids in the CNS (see Johnson, 1972). However, glutamate and aspartate exhibit high affinity components in their uptake by synaptosomes (Logan and Snyder, 1971), while incubation studies with ^{3}H–glutamate at the LM level point to its localization over glial elements (Hökfelt and Ljungdahl, 1972—cerebellar slices; Ehinger and Falck, 1971—retina *in vivo*).

4.3.4 Separating synaptosomal populations

As discussed in previous sections (e.g. 1.2.1, 2.4.2 and 3.4), a range of criteria has been developed for separating synaptic and synaptosomal populations on morphological grounds. Although suggestive, these studies have fallen short of providing readily recognizable criteria by which nerve terminals containing various transmitters can be distinguished from one another. The possibility of using EM autoradiography to label specific neurotransmitters and hence localize them to distinct synaptosomal subfractions raises exciting prospects in this direction. A series of experiments from Snyder's laboratory has provided the groundwork for such an approach.

Initially, Iversen and Snyder (1968) used single regions of the brain labelled with two putative transmitters. Using whole homogenates of striatal slices of rat brain, Iversen and Snyder labelled them with a mixture of ^{14}C–NE and ^{3}H–GABA. Following centrifugation on continuous sucrose density gradients, a clear separation of particle populations was obtained with the peak of ^{14}C–NE at a denser level of sucrose than that of ^{3}H–GABA (Fig. 4.5). A similar separation of ^{14}C–GABA particles and ^{3}H–dopamine particles was also achieved, although they were unable to separate ^{3}H–dopamine particles from ^{14}C–NE ones.

In a parallel study Green *et al.* (1969) examined the subcellular localization of ^{3}H– and ^{14}C–NE in four different brain regions. When slices from different regions were incubated with ^{3}H–NE or ^{14}C–NE, combined, homogenized and centrifuged on continuous sucrose density gradients, different patterns of subcellular localization were observed in hypothalamus, striatum, cerebral cortex and medulla-pons. From these results they concluded that catecholamine-containing nerve terminals from different areas of the brain vary in density and can be separated by density gradient centrifugation. More specifically, these synaptosomes could be ranked in order of increasing sedimentation density, namely, hypothalamus < medulla oblongata-pons < cerebral cortex < striatum (Snyder, 1970).

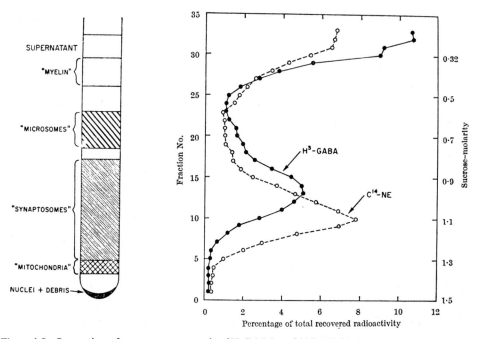

Figure 4.5 Separation of synaptosomes storing ^{3}H-GABA and ^{14}C–NE in the corpus striatum. Slices of tissue were incubated with a Krebs–Henseleit solution to which ^{3}H–GABA and ^{14}C–NE were added; they were then homogenized in sucrose, centrifuged on a continuous linear sucrose density gradient, after which the ^{3}H and ^{14}C labels were determined in 33 fractions. (From Iversen and Snyder, 1968)

Following on from the Iversen and Snyder (1968) study, Kuhar *et al.* (1970) employed crude mitochondrial pellets as their starting point in order to eliminate the cellular debris of whole homogenates. Varying amounts of the crude mitochondrial tissue were layered on continuous sucrose gradients which were centrifuged to density equilibrium. This study confirmed the separation of GABA and catecholamine particles in striatum, and also demonstrated that the extent of separation was dependent on the amount of tissue placed on the gradient but independent of incubation time or isotopic label (Fig. 4.6).

EM observations of the various synaptosomal fractions revealed certain morphological differences between the 'catecholamine' and 'GABA' particles. The area of the gradient with peak catecholamine content contained relatively few synaptosome profiles interspersed with large numbers of free mitochondria, the synaptosomes themselves having a fairly uniform appearance with vesicles 30–40 nm in diameter, a dense cytoplasm in some instances and a visible synaptic junctional region in others. The synaptosomes of the GABA peak were larger although their diameters were highly variable, while adherent

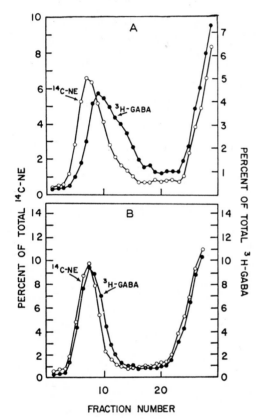

Figure 4.6   Effects of amount of tissue on separation of ^{14}C–NE and ^{3}H–GABA in continuous sucrose gradients. In A, the entire P$_2$ pellet was resuspended and layered on the gradient. In B, the P$_2$ pellet was resuspended and a quarter of it layered on the gradient. (From Kuhar *et al.*, 1970)

postsynaptic membranes were infrequent. There were few free mitochondria in this peak. These results taken in isolation do not constitute sufficient evidence to distinguish between catecholamine and GABA synaptosomes, particularly since there is considerable variation in the number of free mitochondria in the fractions. It is also possible that synaptosomes storing other transmitters exist in the fractions. Nevertheless this approach is a potentially powerful one, opening the way to the classification of synaptosomes into different types with different transmitters.

Following up these observations, Gfeller *et al.* (1971) demonstrated that synaptosomes from denser gradient fractions rich in NE, dopamine, 5–HT and ACh have an increased frequency of adherent postsynaptic elements and intraterminal mitochondria compared with those in lighter portions of the gradients rich in GABA. This distinction may

157

suggest a difference in the macromolecular constitution of the cleft region in the different synaptosomal populations (Jones, 1972). However, even if this is so, it does not answer the question whether it may one day be possible to identify neurotransmitters on the basis of the morphological appearance of synaptosomes, and perhaps ultimately of intact nerve terminals (Gfeller *et al.*, 1971). The case for such morphological distinctness remains to be proved.

The direct application of EM autoradiography is a related approach and the separation of synaptosomes accumulating glycine from those accumulating other amino acids illustrates the progress made to date. Arregui *et al.* (1972) have provided evidence for the existence of a spinal cord synaptosomal fraction selectively accumulating glycine, the particles in this fraction sedimenting to a less-dense portion of the sucrose gradients than particles accumulating neutral, basic, aromatic and acidic amino acids. This fits in with the earlier evidence of Iversen and Johnston (1971) that ^{14}C-glycine and ^{3}H–GABA are probably taken up by different synaptosomes in homogenates of rat spinal cord. The differential labelling of synaptosomes for glycine or GABA, noted by Iversen and Bloom (1972) in their EM autoradiographic study (Section 4.3.3), confirms this separation of synaptosomal populations. It is unfortunate that no clear morphological differences could be detected between the synaptosomes labelled with GABA and glycine. A combination of techniques however, with direct EM autoradiographic study of synaptosomes containing known transmitters may help overcome the present morphological impasse.

4.3.5   Protein turnover in axons and nerve endings

Considerable controversy has surrounded the turnover of proteins in axons and nerve endings, and conflicting interpretations have been rife. Subcellular fractionation techniques have been used extensively in these studies, although the difficulty of obtaining fractions free of contaminants, particularly membranes, has proved a drawback. Autoradiography is therefore a most useful ancillary tool in this situation and its role in these investigations will be briefly reviewed.

Proteins transported at a fast rate from the cell body along the axon have been principally located in the particulate fractions of brain homogenates, principally the synaptosomal fraction (e.g. Barondes, 1969; Cuénod and Schönbach, 1971; Ochs, 1972). The application of EM autoradiography has pinpointed these protein molecules in peripheral regions of axons and within nerve endings themselves. The actual components of these labelled areas include the axolemma, axoplasm and agranular endoplasmic reticulum of the axon (e.g. Schönbach, Schönbach and Cuénod, 1971; Lentz, 1972), and the synaptic vesicles, mitochondria, microfilaments and presynaptic membrane of the nerve ending (e.g. Droz and Barondes, 1969; Koenig and Droz, 1971; Hendrickson, 1972; Droz, Koenig and Di Giamberardino, 1973).

Proteins transported at a slow rate appear in the 'soluble' and 'mitochondrial' fractions on subcellular fractionation (e.g. Barondes, 1969; Cuénod and Schönbach, 1971; Ochs, 1972). Further localization of these proteins with EM autoradiography has confirmed their axonal localization, the axoplasm itself and associated microfilaments, the axolemma, endoplasmic reticulum and mitochondria, being labelled (Droz, 1967; Hendrickson, 1972). What is in dispute is whether any of the slowly moving proteins pass into nerve terminals and contribute towards the renewal of presynaptic components (Droz and Barondes, 1969; Cuénod and Schönbach, 1971; Karlsson and Sjöstrand, 1971). The alternative is that they remain within the axon (Grafstein, 1969; Hendrickson, 1972).

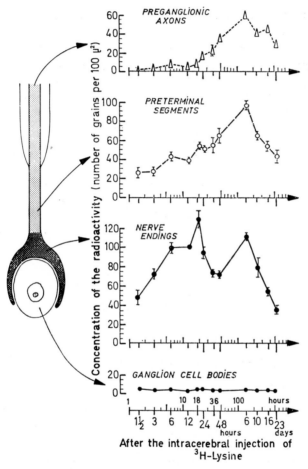

Figure 4.7 Time curves of the concentration of radioactivity in preganglionic axons, preterminal segments, calciform nerve endings and ganglion cell bodies. (From Droz *et al.*, 1973)

This latter issue has recently been reinvestigated by Droz and co-workers (Droz *et al.*, 1973), who have also reviewed current autoradiographic evidence. After the intracerebral injection of ³H–lysine a significant amount of the label begins to appear in nerve terminals after 1–1·5 h, from which it has been estimated that they have migrated along the axons at 288 mm/day. The peak of labelling observed in nerve endings at 18 h (Fig. 4.7) probably reflects the accumulation of labelled protein either transported at a slower rate or synthesized at a later time (Droz *et al.*, 1973). The second peak of radioactivity in preganglionic axons and their terminals (Fig. 4.7) is probably the result of the arrival of

159

proteins transported at a slow rate of 1·5–10 mm/day. According to a kinetic analysis of the movements of these proteins, Droz and Di Giamberardino (1973) have estimated that less than 5% of the slowly moving proteins enter nerve endings.

Within nerve endings, areas rich in synaptic vesicles contain more label than those regions devoid of them from 1·5–18 h after the intracerebral injection of ^{3}H–lysine (Fig. 4.8; Plates 4.9 and 4.10). In the light of these results Droz et al. (1973) conclude that most of the radioactive proteins rapidly transported to these areas are associated with the synaptic vesicles themselves, and this in turn suggests that some macromolecular material rapidly transported along the axons is essential for the maintenance of synaptic vesicles in nerve endings. Following the 18 h peak (Fig. 4.7) the rapid fall of the label, particu-

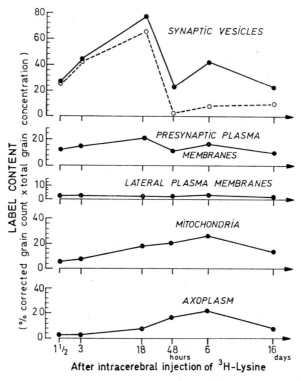

Figure 4.8   Time curves of label content in various components of presynaptic calices, after the intracerebral injection of ^{3}H–lysine. The dotted line corresponds to the radioactivity probably associated with synaptic vesicles. (From Droz et al., 1973)

larly in vesicle-rich areas, points to a high turnover rate (0·1·10^{-2} min^{-1}) of certain protein subunits associated with synaptic vesicles (Droz et al., 1973).

The discussion thus far has assumed that all, or most, of the proteins detected in nerve endings result from their transport along an axonal pathway, rather than from the *in situ* synthesis of new proteins within the nerve endings themselves. Of the mass of evidence, much of it indecisive, a number of observations may be cited as relevant. In ciliary ganglia either incubated *in vitro* in a medium containing labelled amino acids (Droz and Koenig, 1971) or labelled *in vivo* (Droz and Koenig, 1969), the concentration of the radioactivity after 3–4 h is higher in the cell bodies than the nerve terminals. By contrast, only after the intracerebral injection of the labelled amino acid is the distribution reversed. The accumulation of labelled proteins in nerve endings following intracerebral injection does not correspond therefore to the local incorporation of the label (Droz *et al.*, 1973). Allied with this is the further observation that when axonal transport is interrupted a number of nerve terminals are not labelled in spite of the accumulation of label within axons. The migration of proteins along axons would appear therefore to account for the greater proportion of labelled proteins at nerve terminals (e.g. Droz *et al.*, 1973).

One other contentious issue is whether protein molecules present in nerve terminals can move into postsynaptic structures (e.g. Korr, Wilkinson and Chornock, 1967; Globus, Lux and Schubert, 1968; Grafstein, 1969). Care is required to ensure that protein is not being synthesized in the postsynaptic cells, as proteins may be transferred from the presynaptic terminals either as macromolecules or free labelled amino acids (Graftsein, 1971). Even if it is argued that only a limited number of protein or peptide molecules are transferred from one neuron to another, these molecules may still play an important role in the exchange of information between neurons (Droz *et al.*, 1973).

Fractionation studies combined with EM autoradiography have been little used so far in studies of this nature (Droz and Barondes, 1969; Cotman and Taylor, 1971; Di Giamberardino, Bennett, Koenig and Droz, 1973). These studies support those in intact tissue, demonstrating the labelling of synaptosomes and their constituents, the ability of synaptosomal preparations to incorporate label into polypeptides and the association of rapidly labelled protein macromolecules with synaptosomes.

Autoradiographic techniques have also been used to trace labelled glycoproteins along axons to nerve endings following the administration of ^{3}H–fucose and ^{3}H–glucosamine (Bennett, Di Giamberardino, Koenig and Droz, 1973). These workers demonstrated the rapid transport of glycoproteins along axons, with one fraction accumulating as components of synaptic vesicles and presynaptic plasma membranes, and a second one participating in the renewal of axolemmal glycoprotein.

4.4 CYTOCHEMISTRY OF SYNAPSES AND SYNAPTOSOMES

Cytochemical approaches to synaptic organization can be subdivided into two main categories: (a) those employing a dye to demonstrate chemical components and (b) those utilizing enzymic digestions (Jones, 1972). In addition, the area of enzyme cytochemistry or histochemistry should also be mentioned. These general approaches encompass such staining techniques as those utilizing ruthenium red (Luft, 1965, 1966, 1971a, b), PTA (Benedetti and Bertolini, 1963; Pease, 1966), bismuth iodide (Bobtelsky and Cohen, 1960), and periodic acid (Churg, Mautner and Grisham, 1958), as well as those for certain enzymes involved in neurotransmission, namely, AChE, ChAc and GABA. Enzymic digestion studies have principally looked to trypsin, pepsin, pronase, hyaluronidase, neuraminidase and bromalin as the digestive agents (e.g. Leduc and Bernhard, 1961; Monneron and Bernhard, 1966).

Although principally developed for the study of plasma membranes in general, these cytochemical techniques have been successfully adapted for synaptic studies. Their application to synaptosomal preparations is, in a number of instances, in an early stage of development, and where this is the case synaptic results alone will be considered.

4.4.1 Staining of acidic groups

Acidic groups are stained by a number of cationic heavy metal complexes, including uranyl (Watson, 1958), ruthenium red (Luft, 1965, 1966), colloidal iron (Hale, 1946; Mowry, 1958), lanthanum (Doggenweiler and Frenk, 1965) and colloidal thorium dioxide (Revel, 1964). Of these uranyl and ruthenium red will be considered.

As part of an investigation into the staining action of the BIUL method on synaptic junctions, Pfenninger (1971a) analysed the chemistry of uranyl staining. He noted that thin sections of glutaraldehyde-fixed, non-osmicated tissue had virtually no contrast. Section staining this material with either uranyl or lead salts alone had only a minimal effect on contrast, as did lead staining prior to the application of the uranyl salt. A positive effect was obtained however, when the uranyl treatment preceded the lead staining, this combination proving particularly effective on bismuth iodide treated material. These results point to an affinity of lead to uranyl, the uranyl–lead complex reacting with acidic groups (Pfenninger, 1971a; also Hodge and Schmitt, 1960; Huxley and Zubay, 1961; Stoeckenius, 1961), and with the bismuth iodide as well (Pfenninger, 1971a).

A complementary approach to the staining of acidic groups involves the subtraction of possible binding sites of the BIUL components from the total pool of polar tissue residues (Pfenninger, 1971a). This can be accomplished by modifying carboxyl and/or amino groups (Fraenkel–Conrat and Olcott, 1945).

According to Pfenninger (1971a) methylation of carboxyl groups drastically affects uranyl and lead staining of synaptic junctions, but has only a marginal effect on BIUL stained material (Plate 4.11). Acetylation is characterized by its effect on BIUL treated material, the contrast of which decreases markedly. Combined methylation and acetylation leaves little contrast in either BIUL or uranyl and lead stained tissue (Plate 4.11). The methylation result appears to indicate that, in addition to the acidic components which are blocked by methylation as demonstrated by the failure of uranyl and lead staining, basic amino groups are also present at synaptic junctions as demonstrated by the limited effect on contrast in the BIUL material. The reduction in BIUL contrast following the acetylation of amino groups confirms the BIUL affinity for basic amino groups.

The inorganic dye ruthenium red was adapted for EM use by Luft (1964, 1965) who found that it gave good localization in various tissues without resorting to low pHs, and at the same time developed densities in tissues with fine enough granularity to define reliably plasma membrane structure. According to Luft (1971b) ruthenium red stains what are probably acid mucopolysaccharides. With *en bloc* staining, it is mostly excluded by plasma membranes being localized in those extracellular materials having important mechanical functions. Accordingly, it is present intracellularly only when it can penetrate

162

broken membranes, or in exceptional situations such as the T-tubules or sarcoplasmic sacs in certain states of muscle contraction. Luft (1971b) maintains that its exclusion by cell membranes permits the tracing of tortuous cellular invaginations, while the exceptions to its cellular exclusion may be explainable in terms of the function of the cell.

Possible reasons advanced by Luft for the occasional instances of intracellular staining are complex and will not be entered into here. Although Pfenninger (1972) claims to have obtained intracellular deposits on incubating 200 μm thick tissue slices in ruthenium red, the relationship between these deposits and those occasionally observed intracellularly by Luft (1971b) is not clear. Pfenninger (1972) concludes from his observations on tissue slices previously treated with neuraminidase that ruthenium red is a potent agent for the demonstration of anionic groups of every kind.

Turning to synaptic investigations, Bondareff (1967) observed that the granular material within synaptic clefts is stained with ruthenium red, the cleft being filled with its reaction product except for a translucent ridge on either side (Plate 4.12). This intracleft reaction product is continuous with that distributed extracellularly on adjacent plasma membranes. These observations on intact cortical tissue have been repeated with isolated cortical synaptosomes, the reaction product surrounding pre- and postsynaptic components (Jones, 1972, 1974; Plate 4.13). As seen in Plate 4.13 there has been limited penetration of the stain intracellularly, affecting principally the postsynaptic thickening and the cytoplasm between the closely-packed synaptic vesicles. In contrast to these observations based on *en bloc* staining (Luft, 1965), Pfenninger's (1972) staining of tissue slices resulted in more intense staining of these intracellular elements.

Apart from any intracellular localization, the distribution of the reaction product coincides with the position of the external coat of synaptic membranes; the internal coat is visible but largely unstained by the dye while the intermediate coat is electron-translucent (Jones, 1972; Plate 4.13). This reaction has been interpreted by Bondareff (1967) as the existence of a mucopolysaccharide-containing material which (a) adheres closely to the plasma membrane, (b) fills the intercellular gap more or less completely, and (c) is especially dense in synaptic regions. These characteristics make it difficult to distinguish the intercellular space from extensions of the membrane surface (Schmitt and Samson, 1969).

This polysaccharide-rich extracellular coat or 'glycocalyx' (Bennett, 1963) can bind large amounts of water. As the anionic side chains of acid mucopolysaccharides appear to facilitate utilization and transfer of various ions and metabolites (Mathews, 1964; Goldstein, 1969), the intercellular situation of mucopolysaccharides in the neuropil may represent routes for the diffusion of ions and metabolites (cf. the retina—Matsusaka, 1971).

4.4.2 Staining of basic groups

Two principal staining procedures are thought to be capable of staining basic groups, these being the anionic heavy metal complexes, PTA and BIUL. In synaptic studies both are used as *en bloc* stains, although as discussed previously (4.4.1) section staining with uranyl and lead is essential for maximal contrast in the BIUL technique. Non-osmicated, glutaraldehyde-fixed material is mainly used in both cases.

(i) *PTA*. A major consideration with PTA is the specificity of its action, and unfortunately there is not a consensus of opinion on the chemical nature of the reactive groups within tissue sections that are stained by PTA at low pH (for discussion, see Dermer, 1973). For instance Pease (1966) has argued that the material stained by PTA at low pH is probably polysaccharide, the PTA forming hydrogen bonds with hydroxyl radicals common to large complex polysaccharides (Pease, 1970). Similar views have been expressed by Rambourg (1967, 1971), Marinozzi (1968), Rambourg, Hernandez and Leblond (1969), Meyer (1969, 1970) and Dermer (1973).

Over against these views are those of other workers who have presented evidence that at low pH, PTA is anionic and interacts electrostatically with cationic residues, particularly basic protein. Scott and Glick (1971) for example, have shown that with sections exposed to PTA at low pH, hydroxyl groups of sugars can be protonated and interact with PTA. It may be argued therefore that under these conditions PTA does not appear to be specific for polysaccharides. *In vitro* experiments have shown that basic amino acids are precipitated with PTA (Silverman and Glick, 1969; Quintarelli, Cifonelli and Zito, 1971a; Scott, 1971), while decreased PTA staining following deamination (Silverman and Glick, 1969; Quintarelli, Zito, and Cifonelli, 1971b) and amino acetylation (Sheridan and Barrnett, 1967; Quintarelli *et al.*, 1971a) support this contention.

Further evidence in favour of the idea that PTA demonstrates basic amino groups comes from enzyme digestion studies of synaptic junctions. These are dealt with in detail in Section 4.4.4. The findings of Bloom and Aghajanian (1966, 1968) that (a) PTA staining is decreased by amino acetylation and (b) PTA positive material is digested by proteolytic activity and not polysaccharide-degrading enzymes, consitute important evidence in support of this role of PTA.

(ii) *BIUL*. In view of the staining reaction of bismuth iodide impregnation at the ultrastructural level (Pfenninger *et al.*, 1969; Section 1.3.1), a cytochemical study of the reaction was carried out by Pfenninger (1971a). In a series of *in vitro* experiments the chemistry of the bismuth iodide reaction was studied before and after glutaraldehyde fixation. In test tube experiments the addition of bismuth iodide to acidic and neutral polyamino acids produced no visible effect; similarly for hyaluronic and sialic acids. When bismuth iodide was added to basic polyamino acids however, namely polylysine, polyarginine and polyhistidine, there was a prominent precipitate (Plate 4.14a). Electrophoresis yielded a comparable result, the bismuth iodide complex being immobilized and precipitated by the basic polyamino acids tested but not by the neutral or acidic polyamino acids (Plate 4.14b). After glutaraldehyde treatment, polylysine and polyhistidine form the characteristic precipitate, whereas polyarginine together with the acidic and neutral polyamino acids show no reaction.

The bismuth iodide impregnation gives weak contrast, so that in practice it is combined with double staining of the sections with uranyl and lead. The function of the uranyl–lead

164

complex has already been considered (Section 4.4.1). The BIUL complex as a whole appears to be specific for the demonstration of basic tissue components, and without blockade of acidic residues it is a powerful means of demonstrating all polar groups (Pfenninger, 1972). This conclusion points to the overall similarity of the PTA and BIUL techniques especially if the PTA material is section stained with uranyl and lead (Ogawa, Hirano, Saito and Ago, 1970; Pfenninger, 1972).

4.4.3 Staining of carbohydrates

Detailed discussion of the localization of carbohydrates is of little more than peripheral interest for synaptic investigations, except that the cleft material appears to be continuous with the outer 'fuzz' coat of general cell membranes. A detailed examination of relevant techniques will not be entered into here, a succint review of the field having been provided by Pfenninger (1972). (See also Section 4.4.5).

The principal methods of demonstrating polysaccharides depend upon the oxidation of glycols by periodic acid to aldehydes, a number of alternative procedures having been devised at the EM level. Of these only the periodic acid–silver methenamine method has been applied to brain tissue (Rambourg and Leblond, 1967). These investigators concluded that the cell coat consists of material rich in glycoprotein and acidic residues. Lehninger (1968) concluded that the outer 'fuzz' coat of the neuronal membrane contains glycoproteins and glycolipids, these in turn containing gangliosides of which polysialogangliosides may be profuse at nerve endings.

As discussed in the preceding section (4.4.2.), Pease (1966, 1970) has consistently argued for the carbohydrate specificity of aqueous, acidic PTA. Using his 'inert dehydration' preparative technique coupled with aqueous PTA staining of rat cerebral cortex, he described a clearly defined, uniform, densely staining layer of material separated from the adjacent synaptic membranes by translucent bands. This layer, with a width of 16 nm, is probably external to the osmiophilic surface layer of conventionally prepared tissue. Developing this method, Meyer (1969, 1970) obtained a similar picture to Pease (1966) using aqueous acidic PTA. By contrast he noted that anhydrous PTA increased the electron–opacity of the pre- and postsynaptic condensations more than that of the cleft substances which appeared as two parallel lines. He concluded that aqueous, acidic PTA positively points to the presence of polyanionic and polyhydroxyl-containing extracellular substances, whereas affinity for anhydrous PTA demonstrates the presence of basic amino acid-rich proteins which are polycationic in the pre- and postsynaptic cytoplasmic condensations (Jones, 1972).

Pfenninger (1972) has argued that under moderately acidic conditions the PTA anions are bound to basic groups, whereas at very low pH phosphotungstate may become increasingly protonated, the interactions with cationic groups becoming less important and hydrogen bonding to polyalcohols coming to the fore. It is also important to recognize the difference between ethanolic–PTA staining as routinely used in synaptic investigations and acidic–PTA staining. The former does not stain basal laminae, glycogen or the Golgi apparatus, whereas the latter does.

4.4.4   Enzymic digestion

Certain enzymes are characterized by selective degradation properties, a factor which renders enzymic digestion studies of value in analysing the macromolecular components of tissues (Pfenninger, 1972). Developed by Leduc and Bernhard (1961), this technique is a useful, if relatively non-specific, one in a range of studies, including synaptic investigations. As examples of the latter, the principal ones to date are those of Bloom and Aghajanian (1966, 1968), Bondareff and Sjöstrand (1969), Barrantes and Lunt (1970), Pfenninger *et al.* (1970) and Pfenninger (1971b).

Bloom and Aghajanian (1968) found that in tissue blocks stained with PTA and incubated in trypsin the synaptic material with affinity for PTA was largely removed, whereas the membranous components were preserved (Plates 4.16 and 4.17). They interpreted this as demonstrating that synaptic material consists mainly of a protein differing from that of the remainder of the membranes. Pfenninger *et al.* (1970) however, have shown that membrane components contrasted by uranyl and lead are degraded by trypsin, in contrast to the BIUL-positive intracleft lines which show only slight reaction. From these observations they concluded that the dense lines may contain trypsin-labile peptidic components with acidic groups, and the trypsin-resistant membrane components mainly basic groups. This has led Pfenninger (Pfenninger *et al.*, 1970; Pfenninger, 1971b) to propose that the cleft material may maintain the attachment between the apposing neural processes via polyionic binding.

Barrantes and Lunt (1970) performed their trypsin experiments on thin sections subsequently stained with uranyl and lead. Following 10 minutes digestion, the presynaptic area had a netlike appearance, the synaptic cleft was unaffected and the remaining membranous components were extracted. After 1 h, only the subsynaptic web and part of the cleft were visible (Plate 4.15). In terms of this differential extraction they suggested that the composition of the network, dense projections and presynaptic membrane differs from that of the subsynaptic membrane and web. The removal of dense projections by trypsin may point to a relatively high proportion of the basic amino acids, lysine and arginine, in their protein composition.

Pepsin and pronase uniformly prevent the staining of synapses with PTA, BIUL and uranyl–lead alone (Bloom and Aghajanian, 1968; Pfenninger, 1971b), although Barrantes and Lunt (1970) claim that pronase differentially removes the vesicular content of the presynaptic bulb and part of the cleft material. Since pronase has an effect on proteolipids, they speculated that its action depends on the removal of the proteolipids present in the junctional complex.

In PTA and BIUL material digestions with neither hyaluronidase nor neuraminidase have any effect on the staining of the junctions (Bloom and Aghajanian, 1968; Pfenninger, 1971b). These results further implicate the presence of a protein within the material at synaptic contacts. Colloidal iron staining which has been reported to show specificity for acid mucopolysaccharides (Curran, Clark and Lovell, 1965), was found by Bloom and Aghajanian (1968) to have no effect in synaptic material subsequently stained by PTA.

Barrantes and Lunt (1970) extended the range of enzymes used by employing bromalin, which contains at least five different enzymes with distinct proteolytic activities. This resulted in the loss of synaptic vesicles and the appearance of a netlike entity in the presynaptic terminal. They viewed this netlike formation as a probable result of the partial digestion of the protein constituents, thereby rendering them susceptible to the uranyl–lead staining.

The one cytochemical study so far performed on synaptosomes is that by Bondareff and Sjöstrand (1969), in which they demonstrated that some of the sialic acid freed from synaptosomes by incubation in neuraminidase is located extracellularly within the synaptic cleft. Finding that it is gangliosidic in the native state and not associated with mucopolysaccharides, they assumed the cleft material to be mostly protein.

Pfenninger's (1971b) results on intact synaptic junctions confirm Bondareff and Sjöstrand's data and are consistent with the finding of N-acetylneuraminate-bearing glycoproteins and gangliosides in the synaptic area (Brunngraber, Dekirmenjian and Brown, 1967). The neuraminidase-induced loss of acidic groups is much weaker however, in synapses *in situ* than in synaptosomes.

Basic to an understanding of the results of enzymic digestion studies is the method of specimen incubation. For instance tissue blocks may be used and these, in turn, may be fixed or unfixed. Alternatively, thin sections may be employed. Each method has advantages and disadvantages. While unfixed small tissue blocks leave the macromolecules in as natural a state as possible, tissue damage may occur during incubation and penetration of the specimen by the enzyme may be incomplete. Aldehyde-fixed tissue blocks avoid these difficulties as long as potential drawbacks resulting from the aldehyde fixation are considered (see Pfenninger, 1972). Thin sections are useful because cells and cell organelles on the surface of a section are fully exposed to the enzyme solution, while the action of the enzyme is homogeneous throughout the section. A disadvantage follows from the possible retention of substrate fragments *in situ*.

Synaptic connectivity has also been examined by analysing the dissociation of synaptic contacts by incubating them in solutions of high ionic strength prior to fixation (Pfenninger et al., 1970; Pfenninger, 1971b). After incubation in 0·05M or 0·1M–$MgCl_2$, 0·05M or 0·1M–$CaCl_2$, 0·1M–NaCl or 0·1M–$NaClO_4$, BIUL treated synaptic contacts remain intact although sometimes the gap between the intracleft lines appears slightly widened (Plate 4.18d). In higher salt concentrations increasing numbers of presynaptic sites are separated from postsynaptic membranes, but without visible alterations of the external membrane coats (Pfenninger, 1971b; Plate 4.18f; Table 4.8). Incubation in 3M and 5.5M sucrose causes the separation and disruption of many tissue elements, leaving relatively unaltered the majority of synaptic contacts (Plate 4.18c). In some cases the wide separation of pre- and post-synaptic membranes is accompanied by the presence of thin filamentous strands running between the respective external membrane coats (Plate 4.18f). Incubation in high concentrations of EDTA has no discernible effect on synaptic contacts (Plate 4.18e).

These experiments point to a polyionic binding mechanism for synapses, as the dissociation of the cleft can only be brought about by employing polymers of high ionic strength, some of which have a strong affinity for basic amino groups (Ohlenbusch,

167

Table 4.8 Dissociation of synaptic contacts with solutions of high ionic strenth (From Pfenninger, 1971b)

Salt	Concentration (M)	Ionic strength	Effect on synaptic connectivity
NaCl	0·1 –1·0	0·1 –1·0 ⎫	
NaClO$_4$	0·1 –1·0	0·1 –1·0 ⎬ Increasing number of synaptic contacts opened	
MgCl$_2$	0·05–1·0	0·15–3·0 ⎭	
MgCl$_2$	2·0	6·0	Majority of synapses dissociated
CaCl$_2$	0·05–1·5	0·15–4·5	Same as MgCl$_2$
LiBr	2·0	2·0	Majority of synapses dissociated
(NH$_4$)$_2$SO$_4$	2·0	6·0	Majority of synapses dissociated

Olivera, Tuan and Davidson, 1967). If this conclusion is valid the mechanism of synaptic adherence differs from that at desmosome-like junctions (see Pfenninger, 1971b). Furthermore, the material in the synaptic cleft (the 'synaptin' of Schmitt (1969)) differs from the cytoplasmic membrane coat in having a higher membrane content in carbohydrates (Pease, 1966; Meyer, 1969, 1970) and a lower membrane content in stainable noncarboxyl acid residues (Pfenninger, 1971b).

4.4.5 Enzyme cytochemistry

Of the enzymes involved in the ACh system, AChE is the only one to have been investigated in any detail at the histochemical level. The literature is enormous and no attempt will be made here to consider it in anything other than a cursory fashion. ChAc has been histochemically located at the EM level by one or two groups of workers, and interesting as their results are the technique cannot as yet be regarded as routine.

A number of techniques have been employed, with varying degrees of success, to demonstrate the localization of ChE at the ultrastructural level. The principal ones are the azo-dye method (Lehrer and Ornstein, 1959), thiolacetic acid methods (e.g. De Lorenzo, 1961; Barrnett, 1962; Mori, Maeda and Shimizu, 1964; Koelle and Foroglou-Kerameos, 1965; Smith and Treherne, 1965), and thiocholine methods (e.g. Karnovsky, 1964; Brzin, Tennyson and Duffy, 1966; Lewis and Shute, 1966; Shute and Lewis, 1966; Tennyson and Brzin, 1970; Pannese, Luciano, Iurato and Reale, 1971).

Results with the azo-dye techniques were largely disappointing because the reaction product was not sufficiently electron-dense. While more satisfactory, thiolacetic acid methods suffer from a lack of enzyme specificity. Consequently, the thiocholine technique which is highly specific for EM has been modified by various workers to adapt it for different tissues. Among the various methods available are the copper–thiocholine, copper–ferrocyanide thiocholine and gold thiocholine techniques (see for example Bloom and Barrnett, 1966; Davis and Koelle, 1967).

While minor differences exist in the exact localization of AChE in nervous tissue, depending principally on the tissue examined and secondarily on the technique employed, the results as a whole are remarkably clear-cut. Cytoplasmic staining of AChE in cholinergic neurons appears to be confined to the rough endoplasmic reticulum and occasionally to tubules and areas of the nuclear envelope in cell bodies. Mitochondria, lysosomes, the smooth endoplasmic reticulum and most of the plasma membrane are unstained. In cholinergic nerve fibres staining is particularly intense at the axonal membrane, while in synaptic regions staining is usually present around much of the presynaptic terminal, over part of the postsynaptic process and 'in' the synaptic cleft (Lewis and Shute, 1966; Plates 4.19 and 4.20).

Methods for the histochemical localization of ChAc have been developed by Burt (1969, 1970) and Kása, Mann and Hebb (1970a, b). Each of these depends on the precipitation by lead of coenzyme A (Co A) as it is released from acetyl-Co A during the acetylation of choline. The specificity of this technique is increased by using inhibitors of non-specific hydrolysis of the acetyl-Co A (diisopropylphosphorofluoridate, DFP) and of ChAc (e.g. chloroacetylcholine), as demonstrated by Kása *et al.* (1970b) and Kása and Morris (1972).

Unlike the distribution of AChE, ChAc activity occurs in all parts of cholinergic neurons. In the cell body and dendrites, it appears to be connected with ribosomes, vesicles and tubules, with the inner surface of the cell membrane and also free in the cytoplasm (Plates 4.21 and 4.22). In axons, it is attached to axon filaments, the outer surface of vesicles and is also free in the axoplasm. Interestingly, ChAc appears to be localized in a percentage of round synaptic vesicles, but never in flattened vesicles (Kása *et al.*, 1970b; Kása, 1971).

While further refinements are required to these histochemical techniques, particularly the ChAc one, present results point to different localizations of the two enzymes and also different mechanisms for their transport from the cell body to nerve terminal (Kása, 1971; Kása, Mann, Karcsu, Tóth and Jordan, 1973). A postulate of this nature is closely bound up with fractionation studies (Section 4.1.1), and it is therefore disappointing that histochemical techniques have not been exploited in synaptosomal studies. Preliminary investigations however, have demonstrated AChE on the external membrane of both pre- and postsynaptic components of synaptosomes (Teravainen, 1969; Jones, quoted by Whittaker, 1969b; Plate 4.23), although McBride and Cohen (1972) were only able to demonstrate the enzyme on the postsynaptic membrane.

A number of other histochemical techniques deserve mention in relation to synaptic studies, even though at present they are in their infancy. Thiamine pyrophosphat as (TPPase), which with thiamine is essential for the oxidation of lactate and pyruvate (Peters, 1963; McIlwain and Bachelard, 1971) and plays therefore a decisive role in ACh synthesis, can be localized histochemically in synaptic vesicles (Griffith and Bondareff, 1973; Knyihár, László and Csillik, 1973). On further investigation, Csillik, Knyihár, László and Boncz (1974) found that TPPase activity characterizes all synaptic terminals in rat spinal cord, round synaptic vesicles demonstrating the greatest activity with flattened vesicles showing less and DCV failing to react.

Cyclic 3′, 5′-nucleotide phosphodiesterase (PDE) catalyzes the metabolism of cyclic

169

AMP, which in turn mediates catecholamine-induced changes in the excitability of postsynaptic cells (see for example Greengard, McAfee and Kebabian, 1972). PDE is located primarily in synaptosomal fractions (De Robertis *et al.*, 1967b; Weiss and Costa, 1968), while in developing cerebral cortex it is present at birth and increases gradually during the first postnatal month (Weiss, 1971; Schmidt and Lolley, 1973). Histochemical studies of PDE in adult rat cerebral cortex have demonstrated its cytochemical localization at postsynaptic sites on dendritic profiles (Florendo, Barrnett and Greengard, 1971), while in the developing situation Adinolfi and Schmidt (1974) have consistently found reaction product at emerging postsynaptic sites along developing dendrites. This accumulation of reaction product in dendritic profiles prior to morphological synaptic maturation suggests that immature receptor sites may be capable of cyclic nucleotide metabolism.

Bittiger and Schnebli (1974) have investigated the capacity of the plant lectins concanavalin A (con A) and ricin, labelled with ferritin, to bind to synaptosomes. They noted that the synaptic cleft region has the greatest binding capacity for both ferritin–con A and ferritin–ricin, while the cleft region of isolated synaptic junctions is considerably more densely coated with labelled con A. From these results they concluded that the synaptic cleft contains a high density of con A receptors (mannosyl and glucosyl end-groups) and an appreciable number of ricin receptors (galactose end-groups). In addition lectin-binding carbohydrate groups are firmly bound to the cleft region and may be anchored within a part of the postsynaptic web.

4.5 IMMUNOCHEMICAL STUDIES

A number of studies over recent years have demonstrated that antisera against synaptosomes or subsynaptosomal components can be used to investigate the structure of nerve membranes plus various aspects of information transfer between nerve cells. Antisera to synaptosomal preparations (De Robertis, Lapetina, Saavedra and Soto, 1966; Mickey, McMillan, Appel and Day, 1971; Herschmann, Cotman and Matthews, 1972) together with antisera to isolated synaptosomal membranes (Lim and Hsu, 1971; Jarosch and Precht, 1972) have been the methods adopted to date.

An additional dimension is that provided by the histochemical localization of the antigen, an approach attempted by Kornguth *et al.* (1969) and Livett, Rostas, Jeffrey and Austin (1974).

Using this range of techniques it has been possible to investigate a number of parameters, including the detection of brain-specific proteins (Lim and Hsu, 1971), and the effects of synaptosomal or synaptosomal membrane antisera on various aspects of neuronal electrical activity (Wald, Mazzuchelli, Lapetina and De Robertis, 1968; Costin, Cotman, Hafemann and Herschman, 1972; Jarosch and Precht, 1972) and on the permeability of neuronal membranes (Raiteri, Bertollini and La Bella, 1972). In addition, preliminary investigations have been carried out in attempts to gain information about specific components in the pre- and postsynaptic membranes (De Robertis, Lapetina and Wald, 1968; Rostas and Jeffrey, 1973; Livett *et al.*, 1974).

4.5.1 Cerebral electrical activity

Interest in immunological studies of the CNS was aroused by the findings of Mihailović and Janković (1961, 1965) that extracts from certain regions of the cat brain are capable of producing antibodies which, following intraventricular injection, modify cerebral electrical activity. Furthermore, they suggested the antigen was regionally specific. In these, and later studies crude homogenates of various brain regions have been used as antigens to produce antisera, which in turn evoke changes in the electrical activity of the structures for which they are specific (Mihailović and Janković, 1961; Mihailović, Janković, Beleslin, Milošević and Cupić, 1965; Janković, Rakić and Sestović, 1969). These studies however, are limited by the degree of purity of the immunogens used, and it is in an attempt to increase their purity that antisera against synaptosomes, or preferably synaptosomal membranes, have been developed (Wald *et al.*, 1968; Jarosch and Precht, 1972).

Wald *et al.* (1968) in their study using antiserum against synaptosomal membranes from cat cerebral cortex, noted that when applied to mollusc neurons in the presence of complement this antiserum produced a progressive, permanent deterioration of bio-electric activity. This effect was not produced by normal rabbit serum with complement nor by anticollagen serum with or without complement. The need for complement with the membrane antiserum suggested a cytolytic action, a postulate confirmed by ultrastructural findings (De Robertis *et al.*, 1968). This cytolytic action principally affected the limiting membrane of synaptosomes, with loss of axoplasm and synaptic vesicles. In mollusc ganglia the structural damage was mainly of plasma membranes with, in addition, separation of neuronal and glial processes. These studies, plus an earlier preliminary one (De Robertis *et al.*, 1966), suggest that the lytic action of the antiserum is confined to the soma and synaptic region of neurons.

Jarosch and Precht (1972) demonstrated that the electrical activity of the trans-synaptic component of the cerebellar parallel fibre system was suppressed by antisera against cerebellar synaptosomal membranes. The specificity of this reaction was demonstrated by the failure of antisera to water-soluble proteins of rat brain extracts to produce a comparable effect. Unlike the results of De Robertis and co-workers, these electrical effects occurred without complement and were reversible, indicating the absence of any permanent damage. No evidence was presented by Jarosch and Precht however, concerning the site of antibody action.

4.5.2 Immunohistochemical localization of antigens

As was seen in the previous section (4.5.1), De Robertis and co-workers used EM to localize the cell components affected by antiserum in their studies. While this has not as yet been followed up by other workers, a complementary technique is that of immuno-fluorescence histochemistry. Kornguth *et al.*, (1969) noted that, when fluorescent-immune γ-globulin solutions reacted with cerebellar cortex, the primary reactive regions were the plasmalemmae of granule cell and Purkinje cell bodies and dendrites. Additional fluorescent areas near the Purkinje cell dendrites appeared as discrete particles, and may represent synaptic contacts. Comparable results were obtained with cerebral cortex slices. By contrast, the cervical cord did not react, pointing perhaps to the possibility that synapses in different regions of the CNS may be antigenically unique.

In order to eliminate as much antigenic contamination as possible, Rostas and co-workers (Rostas and Jeffrey, 1973; Livett *et al.*, 1974) employed antisera raised against an isolated synaptosomal membrane fraction, which is itself relatively free of intrasynaptosomal and glial contaminants (Cotman and Matthews, 1971; Section 2.5.1). Having obtained this fraction from 1-day-old chick forebrain, antisera were prepared to it. Immunofluorescence histochemistry was carried out on cryostat sections of snap-frozen chick forebrain and cerebellum. In the forebrain the antiserum stained structures 2–3 μm in diameter which, allowing for the enlarging effect of a fluorescence halo, could represent synaptic terminals (Plates 4.24 and 4.25). No components in the cell body were stained, while the specificity of the fluorescence was demonstrated by the fact that neither preimmune nor immune serum absorbed with the membrane fraction gave a positive result.

To confirm that the fluorescence was located in synaptic regions, cerebellum and retina, with their well mapped distributions of cells, were investigated. The antigen was indeed observed in areas rich in synapses and axons. For instance, in the cerebellum the white matter and the molecular layer fluoresced strongly, in distinction to the granular layer with its sparse fluorescence and the Purkinje cells with their lack of reaction (Rostas and Jeffrey, 1973; Plate 4.26). Due to the lack of glial staining, the antiserum employed by these workers appears to be specific for neuronal membranes. The staining of white matter and the improbability of much myelin contamination of the original synaptosomal fraction points to the possibility of a common antigenic determinant in both the synaptic and axonal regions of the neuronal membrane (Livett *et al.*, 1974). Since the antigen is probably not present in cell body or dendritic membranes, it appears to be specific for axonal membranes.

Ulmar and Whittaker (1974b) and Widlund, Karlsson, Winter and Heilbronn (1974) have investigated the immunological characteristics of cholinergic synaptic vesicles and have succeeded in raising specific antisera in rabbits to the membrane proteins of homogeneous preparations of cholinergic synaptic vesicles from *Torpedo*. In another investigation Ulmar and Whittaker (1974a) utilized these antisera to localize vesicular membrane proteins in cholinergic tracts and nerve terminals in *Torpedo* tissues using indirect immunohistofluorescence. In this latter study Ulmar and Whittaker noted strong immunofluorescence immediately cranial to a constriction of electromotor nerve axons, a finding consistent with the proximo-distal flow of cholinergic vesicle membrane proteins and possibly of whole vesicles. They also found a lack of immunological homology between *Torpedo* cholinergic vesicles and a mixed vesicle fraction derived from guinea-pig cerebral cortex.

4.5.3   Specificity of antisynaptosome antibodies

Underlying the foregoing discussion are doubts about the antigenic specificity of the synaptosomal or synaptosomal membrane antisera, employed in the investigations. In particular it has been widely recognized that synaptosomal antisera may well have common antigenic determinants with other subcellular fractions, notably mitochondria and myelin (e.g. De Robertis *et al.*, 1968). Furthermore, as synaptic endings themselves contain mitochondria, axoplasm and synaptic vesicles plus pre- and postsynaptic membranes (associated with axons and dendrites or axons and cell bodies), they are immunologically very complex (De Robertis *et al.*, 1966). Consequently, several antigens may be present in them. These may or may not be common to other parts of the neuron. Yet another relevant consideration is the purity of the synaptosomal fraction itself. Contamination with mitochondria, myelin and nonspecific membranes limits the value of any discussion on antigenic specificity. More recent investigations using synaptosomal membrane preparations and utilizing improved fractionation techniques have minimized these drawbacks.

An important aspect therefore of these immunological investigations, in which synaptosomes and synaptosomal membranes are used as antigens to produce antisera against nerve endings, is the improved characterization of the immunological system. To this end a number of studies have concentrated on the specificity and cross-reactivity of antisynaptosome antibodies (Mickey *et al.*, 1971; Herschmann *et al.*, 1972; Raiteri and Bertollini, 1974).

The results of these preliminary studies are conflicting, although certain general principles are beginning to emerge. Herschmann *et al.* (1972) noted cross-reactivity of their antisynaptosome serum with brain mitochondria. This they interpreted as due to synaptosomal contamination with mitochondria. By contrast, Mickey *et al.* (1971) found that synaptosomes and brain mitochondria have some antigenic determinants in common. However, absorption of their antiserum with myelin and mitochondria resulted in a very small percentage of antisynaptosome antibodies still able to react with synaptosomes.

Raiteri and Bertollini (1974) studied the specificity and cross-reactivity of antisynaptosome sera by absorption with various brain subcellular fractions. Absorptions were followed by complement fixation and by observing the decrease of synaptosomal swelling in glycerol solutions caused by incubation with antiserum and complement (Raiteri *et al.*, 1972). They observed that purified myelin and purified mitochondria absorbed antibodies from the antisynaptosome serum, these and other observations indicating that myelin, mitochondria and external synaptosomal membranes share some antigenic determinants. These results, in turn, suggest that a suitable absorption of the antisynaptosome sera is necessary to improve their specificity and to increase their usefulness as tools in the study of synaptic function (Raiteri and Bertollini, 1974).

Chapter 5: The Release of Transmitter at Synapses

5.1 THE VESICLE HYPOTHESIS

Undoubtedly the most significant event in the recent study of the synapse was the demonstration by Katz and co-workers in the early 1950s that ACh is released in discrete quantal packages at the neuromuscular junction (Fatt and Katz, 1952; del Castillo and Katz, 1956; see also Section 1.1.3). Each quantum or package of ACh was thought by Katz (1966, 1969) to contain in the order of 10^3–10^4 molecules of the transmitter, the quanta themselves being released either singly to generate miniature e.p.p.'s or in large numbers in response to a nerve impulse. The result of the latter event is the generation of an endplate potential.

Remarkable as this conception was, its significance was immeasurably enhanced by the description at much the same time of vesicular profiles within the presynaptic terminals at the neuromuscular junction (Robertson, 1956) and at a variety of central synapses (Palay, 1954; Palade, 1954; De Robertis and Bennett, 1954, 1955; Fernandez-Moran, 1957). These early EM observations were almost too good to be true as these characteristic synaptic vesicles, which were especially densely packed in the vicinity of the presynaptic membrane, occupied just the position expected of the quanta, while their diameter of 40–50 nm fitted in with the anticipated size of the quanta (De Robertis and Bennett, 1955; Del Castillo and Katz, 1955, 1956).

De Robertis and Bennett, who coined the term 'synaptic vesicle', accurately reflected the expectations of their contemporaries when they wrote in 1955: 'there is evidence in the literature that two of the substances pharmacologically active at synapses are associated with particles or viscous droplets as found in the cell. It is not unreasonable to speculate that active compounds of this nature might, under some circumstances, be associated with particles or granules or droplets or vesicles of submicroscopic size'.

The scene was thus set for the formulation of the *vesicle hypothesis*, according to which transmitter substances are stored within synaptic vesicles and conveyed by them to the presynaptic membrane. In its fully-developed form this hypothesis states that the synaptic vesicle and the quantum of chemical transmitter are equivalent (Fig. 5.1), from which it follows that quantal release is equivalent to the release of the contents of one vesicle into the synaptic cleft.* For a discussion of this hypothesis see reviews such as those by Katz (1966), Hubbard (1970), Whittaker (1970) and Pfenninger (1972).

The close correspondence between the ultrastructural characteristics of the subcellular particles as *predicted* by the quantal theory and the *actual* vesicles observed by electron

---

* The term *quantal theory* is used here to denote the concept of transmitter release in quanta as postulated originally by Katz. The term *vesicle hypothesis* refers to the equating of quanta with synaptic vesicles, which therefore become the sole means responsible for the transport and release of the transmitter towards and into the cleft.

microscopists was sufficient to assure rapid adoption of the idea by an overwhelming majority of synaptologists. Furthermore, as improved ultrastructural techniques were employed and as an increasing range of chemical and electrotonic synapses were examined, many other expectations were also fulfilled. The vesicle hypothesis therefore appeared to be strengthened and validated with the passage of time.

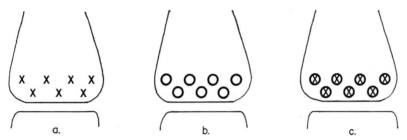

Figure 5.1 Schematic diagram to highlight the relationship between the quantal theory of neurotransmission and the more specific vesicle hypothesis. The 'x's' in (a) represent quantal packets of transmitter in the vicinity of the synaptic cleft. The synaptic vesicles depicted in (b) correspond in size and position to the subcellular particles anticipated by the quantal theory. This is summed up in (c) by the vesicle hypothesis which equates the quantal packets and synaptic vesicles.

In particular, it received immense support from the initial studies carried out by Whittaker in Cambridge and De Robertis in Buenos Aires on the subcellular fractionation of nervous tissue (Whittaker, 1959; Gray and Whittaker, 1960, 1962; De Robertis *et al.*, 1961a, b, 1962a, 1963; Whittaker *et al.*, 1964; Whittaker and Sheridan, 1965). As discussed previously in Section 2.3.1, they succeeded in isolating synaptosomes (Whittaker *et al.*, 1964) from central nervous tissue and convincingly demonstrated the preferential localization within them of ACh and the enzymes of the ACh system, ChAc and AChE. On further subfractionation, the synaptosomes yielded discrete synaptic vesicle and heterogeneous membrane fractions and these revealed that the highest specific concentration of ACh resided in the vesicle fraction and the next highest in the fraction containing disrupted synaptosomes.

The relationship between synaptic vesicles and ACh appeared therefore a close one, and perhaps even a direct one. It is hardly surprising that the conclusion was reached that synaptic vesicles actually correspond to the quanta of transmitter, a necessary equation for the vesicle hypothesis (Fig. 5.1).

This hypothesis represents what may be called the *simple solution* to the problem of neurotransmission. The vesicle hypothesis represents an obvious answer to the demands of the quantal theory. It fits in so nicely with the theory, and fulfils its main prediction in such a neat manner that it may appear sacrilegious even to question it.

This simple solution however, is not as satisfactory as may appear at first glance. It has, for the most part, left unanswered a number of basic questions, the main one of which concerns the *mechanism* of transmitter release. While this was of no major concern during the developmental stage of ideas on neurotransmission, exocytosis being the presumed mode of release, the lack of a satisfactory mechanism came to assume a more important role in people's thinking as exocytosis itself came under fire. In other words, questioning of the presumed mechanism of neurotransmission threw into relief possible inadequacies of the simple solution. This, in turn, reopened the whole issue of the relationship between synaptic vesicles and the quanta of ACh. In order to study this we must first re-examine the various arguments put forward in support of the vesicle hypothesis as well as some of its principal drawbacks. In doing this the essential validity of the quantal theory itself will be assumed. At this stage no attempt is made to deal with those recent studies aimed at analysing exocytosis as a mechanism.

5.2   EVIDENCE CITED IN FAVOUR OF THE VESICLE HYPOTHESIS

Until fairly recently, all the evidence cited in its favour has, of necessity, been circumstantial.* This is necessitated by the lack of a histochemical staining technique for ACh either at the light microscopic or EM levels. The hopes raised by the ZIO technique a few years ago, when it was suggested by Akert and Sandri (1968) that it may be specific for ACh at the EM level, were sadly dashed when it was demonstrated that it stained presumed NE-containing vesicles almost as readily as it stained vesicles in cholinergic terminals (Pellegrino de Iraldi and Gueudet, 1968; Martin et al., 1969; see Section 1.3.4). Even in adrenergic situations, the highly successful fluorescent techniques are at present confined to the light microscopic level, while in autoradiography the grains are large compared with the size of synaptic vesicles and, consequently, this technique is of limited applicability for accurate ultrastructural tracing of neurotransmitter substances.

5.2.1   Subcellular fractionation

The circumstantial evidence provided by subcellular fractionation is in many ways strong. The contribution of these procedures has been a major one and has been further facilitated of late by the isolation of synaptic vesicles from the electric organ of *Torpedo*. This has a purely cholinergic innervation and serves therefore as a source of cholinergic vesicles, in contrast to mammalian brain in which only about 15% of the vesicles are thought to be derived from cholinergic nerve endings (Whittaker, 1966b, 1970; Section 2.4.5).

Fractionation studies initially provided a congenial atmosphere for the reception of the vesicle hypothesis, a necessary phase in the development of any new idea and yet after a while stultifying in the absence of more radical approaches (Sections 2.1.2 and 5.1).

5.2.2   Acetylcholine molecules

An important aspect of the evidence in favour of the vesicle hypothesis revolves around the size of the vesicles. If quanta consist of 10^3–10^4 molecules of ACh as postulated by Katz, vesicles approximately 40 nm in diameter would be filled with almost solid ACh, assuming the higher estimate (Whittaker, 1970). X-ray diffraction studies on vesicle pellets

---

* This may well not be true of Heuser and Reese's (1973) investigation on membrane recycling in neuromuscular junctions (Section 5.4.3).

176

by Whittaker (1970) have not demonstrated the presence of crystalline ACh, rendering this number of molecules (10^4) an unacceptably high one in terms of vesicle size.* Another possibility exists however, and this is that the molecules may be attached to the external wall of the vesicle rather than be accommodated within its core. This appears an unlikely alternative.

Using fractions of synaptic vesicles and tagging the preparations with a known number of polystyrene beads, Whittaker and Sheridan (1965) estimated the number of ACh molecules per cholinergic vesicle at about 2×10^3 (2000). This is close to the number of molecules which would fill a 31 nm diameter vesicle core with isotonic ACh. Convenient at this estimate is, it involves a number of major assumptions, including the percentage of cholinergic synapses in mammalian brain. Corresponding estimates for endings in the electric organ of *Torpedo* are subject to similar difficulties. A tagging procedure similar to that of Whittaker and Sheridan (1965) employed on a vesicle fraction from bovine superior cervical ganglion, a peripheral tissue rich in cholinergic nerve endings (Wilson *et al.*, 1973) gave a mean content of 1630 molecules ACh per vesicle. Comparable estimates from electrophysiological studies range from 10^3 (MacIntosh, 1959) to 10^5 (Krnjević and Mitchell, 1961).

Aware of these and other difficulties Whittaker (1970) is still forced to conclude: 'These results taken as a whole may be regarded as the best direct evidence in favour of the vesicle hypothesis: acetylcholine is indeed present in synaptic vesicles, and in amounts that are not incompatible with the requirements of the quantal hypothesis'.

For comparison, this estimate of the number of ACh molecules per vesicle may be compared with an estimate of 15 000 NE molecules in vesicles of the varicosities of nerve endings in cat gastrocnemius muscle (Folkow and Haggendahl, 1970), and 5000 to 7500 molecules of cyclic AMP per vesicle in mouse brain preparations (Johnson *et al.*, 1973).

5.2.3 Stimulation experiments

If synaptic vesicles are indeed the carriers of the transmitter substance(s) they would be expected to move towards the presynaptic membrane with the arrival of an impulse at the terminal. After releasing the substance into the cleft they may disappear in some way—probably, if exocytosis is the mechanism of release, by fusing with the terminal membrane. The question of the mechanism of release is considered in Sections 5.4 and 5.5. The important point at this juncture is that some change in vesicle numbers should occur with neurotransmission. If such a change does occur it should be detectable on EM examination.

The possibility of detecting morphological changes in terminals during experimental conditions of altered transmitter release or synthesis has proved a spur to investigators using a variety of techniques and experimental models. Among these can be included studies by De Robertis (1958, 1959), Siegesmund, Sances and Larson (1969), Jones and

*Katz (1969) concedes that 10^4 molecules in a 50nm vesicle would give a hypertonic solution, while 10^5 molecules 'would be stretching our imagination a bit too far'. It appears that a more reasonable estimate would be 10^3 molecules.

Kwanbunbumpen (1970), Párducz and Fehér (1970), Párducz, Fehér and Joó (1971a), Jones and Bradford (1971a), Atwood, Lang and Morin (1972), Fehér, Joó and Halász (1972), Korneliussen (1972), Perri, Sacchi, Raviola and Raviola (1972), Pysh and Wiley (1972, 1974), Ceccarelli, Hurlbut and Mauro (1973), Heuser and Reese (1973), Quilliam and Tamarind (1973) and Zimmerman and Whittaker (1973). Unfortunately for the vesicle hypothesis these results have been confusing to say the least. Variations in the precise conditions employed, in the criteria used for analysing vesicle numbers, in the lack of electrophysiological controls in some studies and, of course, variations in the synaptic regions under investigation make assessment difficult. According to a majority of investigators, there is a decrease in the number of synaptic vesicles accompanying electrical stimulation. If however, the vesicles within different regions of the nerve terminal are examined separately it appears the vesicles do not form a homogeneous population. For instance, Perri et al. (1972) noted that vesicle depletion is more pronounced as distance from the synaptic junction increases. In the light of these results they speculated that a trapping mechanism may operate near the synaptic membrane to maintain a high vesicle concentration at the active zone. From this it is but a short step to some results obtained by Jones and Kwanbunbumpen (1970) at the mammalian neuromuscular junction, in which the number of vesicles within 180 nm of the synaptic cleft was estimated. They concluded there was an increase in the number of these vesicles 2 and 4 minutes after stimulation, with an accompanying reduction in synaptic vesicle volume.

Other possibilities to emerge from certain studies include different reactions by different vesicle types (Korneliussen 1972) and by different terminals (Fehér et al., 1972). Needless to say, major difficulties arise when different synaptic types are examined, as is the case with these studies. There is no reason to suppose that exactly the same principle of transmitter release applies in the terminals of neuromuscular junctions, peripheral ganglia and central nervous tissue. For instance, even within the CNS, Fehér et al. (1972) suggest that cortical endings of the specific thalamocortical pathway shows a decrease in vesicle density on stimulation, whereas the endings of the reticulo-cortical neurons contain vesicles which respond by increasing in number.

An interesting sidelight on this controversy was provided by Párducz and co-workers (1971a) with their demonstration that preservation of the normal blood supply to the superior cervical ganglion prevented its exhaustion by electrical stimulation. According to them, the essential element maintaining the density of the synaptic vesicles is choline. Consequently, exhaustive stimulation may be responsible for releasing ACh stored in the synaptic vesicles and also for utilizing the choline which is structurally bound in the presynaptic terminals.

The inhibition of ACh synthesis by HC-3, presumably by competing with choline during its acetylation to form ACh, would be expected to decrease vesicle numbers if applied during stimulation. This indeed appears to be the case, in addition to which there is evidence for a reduction in synaptic vesicle volumes (Elmqvist and Quastel, 1965; Jones and Kwanbunbumpen, 1970; Párducz et al., 1971a). These results provide strong evidence linking synaptic vesicles with ACh stores. The application of HC-3 to unstimulated preparations appears to have little or no effect on vesicle numbers in spite of a depletion in the ACh content of the nerve endings (Hebb, Ling, McGeer and Perkins, 1964; Csillik and Joó, 1967; Rodriguez de Lores Arnaiz et al., 1970). If this release occurs without mobilization of structurally-bound choline, the vesicle numbers may be expected to remain static (Párducz et al., 1971a) as, one imagines, is the balance between the production and disappearance of synaptic vesicles. Consequently, any increase or decrease in the number of synaptic vesicles within presynaptic terminals must be the result of a series of interrelated factors, any one of which may be operative under a given set of circumstances. In view of this, the variable results of stimulation experiments are not surprising. Unfortunately, this lability inherent in the experimental situation makes assessment of the vesicle hypothesis a tenuous exercise.

For instance, Fehér et al. (1972) conclude from their results that the number of vesicles in central and peripheral synaptic endings may rise or fall depending on the functional state of the endings. Even if this statement is valid, its value in terms of confirming or falsifying the vesicle hypothesis is negligible, given the lack of an accurate knowledge of the functional state. Any interpretation can be resorted to as justification for any series of ultrastructural results. Consequently, decrease in synaptic vesicle numbers may demonstrate transmitter release, while an increase may be the result of an excessive supply of new or reconstituted vesicles either from a more proximal portion of the axon or from the terminal itself. And so the possibilities of interpretation can be multiplied. The weakness lies not in the plausibility of these and other interpretations but in the fact that they are merely being used to bolster up the vesicle hypothesis and, consequently, shield it from serious debate.

Stimulation experiments, as noted above, demonstrate unequivocally a relationship between synaptic vesicles and the transmitter substance ACh in the experiments under discussion. This relationship appears to encompass storage of ACh and probably some aspect of its release as well. However, the fate of the vesicles and the origin of the quanta of ACh actually released during neurotransmission remain unanswered queries. These experimental approaches by themselves cannot by their very nature provide solutions to these queries, and in this regard the vesicle hypothesis with its emphasis on the identification of vesicles with quanta remains an elusive theory. Stimulation experiments in isolation from other experimental approaches appear inappropriately designed to provide clear confirmation or refutation of the vesicle hypothesis.

5.2.4   Further experimental tools

The number of synaptic vesicles in nerve terminals can also be reduced by the application of agents such as black widow spider venom (BWSV) and beta bungarotoxin (Chen and Lee, 1970). Of course, BWSV has been investigated in some detail. When applied to neuromuscular preparations it provokes considerable miniature e.p.p. activity and results in a severe depletion of vesicles (Clark, Mauro, Longenecker and Hurlbut, 1970; Longenecker, Hurlbut, Mauro and Clark, 1970; Okamoto, Longenecker, Riker and Song, 1971). A more detailed ultrastructural examination of the events following this increase in miniature e.p.p. frequency was made by Clark, Hurlbut and Mauro (1972). The principal feature noted by them was the conspicuous increase in number of synaptic vesicles in various stages of fusion with the presynaptic membrane, accompanying which was a marked reduction in axoplasmic volume and a possible increase in the surface of the nerve terminal.

These results, like those of stimulation experiments, require explanation in terms of the vesicle hypothesis and, in turn, may cast light on the validity of the hypothesis itself. Unfortunately, as Clark and his co-workers realized, this approach suffers from the same drawback as approaches relying on stimulation, namely, that the miniature e.p.p. activity and the ultrastructural evidence concerning the fusion of the synaptic vesicles with the presynaptic membrane may be separate, unrelated events. In their own words: 'direct, visual proof of the vesicle hypothesis may not be possible'.

Another factor expected to accelerate quantal release is an increase in potassium concentration (Liley, 1956). When a hemidiaphragm is soaked in a solution containing 20mM K^+, as opposed to a normal level of 5mM K^+, a significant reduction in the number of synaptic vesicles adjacent to the synaptic cleft was noted by Hubbard and Kwanbunbumpen (1968). This was part of a general depletion of vesicles, and the fact that this depletion was prevented when magnesium was present argues for a connection between vesicle number and quantal release rate. This connection however, may not be a direct one as the vesicles are involved in a feed-back mechanism by which transmitter synthesis and mobilization are regulated by the demand for transmitter release.

In the light of the possible significance for the vesicle hypothesis of the vesicles close to the presynaptic membrane, a number of workers have concentrated on these. An example has already been encountered in the nerve stimulation experiments of Jones and Kwanbunbumpen (1970), in which they compared vesicle numbers within 180 nm of the synaptic cleft. Quilliam and Tamarind (1973) in similar vein have designated those vesicles within 250 nm of the presynaptic membrane, the 'local vesicle population' (LVP). Following relatively mild stimulation they recorded an increase in the LVP in rat superior cervical ganglia. Replacement of calcium by magnesium had no effect on the LVP, although it did prevent the increase in vesicle numbers following preganglionic stimulation. A reduction in vesicle numbers occurred on the stimulation of ganglia immersed in a high calcium medium or in the presence of drugs such as caffeine, morphine and adrenaline.

These results still do not permit a decision on the vesicle hypothesis, although they strengthen the possibility that the vesicles have a definite role in the process of transmitter release. Quilliam and Tamarind (1973) contend that the decreased LVP in the high calcium medium militates against the possibility that many of the vesicles are 'empty'. This however, is debatable as it fails to account for any recycling of vesicles within the terminal as a whole. Differences in size between 'empty' and 'full' synaptic vesicles, based on evidence from neurosecretory vesicles (Nagasawa, Douglas and Schultz, 1970; Grynszpan–Winograd, 1971), is also used as an argument against the existence of empty vesicles, the contention being that empty agranular vesicles may be too small to recognize (Quilliam and Tamarind, 1973). Interesting as this speculation is, it cannot be tested using available techniques and fails to advance our understanding of this problem.

5.2.5   Status of evidence favouring the vesicle hypothesis

All the evidence just discussed has resulted from investigations directed at confirming the hypothesis itself. Emphasis has been placed on the relationship between the vesicles and quanta, and experiments have been designed with this relationship in mind. As we have seen however, they have been unable to provide an adequate test of the vesicle hypothesis because they have ignored the way in which vesicles release transmitter at the presynaptic membrane, that is, the mechanism of transmitter release. It is only as attention has more recently been directed towards demonstrating the fate of the vesicles and their transmitter that a substantial advance has taken place in this area (Section 5.4.3).

5.3   EVIDENCE DIFFICULT TO HARMONIZE WITH THE VESICLE HYPOTHESIS

5.3.1   Nature of acetylcholine pools

Up to this point the only ACh mentioned has been that found in synaptic vesicles. This belongs to the bound component of ACh described by Whittaker and is associated with the vesicular fraction isolated from brain tissue. In other words, this represents just one of the compartments in which ACh is thought to be situated in nerve terminals (Sections 2.1.2 and 4.1.1).

More specifically the ACh of the neuron exists in three forms, free ACh, labile-bound ACh and stable-bound ACh (Whittaker, 1959; Whittaker et al., 1964; Marchbanks, 1968a). Free ACh exists within the cytoplasm of the neuron, and may be preferentially located within the perikaryon or axon. *Stable-bound* ACh survives hypotonic treatment and is present in synaptic vesicles, whereas the *labile-bound* form fails to survive this treatment and is destroyed in the absence of a ChE inhibitor. Labile-bound ACh occurs predominantly in the cytoplasm of the terminal (Sections 2.1.2, 4.1.1).

The labile-bound or cytoplasmic ACh exchanges with externally applied radioactive ACh (Marchbanks, 1968a), while there is also evidence to suggest that ACh transfer is possible between synaptic vesicles and their surrounding cytoplasm (Chakrin and Whittaker, 1969; Guth, 1969).

The three kinds of ACh differ markedly in their specific radioactivity following injection of radioactive choline *in vivo* (Chakrin and Whittaker, 1969; Whittaker, 1970). It is unlikely therefore, that they can have risen from a single homogeneous pool, pointing towards the validity of thinking in terms of three distinct pools.

The simple solution, with its emphasis solely on the vesicular pool of ACh, fails to consider these other pools. If some form of dynamic interaction between the three pools is assumed therefore, the vesicular pool need not correspond to the final stage in the release of transmitter into the synaptic cleft. Given this assumption, the limitations of the stimulation-based experiment become obvious. Not only this, the simple solution as epitomized by the classic vesicle hypothesis is seen as perhaps one of a number of alternatives. True, the alternatives do not represent straightforward explanations of neuro-transmission, and therefore theoretically stand at a disadvantage as solutions.

Nevertheless, the seeming inability of most workers to devise experimental models to test the simple solution is an important factor in enlarging the range of possible solutions requiring investigation.

This concept of three (or more) compartments housing the ACh within nerve terminals has been elucidated in central synapses. Neuromuscular junctions, which occupy a most important place in discussions on quantal transmission and the vesicle hypothesis, are notoriously difficult to fractionate and it is by no means certain that ACh is similarly distributed within them. Objection to the vesicle hypothesis based upon the compartmentation of ACh therefore may not apply to neuromuscular junctions and their mode of transmission.

5.3.2   Vesicular acetylcholine

The stable-bound ACh associated with synaptic vesicles was regarded initially as a homogeneous store, a concept in line with the simple solution. Further investigation however, has cast doubt upon this, suggesting instead that newly-synthesized ACh is preferentially released (Collier, 1969; Collier and MacIntosh, 1969; Potter, 1970; Whittaker, 1970; Molenaar, Nickolson and Polak, 1971, 1973a; Dunant et al., 1972; Molenaar and Polak, 1973).

In support of this idea Whittaker (1969a, 1970, 1971a) notes that the specific radioactivity of ACh released from the surface of cortex is considerably higher than that of synaptosomes or isolated synaptic vesicles (see also Chakrin, Marchbanks, Mitchell and Whittaker, 1972). From this he concludes (1971a): 'such acetylcholine is released from a small, rapidly turning over store which is not present in synaptic vesicles of the type isolated in fraction D but which may be present in H'.* While this evidence gives no direct clue to the situation of this hot, easily released ACh, its importance lies in the possibility that vesicles which have been regarded as ultrastructurally identical may well be associated with ACh at different stages of the release process. Further relevant evidence is that of Barker et al. (1972) who found that, at short time intervals following the intraventricular administration of labelled choline, synaptosomes contained highly labelled ACh, some of which was readily released from the intact synaptosomes during isolation, the remainder being recovered in fraction H. From these results they suggested that vesicles near the external membrane of synaptosomes become more highly labelled than the rest and are preferentially sedimented into fraction H. Marchbanks and Israël (1971) and Richter and Marchbanks (1971a, b) have reported that vesicle preparations labelled by exposure of tissue blocks to radioactive choline preferentially lose recently synthesized ACh of high specific radioactivity on gel filtration (Section 4.1.1).

Potter (1970), using a neuromuscular preparation, found that newly synthesized ACh was released at least twice as rapidly as preformed stores, while there was a fall-off in the amount of ACh released during unphysiological rates of stimulation until a constant output was reached. These observations have prompted workers to postulate that there exists a small, immediately available fraction of the vesicular ACh, perhaps the of order

* For designations of fractions D and H, see Section 2.3.1.

of 15–20%, which can be released more rapidly than the remainder (see Hubbard, 1971).

Important as these observations and speculations are they do not attempt to resolve the location of the two fractions of vesicular ACh. The obvious proposition is that those vesicles closest to the presynaptic membrane contain the hot, easily released and newly synthesized ACh (cf. Barker *et al.*, 1972), and those more proximally situated the remainder of the vesicular ACh. Tempting as this hypothesis is, ways need to be found of testing it, involving one would imagine the isolation of two populations of cholinergic vesicles. Even if this is accomplished however, questions remain. In terms of this hypothesis the newly synthesized ACh is preferentially located in one group of vesicles, those adjacent to the cleft, and the storage of ACh in another group. If this proves to be the case, is there any communication between the two groups, and if so, what is it and what is its relationship to the functional requirements of the terminal?

These questions are important ones and, until they are resolved, diminish the value of those ultrastructural studies which place great emphasis on vesicles in the vicinity of the presynaptic membrane (e.g. the local vesicle population of Quilliam and Tamarind, 1973). An attempt by Molenaar, Polak and Nickolson (1973b) to locate the subcellular situation of newly-synthesized ACh, enabled them to reach the limited conclusion that the vesicular and cytoplasmic fractions are not identical with the store in the tissue from which this newly synthesized ACh is preferentially released.

Further relevant evidence is provided by examining the *reception* of newly synthesized ACh. It has been found by a number of workers that the vesicular compartment does not preferentially receive newly synthesized ACh (cortical synaptosomes—Marchbanks, 1969; cortical slices—Richter and Marchbanks, 1971b; Collier *et al.*, 1972; *Torpedo* electric organ slices—Marchbanks and Israël, 1971). From these results it may be postulated that a substantial proportion of the ACh released on stimulation comes from the extravesicular component. For instance, Dunant *et al.* (1971) recorded a marked decrease in the extravesicular ACh and little change in the vesicular (bound) ACh on electrical stimulation of slices of *Torpedo* electric organ.

Marchbanks and Israël (1972) argue that this evidence may be compatible with the idea that vesicles filled with recently synthesized ACh are so unstable that they tend to disintegrate when the tissue is homogenized. If this were the case, both extravesicular and released ACh may originate from this labile, vesicular population. Their results show that the monodisperse synaptic vesicle fraction of electric organ contains a small labile compartment of ACh, which is more recently synthesized than the tightly bound ACh of vesicles. However, as they were unable to show that 'membrane-associated vesicles' contain any specific enrichment of the loosely bound component, their results do not support the concept of a discrete population of labile recently filled vesicles (Barker *et al.*, 1970; Whittaker, 1971a).

On the distribution of this loosely bound ACh (Marchbanks and Israël, 1971), these authors (1972) propose that their results are best explained by postulating its existence on or near the surface of all vesicles. According to this concept, all vesicles contain a core of tightly bound ACh and a surface layer of loosely bound ACh, any movement of tightly bound ACh outwards being accompanied by a corresponding movement inwards of the loosely bound form.

The significance of this concept for exocytosis is that as the most recently synthesized ACh probably exists on the surface of vesicles, and as it is this ACh which is released on electrical stimulation, exocytosis would release little of the vesicular ACh (Marchbanks and Israël, 1972). Total exocytosis would only release the core of the vesicles, with its minimal amount of recently synthesized ACh.

A further study of possible relevance to this idea is that of Dowdall and Zimmerman (1974) who describe two pools of ACh in synaptic vesicles isolated from *Torpedo* electric organ. One of them (pool 1) has a high ACh: ATP molar ratio, and is very labile and rapidly lost when the electric organ is stimulated. The other one (pool 2) has a lower ACh: ATP molar ratio. Dowdall and Zimmerman postulate that these pools may correspond respectively with the 'loosely bound' and 'tightly bound' pools of Marchbanks and Israël.

Related to the distribution of ACh within nerve endings is that of the physiologically active amino acids, namely glutamate, GABA and aspartate (Section 4.2). It is of considerable interest that, despite the high sensitivity of the methods available for amino acid detection, none of these amino acids has been found in synaptic vesicle preparations from cerebral cortex after purification by gel filtration (Rassin, 1972; De Belleroche and Bradford, 1973a). This may point to an extravesicular source for released amino acids although in the light of the above discussion on ACh distribution this must remain a tentative conclusion at present. Of the amino acids associated with isolated vesicles, taurine appears to be the most enriched. Its significance is questionable, although it could function as an inhibitory transmitter or could maintain ion gradients in the vesicles (De Belleroche and Bradford, 1973a, b).

5.3.3   Vesicular membrane composition

Although many experiments purporting to favour the vesicle hypothesis are not directly concerned with a mechanism of transmitter release, a mechanism must be postulated and, in most instances, this is exocytosis. There is a detailed discussion of exocytosis in a subsequent section (5.4) and only one aspect of it concerns us here. This is the relative composition of the membrane of vesicles and the external plasma membrane of the terminal.

If the assumption is made that permanent exocytosis occurs, it follows that the enzymatic and chemical composition of isolated vesicles and external membranes should be similar if not identical. The only way of avoiding this conclusion is to postulate a transformation of constituents as exocytosis takes place. This is generally viewed as an unattractive possibility.

According to Whittaker and co-workers (Eichberg *et al.*, 1964; Hosei, 1965; Whittaker, 1966a, 1970) there are a number of major differences in the constituents of presynaptic external synaptosome membranes and synaptic vesicle membranes. (Na^+–K^-)-activated ATPase, AChE, ganglioside, tetanus toxin receptor groups and cholesterol are all low or even absent from vesicle fractions whereas they are present in appreciable quantities in external membrane fractions. These results based on fractionation studies cast doubt on the simple conversion of synaptic vesicles into the external membrane of the terminal, and hence, in turn, on exocytosis and the vesicle hypothesis as traditionally conceived. A similar conclusion may be drawn from the protein studies of Rodriguez de Lores Arnaiz, Alberici de Canal and De Robertis (1971), in which the turnover of protein in the various subcellular fractions of rat cerebral cortex was compared. These workers noted that the protein of the synaptic vesicle fraction had a faster turnover and a higher initial specific radioactivity than that of the external membrane fraction.

Heuser and Reese (1973), aware of these chemical differences between the external plasma membrane and vesicle membrane, postulate that the vesicle membrane may migrate rapidly within the plasma membrane. Rapid mixing of different membranes does occur (Frye and Edidin, 1970), while membranes may be far more fluid than previously thought (Singer and Nicolson, 1972). Whether these considerations are a sufficient defence of the exocytosis model remains to be seen.

5.3.4 Experimental situations

As we have already seen, the concept of quantal neurotransmission was formulated by Katz and associates at the neuromuscular junction, and much of the follow-up biophysical work has been carried out in terms of this model (Martin, 1966; Hubbard, 1970). By contrast, subcellular fractionation studies which have proved so important in the development of these ideas have largely been confined to mammalian central nervous tissue and, more recently, to the electric organ of *Torpedo*. Early EM studies detailing the features of synaptic vesicles were carried out on neuromuscular junctions (Robertson, 1956; Birks *et al.*, 1960) as well as on CNS synapses, and while the vesicles themselves are similar in both situations the synaptic regions differ noticeably. (Compare, for example, the early studies of Andersson–Cedergren, 1959 and Birks, Huxley and Katz, 1960, with that of Gray, 1959a).

A pertinent question therefore, is whether the transmission process is the same in CNS synapses as in neuromuscular junctions. The more specific question concerning the relationship between the process in cholinergic and adrenergic synapses does not concern us here. This is an extremely important consideration when it is borne in mind that quantal neurotransmission has not been demonstrated for either mammalian central or electric organ cholinergic synapses (Whittaker, 1971a). There is however, no reason for thinking that this mode of transmission is confined to the neuromuscular junction as it may not have been observed centrally on account of technical difficulties and nothing more. Katz (1969) concludes that, while the evidence from synapses other than skeletal neuromuscular junctions is fragmentary, it does suggest that the quantal mechanism of transmitter release is widespread and probably applies to all presynaptic terminals in which chemical transmitters are synthesized. In particular, quantal release and spontaneous synaptic potentials have been demonstrated in sympathetic ganglia (Nishi and Koketsu, 1960; Blackman, Ginsborg and Ray, 1963a, b) and at neurons in the stellate ganglion of the squid (Miledi, 1966, 1967). Spontaneous junction potentials have been observed in central neurons of the isolated spinal cord of the frog (Katz and Miledi, 1963) while it also appears that unitary synaptic potentials in mammalian spinal neurons are made up of quantal components (e.g. Kuno, 1964; Eide, Fedina, Jansen, Lundberg and Vyklický, 1967).

As a working hypothesis quantal neurotransmission may be assumed to exist at central cholinergic synapses, until proved otherwise. Minor differences between central and neuromuscular junctions do exist however, and may be significant in determining the manner by which the transmitter substance is liberated into the synaptic cleft. It is possible therefore, that the vesicle hypothesis, as opposed to the more general concept of quantal neurotransmission, may apply to the neuromuscular junction and yet not to central cholinergic synapses. While this is no more than a possibility, it should remind us that findings at the one site are not of necessity applicable at the other, an important point to bear in mind when considering mechanisms of transmitter release.

5.4 MECHANISMS OF TRANSMITTER RELEASE – EXOCYTOSIS

The almost traditional approach to the testing of the vesicle hypothesis, characterized by stimulation experiments, has failed to evaluate the hypothesis adequately on account of its failure to follow the vesicles to the presynaptic membrane. However fully its anticipations may have been met, therefore, in terms of alterations in the number or size of the vesicles, it has proved powerless to fill the hiatus between these observations and the actual release of the transmitter substance. And, unfortunately, this hiatus constitutes the essence of the classic vesicle hypothesis.

An alternative approach is to study the actual mechanism of transmitter release itself, an approach fraught with difficulties because of the highly dynamic nature of the process. If, however, a satisfactory answer is forthcoming this may partially compensate for the inadequacies of the procedures already considered.

By far the most frequently advocated mechanism of transmitter release into the synaptic cleft is *exocytosis*, which may be defined as the release of stored secretory product to the cell exterior without a preliminary discharge into the cytoplasm and without loss of cytoplasmic constituents (Poisner, 1973). This requires detailed consideration therefore, and only in the light of this will alternative theories be analysed. The fact that exocytosis is the generally accepted model to account for glandular secretion and the release of neurohormones from neurosecretory neurons (see Bloom *et al.*, 1970) has greatly facilitated its acceptance as the mode of transmitter release from neurons, although doubts have grown as detailed features have come under investigation.

5.4.1 Underlying ideas

The strongest arguments in favour of exocytosis come from studies of neuromuscular junctions. Katz, since his original work on quantal neurotransmission (Del Castillo and Katz, 1956), has maintained that each packet of ACh is preformed within a synaptic vesicle in the nerve terminal and that release results from a collision between the vesicular and synaptic membranes. Even if it is assumed that the frequency of collisions is high,

Katz argues that the majority of them fail to lead to transmitter release. This difficulty is overcome by postulating that the vesicles and presynaptic membrane are endowed with reactive or receptive sites, and that release occurs only in the statistically improbable event of the reactive site of a vesicle making contact with a reactive site of the presynaptic membrane (Fig. 5.4b). This sets in motion a reaction which causes the colliding barriers to burst open (Katz, 1969). With the arrival of a nerve impulse the number of reactive sites on the membrane is increased, and in a complementary fashion so is the number of vesicles in the vicinity of the membrane. Calcium ions, which are so essential for quantal release, may play some part in the functioning of these reactive sites (see Hubbard, 1970). More specifically, depolarization may open a gate to calcium ions which, as a result, move towards the inside of the axon membrane and so reach the reactive sites. In other words, calcium may be essential for the transient fusion of axon and synaptic membranes, and hence for quantal release (Katz, 1969).

Underlying Katz's ideas is the assumption that vesicles are in random motion, hence the necessity for the presence of reactive sites on both vesicular and presynaptic membrane surfaces. Vesicles, however, do not appear to be randomly distributed within the terminal, particularly in the region of the presynaptic membrane (e.g. Akert et al., 1969; Jones, 1969). Furthermore, random movement is not required to explain the quasi Poisson character of release as Hubbard (1970) explains. Exocytosis as a mechanism though is not imperilled by this difficulty, because the membrane reactive sites may well correspond to those areas of the presynaptic membrane lying between the dense projections and considered by Akert and his group to be the active sites at the synapse. The need for reactive sites on the vesicles is, however, diminished.

5.4.2 Ultrastructural evidence

Exocytosis has typically been identified with the EM appearance of micropits. These are described by some authors as 'fusing' vesicles (Hubbard and Kwanbunbumpen, 1968), and on the assumption that they are involved in transporting material out of the terminal, they correspond to what would be expected of vesicles undergoing exocytosis.

It is precisely this question which is the difficult one. Micropits by themselves give no clue concerning the direction of transport, and the conclusions reached by various workers may simply reflect their sphere of interest. Westrum (1965), for instance, was principally concerned with the origin of synaptic vesicles and hence interpreted micropits in pinocytotic terms. By contrast, Nickel and Potter (1970) in their freeze-etched preparations of Torpedo electric organ were concerned with the vesicle hypothesis and viewed the micropits in exocytotic terms. These and other authors readily concede, however, that the morphology alone fails to distinguish between pinocytosis and exocytosis. It is also interesting that Hubbard and Kwanbunbumpen (1968) noted that none of the experimental treatments used by them in their neuromuscular preparations produced any significant alteration in the number of 'fusing' vesicles. This was in marked contrast to other vesicles in the terminals, including those touching the axoplasmic membrane opposite junctional folds.

In some situations there is direct evidence that vesicles transport material into a cell. Nagasawa *et al.* (1971) described the uptake of horseradish peroxidase by coated and smooth vesicles in neurosecretory terminals of the posterior pituitary gland, while Zacks and Saito (1969), Holtzman, Freeman and Kashner (1971) and Ceccarelli, Hurlbut and Mauro (1972) reported its uptake in neuromuscular junctions. Tracer particles of thorium dioxide (Nagasawa and Douglas, 1972) and ferritin (Smith, 1970) have also been used in the same way.

The evidence for exocytosis is relatively strong in neurosecretory terminals as exocytotic figures are readily identifiable by their content of electron-dense secretory material (Nagasawa and Douglas, 1972), and can be recognized after freeze-fracturing (Dempsey, Bullivant and Watkins, 1973). Work by Douglas, Nagasawa and others suggests that the expansion of the cell surface resulting from exocytosis may be countered by membrane flow, this subtraction of the surface occurring by pinocytosis (Fig. 5.2). This cycle of

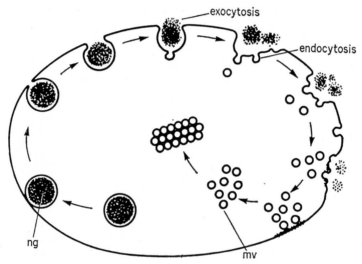

Figure 5.2   A scheme depicting the proposed mechanism of extrusion of posterior pituitary hormones by exocytosis, and formation of microvesicles ('synaptic vesicles') by endocytosis. mv, microvesicles; ng, neurosecretory granules. (Modified from Douglas *et al.*, 1971b)

events is important in two respects: it helps conserve the chemical composition of the cell surface and permits the recapture and conservation of synaptic vesicle membrane and its subsequent re-use (Douglas *et al.*, 1971b). These authors suggest that a similar process may occur in the ordinary neuron, and this is certainly an attractive hypothesis. Whether or not this is the case, however, depends upon the reality of exocytosis as a release mechanism at synapses.

5.4.3   Exocytosis at the neuromuscular junction

We have already discussed the difficulties associated with detecting a dynamic process such as exocytosis using the EM. This has been particularly well illustrated in the case

188

of stimulation experiments. A number of investigators have been led, therefore, to concentrate instead on the recycling of vesicle membrane, working on the postulate that the membrane of synaptic vesicles is incorporated into the terminal membrane and later made available to the terminal in the form of 'new' synaptic vesicles.

Heuser and Reese (1973) in an extensive investigation of the frog neuromuscular junction have tackled the problem from this angle. Stimulation, resulting in a transient depletion of synaptic vesicles, appeared to exert little effect on the total amount of membrane comprising the nerve terminals.* Stimulation of short duration resulted in an increase in external plasma membrane and a small depletion of vesicles, while longer duration stimulation was accompanied by a larger depletion of vesicles and by the appearance of numerous cisternae within the terminals. With rest cisternae disappeared and the vesicle population was reconstituted. In order to fit these events together sequentially horseradish peroxidase was employed as a tracer, from which it was demonstrated that on stimulation the tracer first entered the cisternae. From here it entered the vesicles which were formed from the cisternae during rest. Washing the muscles to remove extracellular horseradish peroxidase and then restimulating the preparation caused the tracer to disappear from the vesicles suggesting that a one-way recycling of synaptic membrane was occurring. One other feature of stimulated junctions noted by these authors was the appearance of coated vesicles close to and often linked with both the plasma membrane and the cisternae.

These results prompted Heuser and Reese to postulate the following sequence of events during transmitter release (Fig. 5.3). Synaptic vesicles discharge their content of trans-

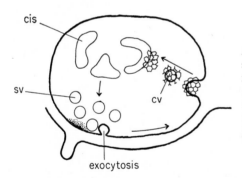

Figure 5.3 Diagrammatic summary of the path of synaptic vesicle membrane recycling as proposed at neuromuscular junctions by Heuser and Reese (1973). After release of the transmitter by exocytosis, the membrane of the vesicles is transported within the terminal membrane to be retrieved via coated vesicles (cv) and cisternae (cis) to form 'new' vesicles (sv).

mitter by coalescing with the external plasma membrane at specific points, that is, by exocytosis. The vesicle membrane incorporated into the plasma membrane enlarges the latter and circulates within it to be retrieved by coated vesicles at a point adjacent to the Schwann sheath. The coated vesicles, in turn, having taken up this vesicle membrane coalesce and form cisternae which appear within the terminal at times of vesicle depletion. The cisternae are then responsible for producing new synaptic vesicles.

The evidence produced by Heuser and Reese (1973) for their hypothesis is strong, although as they themselves admit it is still not possible to visualize directly or to label

* *The total amount of membrane* was calculated to include the external plasma membrane of the terminal, the membrane of the synaptic vesicles plus the membrane of any cisternae.

individual membrane components. It provides evidence, however, for a complete cycle of events and avoids the hiatus always present in stimulation experiments alone. As such it constitutes the most direct evidence yet available for the vesicle hypothesis, especially as their estimate of vesicle depletion at an average end plate (3×10^5 vesicles) after 15 minutes stimulation corresponds in general terms with estimates of 2×10^5 to 5×10^5 quanta released by equivalent stimulation (Martin, 1955; Katz, 1962; Ceccarelli et al., 1972).

It now remains to ask whether these results can be generalized and applied to other synaptic sites, particularly central cholinergic synapses. The distinguishing features of the neuromuscular junction following stimulation are: (a) the expansion of the external plasma membrane, (b) the appearance of coated vesicles, and (c) the appearance of cisternae. Each of these features is essential to Heuser and Reese's hypothesis and substantiates the reality of exocytosis as the release mechanism in this situation. To what extent are these features present in other types of synapse?

Expansion of the plasma membrane of terminals has been described by other workers in crayfish axons (Atwood et al., 1972), frog and rat neuromuscular junctions (Hubbard and Kwanbunbumpen, 1968; Jones and Kwanbunbumpen, 1970; Clark et al., 1972; Ceccarelli et al., 1973), cat superior cervical ganglia (Pysh and Wiley, 1972, 1974) and in Torpedo electric organ (Zimmerman and Whittaker, 1973) during transmitter release. While the emphasis in these studies has been on neuromuscular junctions, Pysh and Wiley's investigations extend the phenomenon further. It remains to be seen whether CNS synapses fit into the same pattern.

An increase in plasma membrane also occurs in secretory cells as an accompaniment of almost undoubted exocytosis, for example, in the adrenal medulla (Grynszpan-Winograd 1971; Nagasawa and Douglas, 1972), the posterior pituitary gland (Nagasawa et al., 1970), the pancreatic exocrine cells (Jamieson and Palade, 1971) and the parotid gland (Amsterdam, Ohad and Schramm, 1969). It would appear then that whenever exocytosis occurs it is accompanied by an observable, if transient, increase in the plasma membrane of the cell concerned. Consequently, such an occurrence should be detectable in central cholinergic synapses if transmission at these synapses is accomplished by means of exocytosis.

The part played by coated vesicles in the formation of synaptic vesicles from the limiting plasma membrane of a cell has been recognized for some time (Roth and Porter, 1962; Palay, 1963; Andrés, 1964; Westrum, 1965; Andrés and During, 1966; Nickel et al., 1967; Kanaseki and Kadota, 1969; Gray and Willis, 1970; Section 1.3.3). What has been unclear is the relationship of the coated vesicles to neurotransmission within nerve terminals. A good illustration of this dilemma is provided by Korneliussen (1972) who, in rat neuromuscular junctions, found that micropits with spikes, coated vesicles and isolated spikes (shells) were abundant in his material. On stimulation she noted a slight, insignificant decrease in the concentration of coated vesicles and complete shells in some experiments. This agreed in general terms with the results of Birks (1966) and Hubbard and Kwanbunbumpen (1968) on neuromuscular junctions and with Jones and Bradford (1971a) using cortical synaptosomes, although at variance with the results of Holtzman *et al.*, (1971) again using neuromuscular junction preparations, and with the neuro-secretory studies of Douglas *et al* (1971b) and Nagasawa *et al.*, (1971). The significance of these observations and thus the role of coated vesicles remains in doubt in the absence of supporting evidence.

Coated vesicles are abundant under certain conditions in CNS synapses (Gray, 1961; Kanaseki and Kadota, 1969; Jones and Bradford, 1971a), and assuming their validity as indicators of membrane flux (see, however, Gray, 1972; Section 1.3.3), their role in neurotransmission should be ascertainable in cholinergic junctions. Even if they are involved, their role may not correspond precisely with that postulated for them in neuromuscular junctions.

The appearance of cisternae after stimulation is a characteristic feature of neuromuscular junctions (e.g. Clark *et al.*, 1972; Korneliussen, 1972; Ceccarelli *et al.*, 1973) and has not been described in central synapses. Jones and Bradford (1971a) commented on the presence of vacuoles in cortical synaptosomes following stimulation, although these bear no resemblance to cisternae. If exocytosis is the principal mechanism responsible for transmitter release in central synapses, therefore, the sequence of steps in membrane transformation must differ in certain respects from that in neuromuscular junctions (see Cooke, Cameron and Jones, 1975 in support of this contention).

5.4.4 Present status of exocytosis

In the light of these combined stimulation and tracer studies on neurosecretory processes and at neuromuscular junctions there appears to be firm evidence for exocytosis in these situations. Equally convincing evidence has not, as yet, been forthcoming for cholinergic synapses, while much of the evidence in its favour at adrenergic synapses is still of a rela-tively indirect nature (see Bloom *et al.*, 1970).

One other point may be mentioned at this juncture, as it has a bearing on the status of exocytosis. This concerns the release of large proteins at synapses. The release of NE at adrenergic synapses is accompanied by the release of *chromogranin A* and *dopamine-β-hydroxylase* (DBO) (Geffen, Livett and Rush, 1969; Gerwirtz and Kopin, 1970; Johnson, Thoa, Weinshilboum, Axelrod, and Kopin, 1971; Smith, 1971), while these same proteins are also released from the adrenal medulla (Viveros, Arqueros and Kirshner, 1968). A low molecular weight protein, provisionally named *vesiculin* (Whittaker, 1971a), has been isolated from synaptic vesicles of *Torpedo* and may represent the counterpart in choliner-gic synapses of chromogranin A which is concerned with the packaging of adrenalin.

As proteins such as those just described do not readily permeate cell membranes, exocytosis provides a mechanism that explains how they may be transferred from the vesicle to the cleft without crossing the vesicle and presynaptic membranes (Bloom *et al.*, 1970). Other large molecules in the axoplasm, for instance, dopadecarboxylase, do not appear to be released.

Caution is required in postulating a single mechanism for hormone and transmitter release, or even for different transmitters. While the apparent unifying thread is the wide-spread requirement for extracellular Ca^{2+} as a prerequisite for hormonal and transmitter

191

release, there are differences (Van der Kloot and Kita, 1974). For instance, catecholamine release from the adrenal medulla is an almost linear function of the extracellular Ca^{2+} concentration (Van der Kloot, Kita and Kita, 1974) whereas ACh release at the neuromuscular junction is a non-linear function of Ca^{2+} concentration (Dodge and Rahaminoff, 1967). Furthermore, colchicine inhibits catecholamine release but has little effect on ACh release (Katz, 1972; Hofmann, Struppler, Weindl and Velho, 1973; Turkanis, 1973).

5.5 MECHANISMS OF TRANSMITTER RELEASE – ALTERNATIVES TO EXOCYTOSIS

5.5.1 Temporary attachment sites

Exocytosis as described above involves a process whereby the vesicle membrane becomes incorporated into the plasma membrane of the cell and is subsequently re-utilized.* In the absence of convincing ultrastructural evidence for exocytosis in central synapses attempts have been directed towards detecting temporary attachment sites (Fig. 5.4d). Important in the search for evidence favouring such sites is the *need* for a mechanism which can circumvent the difficulties inherent in exocytosis. Chief among these difficulties are:

1. the rapidity of transmitter release (Katz and Miledi, 1965) which it is felt is incompatible with the time required for the transformation of membranes involved in exocytosis (Pfenninger, 1972).
2. the existence of different pools of transmitter within the terminal and the preferential release of newly-synthesized transmitter (e.g. Kopin, Breese, Krauss and Weise, 1968; Whittaker, 1970).
3. the low-level release of vesicle protein in some adrenergic endings compared with the rate of release of transmitter (Bloom *et al.*, 1970).
4. the varying composition of vesicle and synaptic membranes (Whittaker, 1966a, 1970; Rodriguez de Lores Arnaiz *et al.*, 1971).
5. the high turnover rate of membranes inherent in the exocytosis concept (Bittner and Kennedy, 1970).

If the concept of the direct release of transmitter from vesicles into the cleft is to be maintained, the temporary attachment of vesicles to the presynaptic membrane provides a useful alternative mechanism to exocytosis. Not only does this overcome the major objections just noted, it also allows for the re-utilization of synaptic vesicles, which, in turn, helps to account for the low-level release of chromogranin A and dopamine-β-hydroxylase (DBO) in adrenergic synapses.

What then is the evidence in favour of such temporary attachment sites for the vesicles? The most positive suggestion concerns the *synaptopores* described in freeze-etched

* Exocytosis as defined here and as commonly envisaged may be regarded as *permanent*, in that particular vesicles are permanently removed from the terminal, and cannot be re-utilized for neurotransmission. This does not preclude re-use of their membrane components in the formation of 'new' vesicles by a recycling process such as that envisaged by Douglas *et al.*, (1971b) and Heuser and Reese (1973). Alternatives to exocytosis incorporate within their schemes the re-use of particular vesicles on a number of occasions, and thus involve *temporary* vesicle attachment.

preparations of CNS synapses by Akert and his group (Akert *et al.*, 1972; Pfenninger, *et al.*, 1972). According to these workers 'synaptopores are synapse-specific, transient attachment sites of the synaptic vesicles to the presynaptic membrane which may represent the morphological basis of transmitter release' (see Pfenninger, 1972).

As previously discussed in Section 1.3.2, synaptopores appear as small protuberances or as micropits (20 nm in diameter) of the presynaptic membrane, depending upon which face of a leaflet is being examined. They are arranged in groups of 10 to 20, and probably occupy a varying proportion of nodal points of a hexagonal pattern. Because the intervals of this lattice are shorter (47–58nm) than those between dense projections (60–80nm),

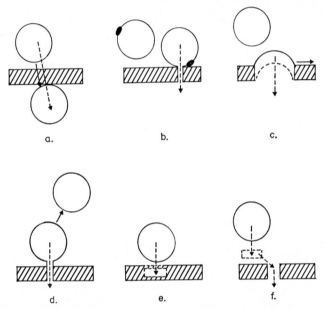

Figure 5.4 Summary of postulated mechanisms of transmitter release into the synaptic cleft. The hatched bars represent presynaptic membranes separating presynaptic terminals above from clefts below. The solid arrows represent the direction of membrane transport and the broken arrows movement of the transmitter.
(a) discharge of entire vesicle; (b) temporary fusion of vesicle and synaptic membrane resulting from the collision of reactive sites (black dots) as envisaged by del Castillo and Katz (1957); (c) exocytosis followed by incorporation of the vesicle membrane into the synaptic membrane; (d) temporary attachment of the vesicle to the synaptic membrane followed by recirculation of the vesicle within the presynaptic terminal; (e) release of transmitter into a membrane store; (f) release of transmitter into a cytoplasmic store and thence through membrane 'gates'.

Akert *et al.*, (1972) put forward the suggestion that synaptopores exist between dense projections, corresponding in position to the synaptic vesicles at the presynaptic membrane. They resemble in some respects the appearance of freeze-etched plasmalemmal vesicle fission or fusion sites (Nickel and Grieshaber, 1969), although there are differences of size and fracturing between the two (Pfenninger, 1972).

In spite of this, synaptopores could still represent sites of fusion or fission of the vesicle and presynaptic membrane (exocytosis), rather than temporary attachment sites. The arguments put forward by Pfenninger *et al.*, (1972) in favour of the latter include the size requirements of exocytosis which are not met by these sites, and the nature of the tip of the protuberances which correspond to the expectations of attachment sites but not of exocytotic stomata.

The temporary nature of these attachment sites is suggested by differences in the numbers of synaptopores per unit area of presynaptic membrane when active and resting synapses are compared (see Pfenninger, 1972). Animals which had received pentobarbital for 20 minutes before being killed (anaesthetized) were examined alongside unanaesthetized animals, their spinal cords being analysed after freeze-etching (Streit *et al.*, 1972). Craters on the presynaptic membrane varied from closed to open, while the number of 'liftings, wrinklings and craters' of the presynaptic membrane depended upon the anaesthetized state of the animals. The authors interpreted these results as supporting exocytosis, and as reinforcing the vesicle hypothesis.

From this it appears that the evidence in favour of synaptopores as *temporary* attachment sites is slim. The most that can be said is that they, in line with the presynaptic membrane as a whole, may undergo conformational changes. Far more evidence is required, however, before this suggestion can be viewed in broader terms and related directly to the processes of neurotransmission.

5.5.2 Actomyosin-like protein in nerve terminals

W hether or not exocytosis is of a permanent or transient nature, the release of transmitte from its store in the vesicle must still involve the interaction of two sets of membranes, that of the vesicle and that of the terminal. If such a process occurs by a mechanochemical interaction between the membranes, the biological model of immediate relevance is the actomyosin system of muscle (Berl, Puszkin and Nicklas, 1973). The isolation, therefore, of actomyosin-like proteins from mammalian brain is of considerable interest. More specifically, the proteins isolated have actomyosin-like, actin-like and myosin-like properties and have been designated neurostenin, neurin and stenin respectively (Puszkin Berl, Puszkin and Clarke, 1968; Berl and Puszkin, 1970; Puszkin and Berl, 1972). The equating of neurostenin with synaptosomal fractions (Puszkin, Nicklas and Berl, 1972) and the demonstration of actin in cultures of chick sympathetic ganglia (Fine and Bray, 1971) strongly suggest the presence of these proteins in nerve terminals.

Subfractionation of the synaptosomal fraction to obtain vesicular and membrane fractions has enabled further characterization of the proteins. Of the two main protein bands resulting, the one having myosin-like properties is associated with the vesicle fraction and that with actin-like properties with the membrane fraction (Puszkin *et al.*, 1972). Furthermore, the former exhibits Ca^{2+}-stimulated ATPase activity.

Working from these data, Berl and co-workers (1973) have put forward a mechanism for transmitter release involving transient exocytosis (Fig. 5.5). According to this postulated mechanism the neurin of the presynaptic membrane combines with the stenin of the vesicle membrane causing conformational changes in the membrane. These result in transient opening of the vesicle and the release of transmitter into the cleft. Following this, the vesicle separates from its synaptic site and can either be replenished or metabolized.

A mechanism such as this is attractive in terms of a transient attachment concept from which it derives its rationale. The significance of neurin and stenin, however, especially in regard to their respective locations, may be even greater in terms of postulating a mechanism for drawing vesicles towards the presynaptic membrane. A hypothesis framed

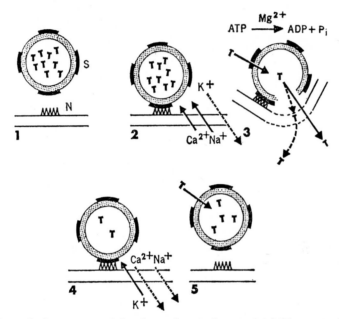

Figure 5.5   Schematic diagram to explain release of transmitter material (T) as a result of interaction between neurin (N) associated with synaptic membranes and stenin (S) associated with vesicle membranes. Stages 1–3 depict movement of the vesicle towards the presynaptic membrane, opening of the membranes in response to the influx of Ca^{2+} and consequent release of transmitter into the cleft. Stage 4 represents termination of the action by efflux of Ca^{2+}, and stage 5 separation of the vesicle from the membrane. (From Berl *et al.*, 1973).

in relation to neurin and stenin would add a biochemical dimension to current morphological concepts of vesicular mobility based on dense projections, presynaptic network and presynaptic vesicular grid (Gray, 1966; Akert *et al.*, 1969; Jones and Revell, 1970b).

5.5.3   Membrane diffusion and control

Once an exocytosis model is discarded, the responsibility for the quantal control of neurotransmission is shifted from the vesicles, which are the obvious source of control. In practice, there is no one dominant alternative, but instead a range of possibilities which are usually fitted together in a number of combinations.

Release of the transmitter from the vesicles may not be directly into the cleft as envisaged in the classical quantal theory but either into the cytoplasm in the vicinity of the presynaptic membrane or into the presynaptic membrane itself (Fig. 5.4e, f). Either of these latter possibilities presumes that the vesicles are primarily storage sites of transmitter, whereas the actual transmitter released at any one time originates from the cytoplasm or membrane. Stimulation of the tissue would still be expected to affect the number of vesicles, as they would be replacing the free or membrane transmitter stores. A number of workers have suggested that the active molecules are those of the ACh (Nachmansohn, 1971) or NE (Kopin, 1968; Von Euler, 1971) stored in the membrane, while Dunant, Gautron, Israël, Lesbats and Manaranche (1971) using subcellular fractions of electric organs observed that the free transmitter pool is decreased when specimens from stimulated tissue are examined.

If either of these mechanisms is allowed, the responsibility for the quantitation of transmitter release is shifted onto the presynaptic membrane. Some form of membrane control theory is thus required, with its demand for a *gating mechanism* in the membrane (Fig. 5.4f). On theoretical grounds, this is an unsatisfactory proposition, necessitating as it does a mechanism in lieu of the vesicles which are thereby rendered redundant as quantal units. Following on from this, the size of a quantum would be governed by the duration of a process in the axon membrane, namely the time during which the gate is open (Katz, 1966). Unfortunately for this theory, the size of the ACh packet is not affected by the membrane change associated with the nerve impulse (e.g. del Castillo and Katz, 1954) but by the probability of the quantal event. Furthermore, there are no data at present in support of a gating mechanism, while the difficulty experienced in releasing cytoplasmically-situated monoamines from reserpine-treated terminals (Malmfors, 1969) argues against it.

Even if the vesicles are storage rather than directly-transmitting units, they must be intimately involved in controlling the amount of transmitter released into the cleft, whether this be by direct or indirect means. One would like to know, therefore, what is the nature of the interaction between the vesicles and any cytoplasmic or membrane compartments which may be directly involved in transmitter release.

A gating mechanism, moreover, demands a relatively labile architecture in the vicinity of the presynaptic membrane, a reasonable expectation in the light of conventionally prepared EMs although more difficult to envisage in terms of the presynaptic vesicular grid of Akert and co-workers. Alternatively, storage vesicles may be relatively static, whether alongside the presynaptic membrane or more proximally situated in the terminal. In this instance, the architecture of the terminal need not be particularly labile. Furthermore, this concept of static storage vesicles may be correlated with the life span of vesicles (20–30 days; Von Hungen. Mahler and Moore, 1968; Blakely, Brown and Geffen, 1969) in that after the vesicles have been utilized on a certain number of occasions, they become incorporated into the terminal membrane.

However attractive one or more of these ideas may be, it is important to realize that they are largely unsubstantiated and that the manner in which they are formulated may not lend them to ready experimental refutation. Furthermore, their relevance is largely confined to central synapses.

Addendum

The following papers appeared subsequent to the completion of the manuscript in June 1974, and were compiled at the end of 1974. Although they are entered under chapter headings, many of them are relevant to the discussions in more than one chapter.

CHAPTER 1

BLANKS, J. C., ADINOLFI, A. M. and LOLLEY, R. N. (1974) Photoreceptor degeneration and synaptogenesis in retinal-degenerative (rd) mice. *J. Comp. Neurol.*, **156**, 95–106.

BLANKS, J. C., ADINOLFI, A. M. and LOLLEY, R. N. (1974) Synaptogenesis in the photoreceptor terminal of the mouse retina. *J. Comp. Neurol.*, **156**, 81–94.

BLOOM, F. E. (1974) Dynamics of synaptic modulation: perspectives for the future. In *The Neurosciences: Third Study Program*, ed. Schmitt, F. O. and Worden, F. G. Pp. 989–999. Cambridge: MIT Press.

COOKE, C. T., CAMERON, P. U. and JONES, D. G. (1975) Stimulation-induced uptake of horseradish peroxidase by rat cortical neurons. Unpublished.

COUTEAUX, R. and PÉCOT-DECHAVASSINE, M. (1973) Données ultrastructurales et cytochimiques sur le méchanisme de libération de l'acéylcholine dans la transmission synaptique. *Arch. ital. Biol.*, **111**, 231–62.

COUTEAUX, M. R. and PÉCOT-DECHAVASSINE, M. (1974) Les zones spécialisées des membranes présynaptiques. *C.R. Acad. Sc. Paris*, **278**, 291–3.

CRAGG, B. G. (1974) Plasticity of synapses. *Brit. Med. Bull.*, **30**, 141–5.

DREIFUSS, J. J., AKERT, K., SANDRI, C. and MOOR, H. (1974) Neurosecretion from the posterior pituitary lobe. In *Electron Microscopy 1974*, **2**, *8th International Congress on Electron Microscopy, Canberra*, pp. 278–9. Australian Academy of Science, Canberra.

GAMBETTI, P., AUTILIO-GAMBETTI, L., RIZZUTO, N., SHAFER, B. and PFAFF, L. (1974) Synapses and malnutrition: quantitative ultrastructural study of rat cerebral cortex. *Exptl. Neurol.*, **43**, 464–73.

GRAY, E. G. (1974) Synaptic morphology with special reference to microneurons. In *Essays on the Nervous System*, ed. Bellairs, R. and Gray, E. G. Pp. 155–78. Oxford: Clarendon Press.

GRAY, E. G. and PAULA-BARBOSA, M. (1974) Dense articles within synaptic vesicles fixed with acid-aldehyde. *J. Neurocytol.*, **3**, 497–512.

JONES, D. G. and ELLISON, L. T. (1975) Personal observations.

KAMIYA, H., KADOTA, K. and KADOTA, T. (1974) Distribution of choline and acetylcholine in coated vesicles and plain synaptic vesicles. *Brain Res.*, **76**, 367–70.

KÁSA, P., JANCSÓ, G., KARCSU, S. and TÓTH, L. (1974) Analysis of synaptic vesicles in F-type axon terminals. *Acta histochem.*, **49**, 46–50.

KIM, S. U. and TUNNICLIFF, G. (1974) Morphological and biochemical development of chick cerebrum cultured in vitro. *Exptl. Neurol.*, **43**, 515–26.

LANDIS, D. M. D. and REESE, T. S. (1974) Differences in membrane structure between excitatory and inhibitory synapses in the cerebellar cortex. *J. Comp. Neurol.*, **155**, 93–125.

LANDIS, D. M. D., REESE, T. S. and RAVIOLA, E. (1974) Differences in membrane structure between excitatory and inhibitory components of the reciprocal synapse in the olfactory bulb. *J. Comp. Neurol.,* **155,** 67–92.

MIZUNO, N., NAKAMURA, Y. and IWAHORI, N. (1974) An electron microscope study of the dorsal cap of the inferior olive in the rabbit, with special reference to the pretecto-olivary fibers. *Brain Res.,* **77,** 385–95.

PAULA-BARBOSA, M. and GRAY, E. G. (1974) The effects of various fixatives at different pH on synaptic coated vesicles, reticulosomes and cytonet. *J. Neurocytol.,* **3,** 471–86.

PFENNINGER, K., BUNGE, M. B. and BUNGE, R. P. (1974) Nerve growth cone plasmalemma – its structure and development. In *Electron Microscopy 1974,* **2,** *8th International Congress on Electron Microscopy, Canberra,* pp. 234–35. Australian Academy of Science, Canberra.

TANAKA, R. (1974) Atpases of plain synaptic vesicle fraction and coated vesicle fraction of rat brain. *Fed. Proc.* **33,** 1550.

VRENSEN, G. and DE GROOT, D. (1974) Osmium-zinc iodide staining and the quantitative study of central synapses. *Brain Res.,* **74,** 131–42.

CHAPTER 2

BANKER, G., CHURCHILL, L. and COTMAN, C. W. (1974) Proteins of the post-synaptic density. *J. Cell Biol.* **63,** 456–65.

BARONDES, S. H. (1974) Synaptic macromolecules: identification and metabolism. *Ann. Rev. Biochem.,* **43,** 147–68.

BRETZ, U., BAGGIOLINI, M., HAUSER, R. and HODEL, C. (1974) Resolution of three distinct populations of nerve endings from rat brain homogenates by zonal isopycnic centrifugation. *J. Cell Biol.,* **61,** 466–80.

COTMAN, C. W., BANKER, G., CHURCHILL, L. and TAYLOR, D. (1974) Isolation of post-synaptic densities from rat brain. *J. Cell Biol.,* **63,** 441–55.

DETER, R. L. (1973) Electron microscopic evaluation of subcellular fractions obtained by ultracentrifugation. In *Principles and Techniques of Electron Microscopy: Biological Applications,* ed. Hayat, M. A. Vol. 3, pp. 199–235. New York: Van Nostrand Reinhold Co.

GOODKIN, P. and HOWARD, B. D. (1974) Studies on acetylcholinesterase of rat brain synaptosomal plasma membranes. *J. Neurochem.,* **22,** 129–36.

ISRAËL, M. and TUCEK, S. (1974) Utilization of acetate and pyruvate for the synthesis of 'total', 'bound' and 'free' acetylcholine in the electric organ of *Torpedo. J. Neurochem.,* **22,** 487–91.

MILLER, R. N., MILLER, E., CAINE, J. and STABLER, M. (1974) Synaptosomes, a possible system for the study of synaptic transmission. *Anesthesia and Analgesia,* **53,** 132–41.

MORGAN, I. G., BRECKENRIDGE, W. C., VINCENDON, G. and GOMBOS, G. (1973) The proteins of nerve-ending membranes. In *Proteins of the Nervous System,* ed. Schneider, D. J., Angeletti, R. H., Bradshaw, R. A. and Grasso, A. Pp. 171–92. New York: Raven Press.

NAGATA, Y., MIKOSHIBA, K. and TSUKADA, Y. (1974) Neuronal cell body enriched and glial cell enriched fractions from young and adult rat brains: preparation and morphological and biochemical properties. *J. Neurochem.,* **22,** 493–503.

TAMIR, H., RAPPORT, M. M. and ROIZIN, L. (1974) Preparation of synaptosomes and vesicles with sodium diatrizoate. *J. Neurochem.,* **23,** 943–49.

CHAPTER 3

BERNAL, A., MORALES, M., FERIA-VELASCO, A., CHEW, S. and ROSADO, A. (1974) Effect of intrauterine growth retardation on the biochemical maturation of brain synaptosomes in the rat. *J. Nutrition,* **104,** 1157–64.

HERVONEN, A., KANERVA, L., TISSARI, A. H. and SUURHASKO, B. V. A. (1974) Ultrastructure of synaptosomes from one-day old rabbit brain stem. *Cell Tiss. Res.* **148**, 535–50.

WHITTAKER, V. P. (1973) The structural and chemical properties of synaptic vesicles. In *Proteins of the Nervous System*, ed. Schneider, D. J., Angeletti, R. H., Bradshaw, R. A. and Grasso, A. Pp. 155–70. New York: Raven Press.

CHAPTER 4

BOCK, E., JØRGENSEN, D. S. and MORRIS, S. J. (1974) Antigen–antibody crossed electrophoresis of rat brain synaptosomes and synaptic vesicles: correlation to water-soluble antigens from rat brain. *J. Neurochem.*, **22**, 1013–17.

COTMAN, C. W. and TAYLOR, D. (1974) Localization and characterization of concanavalin A receptors in the synaptic cleft. *J. Cell Biol.*, **62**, 236–41.

CURTIS, D. R. (1974) Amino acid transmitters and the brain. *Med. J. Aust.*, **2**, 723–31.

DE FEUDIS, F. V. (1974) Preferential 'binding' of γ-aminobutyric acid and glycine to synaptosome-enriched fractions of rat cerebral cortex and spinal cord. *Can. J. Physiol. Pharmacol.* **52**, 138–47.

DOWDALL, M. J., BOYNE, A. F. and WHITTAKER, V. P. (1974) ATP a constituent of cholinergic synaptic vesicles. *Biochem. J.*, **140**, 1–12.

GAREY, R. E. and HEATH, R. G. (1974) Uptake of catecholamines by human synaptosomes. *Brain Res.*, **79**, 520–23.

HONEGGER, C. G., KREPELKA, L. M., STEINMANN, V. and VON HAHN, H. P. (1974) Distribution of H^3-glycine and H^3-L-glutamate in synaptosomal sub-populations after in vitro uptake in cat dorsal and ventral spinal cord slices. *Experentia*, **30**, 369–71.

HODINA, P. D. (1974) Metabolism of brain acetylcholine and its modification by drugs. *Drug Metabolism Reviews*, **3**, 89–129.

KUHAR, M. J. and ROMMELSPACHER, H. (1974) Acetylcholinesterase-staining synaptosomes from rat hippocampus: relative frequency and tentative estimation of internal concentration of free or 'labile bound' acetylcholine. *Brain Res.*, **77**, 85–96.

KUHAR, M. J. and SIMON, J. R. (1974) Acetylcholine uptake: lack of association with cholinergic neurons. *J. Neurochem.*, **22**, 1135–37.

LEVI, G., BERTOLLINI, A., CHEN, J. and RAITERI, M. (1974) Regional differences in the synaptosomal uptake of ^{3}H-γ-aminobutyric acid and ^{14}C-glutamate and possible role of exchange processes. *J. Pharmac. Exp. Ther.*, **188**, 429–38.

LEVI, G. and RAITERI, M. (1974) Exchange of neurotransmitter amino acid at nerve endings can stimulate high affinity uptake. *Nature, Lond.*, **250**, 735–7.

MCLAUGHLIN, B. J., WOOD, J. G., SAITO, K., BARBER, R., VAUGHN, J. E., ROBERTS, E. and WU, J-Y (1974) The fine structural localization of glutamate decarboxylase in synaptic terminals of rodent cerebellum. *Brain Res.*, **76**, 377–91.

ORREGO, F., JANKELEVICH, J., CERUTI, L. and FERRERA, C. (1974) Differential effects of electrical stimulation on release of ^{3}H-noradrenaline and ^{14}C-α-aminoisobutyrate from brain slices. *Nature, Lond.*, **251**, 55–7.

RAITERI, M., ANGELINI, F. and FEDERICO, A. (1973) Quantitative evaluation of antigen antibody interactions at the external surface of the nerve ending membrane. *Neurobiology, Copenh.*, **3**, 225–31.

ROMMELSPACHER, H. and KUHAR, M. J. (1974) Effects of electrical stimulation on acetylcholine levels in central cholinergic nerve terminals. *Brain Res.*, **81**, 243–51.

SAITO, K., BARBER, R., WU, J-Y, MATSUDA, T., ROBERTS, E. and VAUGHN, J. E. (1974) Immunohistochemical localization of glutamate decarboxylase in rat cerebellum. *Proc. Aat. Ncad. Sci. U.S.A.*, **71**, 269–73.

199

SPARF, B. (1973) On the turnover of acetylcholine in the brain. *Acta physiol. Scand.*, Suppl. **397**, 1–47.

SZAMIER, R. B. (1974) Enzymatic digestion of presynaptic structures in electroreceptors of elasmobranchs. *Amer. J. Anat.,* **139**, 567–74.

WENTHOLD, R. J., MAHLER, H. R. and MOORE, W. J. (1974) The half-life of acetylcholinesterase in mature rat brain. *J. Neurochem.,* **22**, 941–43.

WIDLUND, L. and HEILBRONN, E. (1974) Uptake of acetylcholine and choline into rat brain cortical slices and synaptosomes as related to ^{32}Pi incorporation into their phospholipids. *J. Neurochem.,* **22**, 991–98.

WOOD, J. G., MCLAUGHLIN, B. J. and BARBER, R. P. (1974) The visualization of concanavalin A binding sites of Purkinje cell somata and dendrites of rat cerebellum. *J. Cell Biol.,* **63**, 541–49.

CHAPTER 5

EINHORN, V. F. and HAMILTON, R. (1973) Transmitter release by red back spider venom. *J. Pharmacy Pharmacology,* **25**, 824–26.

HEUSER, J. E. and REESE, T. S. (1974) Morphology of synaptic vesicle discharge and reformation at the frog neuromuscular junction. In *Synaptic Transmission and Neuronal Interaction*, ed. Bennett, M. V. L. Pp. 59–77. New York: Raven Press.

HEUSER, J. E., REESE, T. S. and LANDIS, D. M. D. (1974) Functional changes in frog neuromuscular junctions studied with freeze-fracture. *J. Neurocytol.,* **3**, 109–31.

JORGENSEN, O. S. and MELLERUP, E. T. (1974) Endocytotic formation of rat brain synaptic vesicles. *Nature, Lond.,* **249**, 770–71.

ORCI, L. and PERRELET, A. (1973) Membrane-associated particles: increase at sites of pinocytosis demonstrated by freeze-etching. *Science,* **181**, 868–69.

PFENNINGER, K. H. and ROVAINEN, C. M. (1973) Increased vesicle attachment to the presynaptic membrane in stimulated spinal cord. *Anat. Rec.,* **175**, 412A.

PFENNINGER, K. H. and ROVAINEN, C. M. (1974) Stimulation- and calcium-dependence of vesicle attachment sites in the presynaptic membrane. A freeze-cleave study on the lamprey spinal cord. *Brain Res.,* **72**, 1–23.

SCHLAPFER, W. T., WOODSON, P. B. J., TREMBLAY, J. P. and BARONDES, S. H. (1974) Depression and frequency facilitation at a synapse in *Aplysia californica*: evidence for regulation by availability of transmitter. *Brain Res.,* **76**, 267–80.

TURNER, P. T. and HARRIS, A. B. (1973) Ultrastructure of synaptic vesicle formation in cerebral cortex. *Nature, Lond.,* **242**, 57–59.

TURNER, P. T. and HARRIS, A. B. (1974) Ultrastructure of exogenous peroxidase in cerebral cortex. *Brain Res.,* **74**, 305–26.

WHITTAKER, V. P. and ZIMMERMAN, H. (1974) Biochemical studies on cholinergic synaptic vesicles. In *Synaptic Transmission and Neuronal Interaction*, ed. Bennett, M. V. L. Pp. 217–38. New York: Raven Press.

ZIMMERMAN, H. and WHITTAKER, V. P. (1974) Different recovery rates of the electrophysiological, biochemical and morphological parameters in the cholinergic synapses of the *Torpedo* electric organ after stimulation. *J. Neurochem.,* **22**, 1109–14.

ZIMMERMAN, H. and WHITTAKER, V. P. (1974) Effect of electrical stimulation on the yield and composition of synaptic vesicles from the cholinergic synapses of the electric organ of *Torpedo*: a combined biochemical, electrophysiological and morphological study. *J. Neurochem.,* **22**, 435–50.

References

ABDEL-LATIF, A. A. (1966) A simple method for isolation of nerve-ending particles from rat brain. *Biochim. Biophys. Acta*, **121**, 403–406.

ABDEL-LATIF, A. A. (1972) In *Methods in Neurochemistry*, R. L. Fried (ed.), Vol. **4** Marcel Dekker.

ABDEL-LATIF, A. A. and ABOOD, L. G. (1964) Biochemical studies on mitochondria and other cytoplasmic fractions of developing rat brain. *J. Neurochem.*, **11**, 9–15.

ABDEL-LATIF, A. A. and ABOOD, L. G. (1965) Incorporation of ortho [^{32}P] phosphate into the subcellular fractions of developing rat brain. *J. Neurochem.*, **12**, 157–166.

ABDEL-LATIF, A. A., BRODY, J. and RAMAHI, H. (1967) Studies on sodium–potassium adenosine triphosphatase of the nerve endings and appearance of electrical activity in developing rat brain. *J. Neurochem.*, **14**, 1133–1141.

ABDEL-LATIF, A. A. and SMITH, J. P. (1970) *In vivo* incorporation of choline, glycerol and orthophosphate into lecithin and other phospholipids of subcellular fractions of rat cerebrum. *Biochim. Biophys. Acta*, **218**, 134–140.

ABDEL-LATIF, A. A., SMITH, J. P. and ELLINGTON, E. P. (1970) Subcellular distribution of sodium–potassium adenosine triphosphatase, acetylcholine and acetylcholinesterase in developing brain. *Brain Res.*, **18**, 441–450.

ABDEL-LATIF, A. A., YAMAGUCHI, T., YAMAGUCHI, M. and CHANG, F. (1968) Studies on [^{32}P] orthophosphate incorporation into nucleotides, phospholipids and phosphoproteins of isolated nerve endings from developing rat brain. *Brain Res.*, **10**, 307–321.

ABOOD, L., CAVANAUGH, M., TSCHIRGI, R. D. and GERARD, R. W. (1951) Metabolic and pharmacologic studies in glia and nerve cells and components. *Fed. Proc.*, **10**, 3.

ABOOD, L. G., GERARD, R. W., BANKS, J. and TSCHIRGI, R. D. (1952) Substrate and enzyme distribution in cells and cell fractions of the nervous system. *Amer. J. Physiol.*, **168**, 728–738.

ABOOD, L. G., KURAHASI, K. and PEREZ DEL CERRO, M. (1967) Biochemical studies on isolated nerve endings and other particulates of bullfrog brain. *Biochim. Biophys. Acta.*, **136**, 521–532.

ADINOLFI, A. M. (1969) The fine structure of neurons and synapses in the entopeduncular nucleus of the cat. *J. Comp. Neurol.*, **135**, 225–248.

ADINOLFI, A. M. (1971a) The organization of synaptic junctions in cat putamen. *Brain Res.*, **32**, 53–67.

ADINOLFI, A. M. (1971b) The postnatal development of synaptic contacts in the cerebral cortex. In *Brain Development and Behavior*, Sterman, M. B., McGinty, D. J. and Adinolfi, A. M. (ed.) Pp. 73–89. New York: Academic Press.

ADINOLFI, A. M. (1972a) Morphogenesis of synaptic junctions in layers 1 and 11 of the somatic sensory cortex. *Exptl. Neurol.*, **34**, 372–382.

ADINOLFI, A. M. (1972b) The organization of paramembranous densities during postnatal maturation of synaptic junctions in the cerebral cortex. *Exptl. Neurol.*, **34**, 383–393.

ADINOLFI, A. M. and SCHMIDT, S. Y. (1974) Cytochemical localization of cyclic nucleotide phosphodiesterase activity at developing synapses. *Brain Res.*, **76**, 21–31.

AGHAJANIAN, G. K. and BLOOM, F. E. (1966) Electron microscopic autoradiography of rat hypothalamus after intraventricular ^{3}H-norepinephrine. *Science*, **153**, 308–310.

AGHAJANIAN, G. K. and BLOOM, F. E. (1967a) Electron microscopic localization of tritiated norepinephrine in rat brain: effect of drugs. *J. Pharmac. Exp. Ther.*, **156**, 407–416.

AGHAJANIAN, G. K. and BLOOM, F. E. (1967b) Localization of tritiated serotonin in rat brain by electron microscopic autoradiography. *J. Pharmacol. Exp. Ther.*, **156**, 23–30.

AGHAJANIAN, G. K. and BLOOM, F. E. (1967c) The formation of synaptic junctions in developing rat brain: a quantitative electron microscopic study. *Brain Res.*, **6**, 716–727.

AGRAWAL, H. C., DAVISON, A. N. and KACZMAREK, L. (1971) Subcellular distribution of taurine and cysteine-sulphinate decarboxylase in developing rat brain. *Biochem. J.*, **122**, 759–763.

AKERT, K. (1969) The mammalian subfornical organ. *J. Neuro-Visc. Relts., Suppl. IX*, 78–93.

AKERT, K. (1971) Struktur und Ultrastruktur von Nervenzellen und Synapsen. *Klin. Wschr.*, **49**, 509–519.

AKERT, K. (1973), Dynamic aspects of synaptic ultrastructure. *Brain Res.*, **49**, 511–518.

AKERT, K., CUÉNOD, M., and MOOR, H. (1971) Further observations on the enlargement of synaptic vesicles in degenerating optic nerve terminals of the avian tectum. *Brain. Res.*, **25**, 255–263.

AKERT, K., KAWANA, E., and SANDRI, C. (1971) ZIO-positive and ZIO-negative vesicles in nerve terminals *Prog. Brain Res.*, **34**, 305–317.

AKERT, K., MOOR, H., PFENNINGER, K. and SANDRI, C. (1969) Contributions of new impregnation methods and freeze etching to the problems of synaptic fine structure. *Prog. Brain Res.*, **31**, 223–240.

AKERT, K., and PFENNINGER, K. (1969) Synaptic fine structure and neural dynamics. In *Cellular Dynamics of the Neuron, I.S.C.B. Symposium* Vol. 8, ed. Barondes, S. H. Pp. 245–260. Academic Press: New York.

AKERT, K., PFENNINGER, K. and SANDRI, C. (1967) The fine structure of synapses in the subfornical organ of the cat. *Z. Zellforsch.*, **81**, 537–556.

AKERT, K., PFENNINGER, K., SANDRI, C. and MOOR, H. (1972) Freeze-etching and cytochemistry of vesicles and membrane complexes in synapses of the central nervous system. In *Structure and Function of Synapses*, ed. Pappas, G. D. and Purpura, D. P. Pp. 67–86. New York: Raven Press.

AKERT, K. and SANDRI, C. (1968) An electron microscopic study of zinc iodide-osmium impregnation of neurons. I. Staining of synaptic vesicles at cholinergic junctions. *Brain Res.*, **7**, 286–295.

AKERT, K. and SANDRI, C. (1970) Identification of the active synaptic region by means of histochemical and freeze-etching techniques. In *Excitatory Synaptic Mechanisms*, ed. Andersen, P. and Jansen, J. K. S. Pp. 27–41. Oslo: Universitatsforlaget.

ALDRIDGE, W. N., EMERY, R. C. and STREET, B. W. (1960) A tissue homogenizer. *Biochem. J.*, **77**, 326–327.

ALDRIDGE, W. N. and JOHNSON, M. K. (1959) Cholinesterase, succinic dehydrogenase, nucleic acids, esterase and glutathione reductase in subcellular fractions from rat brain. *Biochem. J.*, **73**, 270–276.

ALLEY, K. E. (1973) Quantitative analysis of the synaptogenic period in the trigeminal mesencephalic nucleus. *Anat. Rec.*, **177**, 49–60.

ALTMAN, J. (1971) Coated vesicles and synaptogenesis. A developmental study in the cerebellar cortex of the rat. *Brain Res.*, **30**, 311–322.

AMSTERDAM, A., OHAD, I. and SCHRAMM, M. (1969) Dynamic changes in the ultrastructure of the acinar cell of the rat parotid gland during the secretory cycle. *J. Cell Biol.*, **41**, 753–773.

ANDERSEN, P., ECCLES, J. C. and LOYNING, Y. (1963a) Recurrent inhibition in the hippocampus with identification of the inhibitory cell and its synapses. *Nature, Lond.*, **198**, 541–542.

ANDERSEN, P., ECCLES, J. C. and VOORHOEVE, P. E. (1963b) Inhibitory synapses on somas of Purkinje cells in the cerebellum. *Nature, Lond.*, **199**, 655–656.

ANDERSON, C. A. and WESTRUM, L. E. (1972) An electron microscopic study of the normal synaptic relationships and early degenerative changes in the rat olfactory tubercle. *Z. Zellforsch.*, **127**, 462–482.

ANDERSON, N. G. (1966) An introduction to particle separations in zonal centrifuges. In *The Development of Zonal Centrifuges and Ancillary Systems for Tissue Fractionation and Analysis*, ed. Anderson, N. G. *Natl. Cancer Inst. Monograph*, **21**, 9–39.

ANDERSON, N. G., NUNLEY, C. E. and RANKIN, C. T. (1969) Analytical techniques for cell fractions. XI. Rotor B-XXIX—A new high-resolution zonal centrifuge rotor for virus isolation and cell fractionation. *Analyt. Biochem.*, **31**, 255–271.

ANDERSON, N. G., PRICE, C. A., FISHER, W. D., CANNING, R. E. and BURGER, C. L. (1964) Analytical techniques for cell fractions. IV. Reorienting gradient rotors for zonal centrifugation. *Analyt. Biochem.*, **7**, 1–9.

ANDERSON, N. G., WATERS, D. A., FISHER, W. D., CLINE, G. B., NUNLEY, C. E., ELROD, L. H., and RANKIN, C. T. (1967) Analytical techniques for cell fractions. V. Characteristics of the B-XIV and B-XV zonal centrifuge rotors. *Analyt. Biochem.*, **21**, 235–252.

ANDERSSON-CEDERGREN, E. (1959) Ultrastructure of motor end plate and sarcoplasmic components of mouse skeletal muscle fiber. *J. Ultrastruct. Res.*, suppl. **1**, 1–191.

ANDREOLI, V., CECCARELLI, B., CERATI, E., DEMONTE, M. L. and CLEMENTI, F. (1970) Subcellular fractionation of hypothalamus and pituitary stalk of the bull. Morphologic study and serotonin-norepinephrine distribution. *Exp. Brain. Res.*, **11**, 17–28.

ANDRÉS, K. H. (1964) Mikropinozytose um Zentralnerven-system. *Z. Zellforsch.*, **64**, 63–73.

ANDRÉS, K. H. and DURING, M. (1966) Mikropinozytose in motorischen Endplatten. *Naturwissenschaften*, **53**, 615–616.

ANSELL, G. B. and SPANNER, S. (1972) The application of zonal centrifugation to the study of some brain subcellular fractions. *Prog. Brain Res.*, **36**, 3–11.

APPEL, S. H., DAY, E. D. and MICKEY, D. D. (1972) Cellular and subcellular fractionation. *In Basic Neurochemistry*, ed. Albers, R. W., Siegel, G. J., Katzman, R. and Agranoff, B. W. Pp. 425–448. Boston: Little, Brown and Co.

ARMSTRONG-JAMES, M. and JOHNSON, R. (1970) Quantitative studies of postnatal changes in synapses in rat superficial motor cerebral cortex. An electron microscopical study. *Z. Zellforsch.*, **110**, 559–568.

ARREGUI, A., LOGAN, W. J., BENNETT, J. P. and SNYDER, S. H. (1972) Specific glycine-accumulating synaptosomes in the spinal cord of rats. *Proc. Nat. Acad. Sci., U.S.A.*, **69**, 3458–3489.

ATWOOD, H. L., LANG, F. and MORIN, W. A. (1972) Synaptic vesicles. Selective depletion in crayfish excitatory and inhibitory axons. *Science*, **176**, 1353–1355.

AUSTIN, L., ROSTAS, J. A., LIVETT, B. G. and JEFFREY, P. L. (1973) Disruption and antigenicity of synaptosomal membranes. *Abstracts of Fourth International Neurochemistry Meeting, Tokyo*, 162.

AUTILIO, L. A., APPEL, S. H., PETTIS, P. and GAMBETTI, P. L. (1968) Biochemical studies of synapses in vitro. I. Protein synthesis. *Biochemistry*, **7**, 2615–2622.

AUTILIO, L. A., NORTON, W. T. and TERRY, R. D. (1964) The preparation and some properties of purified myelin from the central nervous system. *J. Neurochem.*, **11**, 17–27.

BACQ, Z. M. (1935) Recherches sur la physiologie et la pharmacologie du système nerveux autonome. XVII. Les esters de la choline dans les extraits de tissus des invertébrés. *Archs int. Physiol.*, **42**, 24–42.

BACQ, Z. M. and MAZZA, F. P. (1935) Recherches sur la physiologie et la pharmacologie du système nerveux autonome. XVIII. Isolement de chloraurate d'acétylcholine a partir d'un extrait de cellules nerveuses d'*Octopus vulgaris*. *Arch. int. Physiol.*, **42**, 43–46.

BALÁZS, R., DAHL, D. and HARWOOD, J. R. (1966) Subcellular distribution of enzymes of glutamate metabolism in rat brain. *J. Neurochem.*, **13**, 897–905.

BALDESSARINI, R. J. and VOGT, M. (1971) Uptake and release of norepinephrine by rat brain tissue fractions prepared by ultra-filtration. *J. Neurochem.*, **18**, 951–962.

BALFOUR, D. J. K. and GILBERT, J. C. (1970) Studies on the respiration of synaptosomes. *Biochem. Pharmac.*, **20**, 1151–1156.

BANDHUIN, P., EVRARD, P. and BERTHET, J. (1967) Electron microscopic examination of subcellular fractions. *J. Cell Biol.*, **32**, 181–191.

BANIK, N. L. and DAVISON, A. N. (1969) Enzyme activity and composition of myelin and subcellular fractions in the developing rat brain. *Biochem. J.*, **115**, 1051–1062.

BARBER, V. C. (1966) The fine structure of the statocyst of *Octopus vulgaris*. *Z. Zellforsch.*, **70**, 91–107.

BARBER, V. C. (1967) A neurosecretory tissue in *Octopus*. *Nature, Lond.*, **213**, 1042–1043.

BARBER, V. C. and GRAZIADEI, P. (1966) Cephalopod synaptic organisation. *Proc. 6th Int. Congr. Electron Microsc., Kyoto*, Tokyo, Maruzen. Pp. 433–434.

BARER, R., HELLER, H. and LEDERIS, K. (1963) The isolation, identification and properties of the hormonal granules of the neurohypophysis. *Proc. Roy. Soc. Lond. B.*, **158**, 388–416.

BARKER, J. L. and GAINER, H. (1973) Pentobarbital: selective depression of excitatory postsynaptic potentials. *Science*, **182**, 720–722.

BARKER, L. A., DOWDALL, M. J., ESSMAN, W. B. and Whittaker, V. P. (1970) The compartmentation of acetylcholine in cholinergic nerve terminals. In *Drugs and Cholinergic Mechanisms in the CNS*, ed. Heilbronn, E. and Winter, A. Pp. 193–223. Stockholm: Almqvist and Wiksell.

BARKER, L. A., DOWDALL, M. J. and WHITTAKER, V. P. (1972) Choline metabolism in the cerebral cortex of guinea pigs. *Biochem. J.*, **130**, 1063–1080.

BARLOW, J. and MARTIN, R. (1971) Structural identification and distribution of synaptic profiles in the *Octopus* brain using the zinc iodide–osmium method. *Brain Res.*, **25**, 241–253.

BARONDES, S. H. (1966) On the site of synthesis of the mitochondrial protein of nerve endings. *J. Neurochem.*, **13**, 721–727.

BARONDES, S. H. (1968) Further studies of the transport of protein to nerve endings. *J. Neurochem.*, **15**, 343–350.

BARONDES, S. H. (1969) Axoplasmic transport. In *Handbook of Neurochemistry*, Lajtha, A. (ed.) Vol. **2**, pp. 435–445. New York: Plenum Press.

BARRANTES, F. J. and LUNT, G. G. (1970) Enzymic dissection of cerebral cortex synapses. *Brain. Res.*, **23**, 305–313.

BARRNETT, R. J. (1962) The fine structural localization of acetylcholinesterase at the myoneural junction. *J. Cell Biol.*, **12**, 247–262.

BASS, N. H., NETSKY, M. G. and Young E. (1970) Effect of neonatal malnutrition on developing cerebrum. 1. Microchemical and histologic study of cellular differentiation in the rat. *Archs. Neurol., Chicago*, **23**, 289–302.

BEANI, L., BIANCHI, C., MEGAZZINI, P., BALLOTTI, L. and BERNARD, G. (1969) Drug induced changes in free, labile and stable acetylcholine of guinea-pig brain. *Biochem. Pharmac.*, **18**, 1315–1324.

BELOFF-CHAIN, A., CANTANZARO, R., CHAIN, E. B., MASI, I. and POCCHIARI, F. (1955) Fate of uniformly labelled ^{14}C-glucose in brain slices. *Proc. Roy. Soc. Lond. B.*, **144**, 22–28.

204

BENEDETTI, E. L. and BERTOLINI, B. (1963) The use of the phosphotungstic acid (PTA) as a stain for the plasma membrane. *J. Roy. Microsc. Soc.*, **81**, 219–222.

BFNEDETTI, E. L. and EMMELOT, P. (1968) Structure and function of plasma membranes isolated from liver. In *The Membranes*, ed. Dalton, A. J. and Haguenau, F. Pp. 33–120. New York: Academic Press.

ƷENNETT, E. L., DIAMOND, M. C., KRECH, D. and ROSENZWEIG, M. R. (1964) Chemical and anatomical plasticity of brain. *Science*, **146**, 610–619.

BENNETT, G. W. and EDWARDSON, J. A. (1973), Ca^{2+} dependent release of hypophysiotropic substances from hypothalamic synaptosomes, *J. Endocrinol.*, **59**, XV.

BENNETT, G., DI GIAMBERARDINO, L., KOENIG, H. L. and DROZ, B. (1973) Axonal migration of protein and glycoprotein to nerve endings. II. Radioautographic analysis of the renewal of glycoproteins in nerve endings of chicken ciliary ganglion after intracerebral injection of [^{3}H]-fucose and [^{3}H]-glucosamine, *Brain Res.* **60**, 129–146.

BENNETT, H. S. (1963) Morphological aspects of extracellular polysaccharides. *J. Histochem Cytochem.*, **11**, 14–23.

BENNETT, M. V. L. (1972) Comparison of electrically and chemically mediated synaptic transmission. In *Structure and Function of Synapses*, ed. Pappas, G. D. and Purpura, D. P. Pp. 221–256. New York: Raven Press.

BENNETT, M. V. L., ALJURE, E., NAKAJIMA, Y. and PAPPAS, G. D. (1963) Electrotonic junctions between teleost spinal neurons: electrophysiology and ultrastructure. *Science*, **141**, 262–264.

BENNETT, M. V. L., PAPPAS, G. D., GIMÉNEZ, M. and NAKAJIMA, Y. (1967) Physiology and ultrastructure of electrotonic junctions. IV. Medullary electromotor nuclei in Gymnotid fish. *J. Neurophysiol.*, **30**, 236–300.

BENSLEY, R. R., and HOERR, N. L. (1934) Studies on cell structure by the freezing-drying method. VI. The preparation and properties of mitochondria. *Anat. Rec.*, **60**, 449–455.

BERL, S. and PUSZKIN, S. (1970) Mg^{2+}–Ca^{2+}-activated adenosine triphosphatase system isolated from mammalian brain. *Biochemistry*, **9**, 2058–2067.

BERL, S., PUSZKIN, S. and NICKLAS, W. J. (1973) Actomyosin-like protein in brain. *Science*, **179**, 441–446.

BERNSTEIN, J. J. and Bernstein, M. E. (1973) Neuronal alteration and reinnervation following axonal regeneration and sprouting in mammalian spinal cord. *Brain, Behav. Evol.*, **8**, 135–161.

BERTHET, J. and DE DUVE, C. (1951) Tissue fractionation studies. I. The existence of a mitochondria-linked, enzymically inactive form of acid phosphatase in rat-liver tissue. *Biochem. J.*, **50**, 174–181.

BINDLER, E., LABELLA, F. S., and SANWAL, M. (1967), Isolated nerve endings (neuro-secretosomes) from the posterior pituitary. *J. Cell Biol.*, **34**, 185–205.

BIRKS, R. I. (1966) The fine structure of motor nerve endings at frog myoneural junction. *Ann. N. Y. Acad. Sci.*, **135**, 8–19.

BIRKS, R., HUXLEY, H. E. and KATZ, B. (1960) The fine structure of the neuromuscular junction of the frog. *J. Physiol., Lond.*, **150**, 134–144.

BIRKS, R. I., KATZ, B. and MILEDI, R. (1960b) Physiological and structural changes at the amphibian myoneural junction in the course of nerve degeneration. *J. Physiol., Lond.*, **150**, 145–168.

BISBY, M. A. and FILLENZ, M. (1969) Isolation of peripheral synaptosomes from a sympathetically innervated tissue. *J. Physiol., Lond.*, **204**, 105P–106P.

BISCHOFF, A. and MOOR, H. (1967) Ultrastructural differences between the myelin sheaths of peripheral nerve fibres and CNS white matter. *Z. Zellforsch.*, **81**, 303–310.

BITTIGER, H. and SCHNEBLI, H. P. (1974) Binding of concanavalin A and ricin to synaptic junctions of rat brain. *Nature, Lond.*, **249**, 370–371.

BITTNER, G. D. and KENNEDY, D. (1970) Quantitative aspects of transmitter release. *J. Cell Biol.*, **47**, 585–592.

BJÖRKERUD, S. (1963) The isolation of lipofuscin granules from bovine cardiac muscle, with observations on the properties of the isolated granules on the light and electron microscopic levels. *J. Ultrastruct. Res.*, supp,. **5**, 1–49.

BLACKMAN, J. G., GINSBORG, B. L. and RAY, C. (1963a) Spontaneous synaptic activity in sympathetic ganglion cells of the frog. *J. Physiol. Lond.*, **167**, 389–401.

BLACKMAN, J. G., GINSBORG, B. L. and RAY, C. (1963b) On the quantal release of the transmitter at a sympathetic synapse. *J. Physiol. Lond.*, **167**, 402–415.

BLACKSTAD, T. W. and FLOOD, P. R. (1963) Ultrastructure of hippocampal axo-somatic synapses. *Nature, Lond.*, **198**, 542–543.

BLAKELEY, A. G., BROWN, L. and GEFFEN, L. B. (1969) Uptake and re-use of sympathetic transmitter in the cat's spleen. *Proc. Roy. Soc. Lond. B.*, **174**, 51–68.

BLASCHKO, H. (1959) The development of current concepts of catecholamine formation. *Pharmacol. Rev.*, **11**, 307–316.

BLASHKO, H., HAGEN, J. M. and HAGEN, P. (1957) Mitochondrial enzymes and chromaffin granules. *J. Physiol. Lond.*, **139**, 316–322.

BLASHKO, H., HAGEN, P. and WELSCH, A. D. (1955) Observations on the intracellular granules of the adrenal medulla. *J. Physiol. Lond.*, **129**, 27–49.

BLASCHKO, H. and WELSCH, A. D. (1953) Localization of adrenaline in cytoplasmic particles of the bovine adrenal medulla. *Arch. exp. Path. Pharmak.*, **219**, 17–22.

BLAUSTEIN, M. P., JOHNSON, E. M. and NEEDLEMAN, P. (1972) Calcium-dependent norepinephrine release from presynaptic nerve endings *in vitro*. *Proc. natn. Acad. Sci., U.S.A.*, **69**, 2237–2240.

BLAUSTEIN, M. P. and WEISMANN, N. W. P. (1970) Potassium ions and calcium ion influxes in isolated nerve terminals. In *Drugs and Cholinergic Mechanisms in the CNS*, ed. Heibronn, E. and Winter, A. Pp. 291–307. Stockholm: Research Institute of National Defence.

BLOMSTRAND, C. and HAMBERGER, A. (1969) Protein turnover in cell-enriched fractions from rabbit brain. *J. Neurochem.*, **16**, 1401–1407.

BLOOM, F. E. (1972a) Localization of neurotransmitters by electron microscopy. In *Neurotransmitters*, Research Publication, Association for Research in Nervous and Mental Disease, Vol. **50**, pp. 25–57.

BLOOM, F. E. (1972b) The formation of synaptic junctions in developing rat brain. In *Structure and Function of Synapses*, ed. Pappas, G. D. and Purpura, D. P. Pp. 101–120. New York: Raven Press.

BLOOM, F. E. and AGHAJANIAN, G. K. (1966) Cytochemistry of synapses: a selective staining method for electron microscopy. *Science*, **154**, 1575–1577.

BLOOM, F. E. and AGHAJANIAN, G. K. (1968) Fine structural and cytochemical analysis of the staining of synaptic junctions with phosphotungstic acid. *J. Ultrastruct. Res.*, **22**, 361–375.

BLOOM, F. E. and BARRNETT, R. J. (1966) Fine structural localization of noradrenaline in vesicles of autonomic nerve endings. *Nature, Lond.*, **210**, 599–601.

BLOOM, F. E. and IVERSEN, L. L. (1971) Localizing ^{3}H-GABA in nerve terminals of rat cerebral cortex by electron microscopic autoradiography. *Nature, Lond.*, **229**, 628–630.

BLOOM, F. E., IVERSEN, L. L. and SCHMITT, F. O. (1970) Macromolecules in Synaptic Function. *Neurosci. Res. Program Bull.*, **8**, 325–455.

BOBTELSKY, M. and COHEN, M. M. (1960) Reactions between alcaloids and bismuth iodide, the compounds formed and their analytical application. A heterometric study. *Anal. Chim. Acta.*, **22**, 270–283.

BOCCI, V. (1966) Enzyme and metabolic properties of isolated neurones. *Nature, Lond.*, **212**, 826–827.

BODIAN, D. (1942) Cytological aspects of synaptic function. *Physiol. Rev.*, **22**, 146–169.

BODIAN, D. (1966a) Development of fine structure of spinal cord in monkey fetuses. I. The motoneuron neuropil at the time of onset of reflex activity. *Bull. Johns Hopkins Hosp.*, **119**, 129–149.

BODIAN, D. (1966b) Electron microscopy: two major synaptic types on spinal motoneurons. *Science*, **151**, 1093–1094.

BODIAN, D. (1968) Development of fine structure of spinal cord in monkey fetuses. II. Pre-reflex period to period of long intersegmental reflexes. *J. Comp. Neurol.*, **133**, 113–166.

BODIAN, D. (1970) An electron microscopic characterization of classes of synaptic vesicles by means of controlled aldehyde fixation. *J. Cell. Biol.*, **44**, 115–124.

BOGDANSKI, D. F., TISSARI, A. and BRODIE, B. B. (1968) The role of sodium, potassium, ouabain and reserpine in uptake, storage and metabolism of biogenic amines in synaptosomes. *Life Sci.*, **7**, 419–428.

BONDAREFF, W. (1967) An intercellular substance in rat cerebral cortex: submicroscopic distribution of ruthenium red. *Anat. Rec.*, **157**, 527–536.

BONDAREFF, W. and GORDON, B. (1966) Submicroscopic localization of norepinephrine in sympathetic nerves of rat pineal. *J. Pharmacol. Exp. Ther.*, **153**, 42–47.

BONDAREFF, W. and HYDÉN, H. (1969) Submicroscopic structure of single neurons isolated from rabbit lateral vestibular nucleus. *J. Ultrastruct. Res.*, **26**, 399–411.

BONDAREFF, W. and SJÖSTRAND, J. (1969) Cytochemistry of synaptosomes. *Exptl. Neurol.*, **24**, 450–458.

BOSMAN, H. B. and HEMSWORTH, B. A. (1970) Incorporation of amino acids and monosaccharides into macromolecules by isolated synaptosomes and synaptosomal mitochondria. *J. Biol. Chem.*, **245**, 363–371.

BOWERS, B. (1964) Coated vesicles in the pericardial cells of the aphid (*Myzus persicae Sulz*). *Protoplasma*, **59**, 351–367.

BOWERY, N. G. and BROWN, D. A. (1972) γ-aminobutyric acid uptake by sympathetic ganglia. *Nature, New Biol.*, **238**, 89–91.

BRADFORD, H. F. (1967) Metabolism of nerve ending particles. *Abstr. 1st Int. Neurochem. Congr.*, 30.

BRADFORD, H. F. (1969) Respiration *in vitro* of synaptosomes from mammalian cerebral cortex. *J. Neurochem.*, **16**, 675–684.

BRADFORD, H. F. (1970) Metabolic response of synaptosomes to electrical stimulation: release of amino acids. *Brain Res.*, **19**, 239–247.

BRADFORD, H. F. (1971) Membrane potentials and metabolic performance in mammalian synaptosomes. In *Defects in Cellular Organelles and Membranes in Relation to Mental Retardation*, ed. Benson, P. F. Pp. 1–15. London: Churchill.

BRADFORD, H. F., BENNETT, G. W. and THOMAS, A. J. (1973) Depolarizing stimuli and the release of physiologically active amino acids from suspensions of mammalian synaptosomes. *J. Neurochem.*, **21**, 495–505.

BRADFORD, H. F., BROWNLOW, E. K. and GAMMACK, D. B. (1966) The distribution of cation stimulated adenosine triphosphatase in subcellular fractions from bovine cerebral cortex. *J. Neurochem.*, **13**, 1283–1297.

BRADFORD, H. F., CHEIFETZ, P. N. and EDWARDSON, J. A. (1972) Release of corticotrophin releasing factor (CRF) following the electrical stimulation of nerve-endings isolated from the sheep hypothalamus. *J. Physiol., Lond.*, **222**, 52P–53P.

BRADFORD, H. F., JONES, D. G., and BOOHER, J. (1975) Biochemical and morphological studies of the short and long term survival of isolated nerve-endings. Unpublished.

BRADFORD, H. F. and THOMAS, A. J. (1969) Metabolism of glucose and glutamate by synaptosomes from mammalian cerebral cortex. *J. Neurochem.*, **16**, 1495–1504.

BRANTON, D. (1966) Fracture faces in frozen membranes. *Proc. Natl. Acad. Sci. U.S.A.*, **55**, 1048–1056.

BRANTON, D. (1967) Fracture faces of frozen myelin. *Exp. Cell Res.*, **45**, 703–707.

BRANTON, D. (1969) Membrane structure. *Ann. Rev. Plant Physiol.*, **20**, 209–238.

BRENNER, S. and HORNE, R. W. (1959) A negative staining method for high resolution electron microscopy of viruses. *Biochim. Biophys. Acta.*, **34**, 103–110.

BRODKIN, E. and ELLIOTT, K. A. C. (1953) Binding of acetylcholine. *Am. J. Physiol.*, **173**, 437–442.

BRODY, T. M. and BAIN, J. A. (1951) Effect of barbiturates on oxidative phosphorylation. *Proc. Soc. Exp. Biol. Med.*, **77**, 50–53.

BRODY, T. M. and BAIN, J. A. (1952) A mitochondrial preparation from mammalian brain. *J. Biol. Chem.*, **195**, 685–696.

BROWN, G. L., DALE, H. H. and FELDBERG, W. (1936) Reactions of the normal mammalian muscle to acetylcholine and to eserine. *J. Physiol., Lond.*, **87**, 394–424.

BRUNI, C. and PORTER, K. R. (1965) The fine structure of the parenchymal cell of the normal rat liver. *Am. J. Pathol.*, **46**, 691–755.

BRUNNGRABER, E. G., DEKIRMENJIAN, H. and BROWN, B. D. (1967) The distribution of protein-bound *N*-Acetylneuraminic acid in subcellular fractions of rat brain. *Biochem., J.*, **103**, 73–78.

BRZIN, M., TENNYSON, V. M. and DUFFY, P. E. (1966) Acetylcholinesterase in frog sympathetic and dorsal root ganglia. A study by electron microscope cytochemistry and microgasometric analysis with the magnetic diver. *J. Cell Biol.*, **31**, 215–242.

BUNEŠOVÁ, O. and BUREŠ, J. (1969) Can the brain be improved? *Endeavour*, **28**, 139–145.

BUNGE, R. P. (1968) Glial cells and the central myelin sheath. *Physiol. Rev.*, **48**, 197–251.

BUNGE, M. B., BUNGE, R. P. and PETERSON, E. R. (1967) The onset of synapse formation in spinal cord cultures as studied by electron microscopy. *Brain Res.*, **6**, 728–749.

BUNT, A. H. (1969) Formation of coated and 'synaptic' vesicles within neurosecretory axon terminals of the crustacean sinus gland. *J. Ultrastruct. Res.*, **28**, 411–421.

BURDICK, C. J. and STRITTMATTER, C. F. (1965) Appearance of biochemical components related to acetylcholine metabolism during the embryonic development of chick brain. *Arch. Biochem.*, **109**, 293–301.

BURN, J. H. and RAND, M. J. (1959) Sympathetic postganglionic mechanism. *Nature, Lond.*, **184**, 163–165.

BURN, J. H. and RAND, M. J. (1965) Acetylcholine in adrenergic transmission. *Ann. Rev. Pharmacol.*, **5**, 163–182.

BURNSTOCK, G. (1970) Structure of smooth muscle and its innervation. In *Smooth Muscle*, ed. Bülbring, E., Brading, H. and Jones, A. Pp. 1–69. London: Arnold.

BURT, A. M. (1969) The histochemical demonstration of choline acetyltransferase activity in the spinal cord of the rat. *Anat. Rec.*, **163**, 162.

BURT, A. M. (1970) A histochemical procedure for the localization of choline acetyltransferase activity. *J. Histochem. Cytochem.*, **18**, 408–415.

BURTON, R. M. HOWARD, R. E. and GIBBONS, J. M. (1964) Ganglioside and acetylcholine-containing synaptic vesicles of rat brain. *Abstracts of Sixth International Meeting of Biochemistry*, V.E–97.

CALEY, D. W. and MAXWELL, D. S. (1968a) An electron microscopic study of neurons during postnatal development of the rat cerebral cortex. *J. Comp. Neurol.*, **133**, 17–44.

CALEY, D. W. and MAXWELL, D. S. (1968b) An electron microscopic study of the neuroglia during postnatal development of the rat cerebrum. *J. Comp. Neurol.*, **133**, 45–70.

CALEY, D. W. and MAXWELL, D. S. (1970) Development of the blood vessels and extracellular spaces during postnatal maturation of rat cerebral cortex. *J. Comp. Neurol.*, **138**, 31–48.

CALEY, D. W. and MAXWELL, D. S. (1971) Ultrastructure of the developing cerebral cortex in the rat. In *Brain Development and Behavior*, ed. Sterman, M. B., McGinty, D. J. and Adinolfi, A. M. Pp. 91–107. New York: Academic Press.

CANNON, W. B. and BACQ, Z. M. (1931) Studies on the conditions of activity in endocrine organs. XXVI. A hormone produced by sympathetic action on smooth muscle. *Am. J. Physiol.*, **96**, 392–412.

CARLINI, E. A. and GREEN, J. P. (1963) The subcellular distribution of histamine, slow reaching substance and 5-hydroxytryptamine in the brain of the rat. *Brit. J. Pharmacol.*, **20**, 264–277.

CECCARELLI, B., HURLBUT, W. P. and MAURO, A. (1972) Depletion of vesicles from frog neuromuscular junctions by prolonged tetanic stimulation. *J. Cell Biol.*, **54**, 30–38.

CECCARELLI, B., HURLBUT, W. P. and MAURO, A. (1973) Turnover of transmitter and synaptic vesicles at the frog neuromuscular junction. *J. Cell Biol.*, **57**, 499–524.

CECCARELLI, B. and PENSA, P. (1968) Morphological aspects of synaptic vesicles after different aldehyde fixations. In *Electron Microscopy 1968*, ed. Bocciarelli, D. S. Vol. 2. Pp. 545–546. Rome: Tipografia Poliglotta Vaticana.

CHAKRIN, L. W., MARCHBANKS, R. M., MITCHELL, J. F. and WHITTAKER, V. P. (1972) The origin of the acetylcholine released from the surface of the cortex. *J. Neurochem.*, **19**, 2727–2736.

CHAKRIN, L. W. and WHITTAKER, V. P. (1969) The subcellular distribution of [N-Me-^{3}H]-acetylcholine synthesized by brain *in vivo*. *Biochem. J.*, **113**, 97–107.

CHALAZONITIS, N. (1969) Differentiation of membranes in axonal endings in the neuropile of *Helix*. In *Cellular Dynamics of the Neuron*, ed. Barondes, S. H. Pp. 229–243. New York: Academic Press.

CHARLTON, B. T. and GRAY, E. G. (1966) Comparative electron microscopy of synapses in the vertebrate spinal cord. *J. Cell Sci.*, **1**, 67–80.

CHEN, I. and LEE, C. Y. (1970) Ultrastructural changes in the motor nerve terminals caused by β-bungarotoxin. *Virchows Arch. Abt. B. Zellpathol.*, **6**, 318–325.

CHURCHILL, L. and COTMAN, C. W. (1973) Analytical zonal centrifugation of synaptosomes and mitochondria from rat brain homogenates. *Neurobiology*, **3**, 311–319.

CHURG, J., MAUTNER, W. and GRISHMAN, E. (1958) Silver impregnation for electron microscopy. *J. biophys. biochem. Cytol.*, **4**, 841–842.

CLARK, A. W., HURLBUT, W. P. and MAURO, A. (1972) Changes in the fine structure of the neuromuscular junction of the frog caused by black widow spider venom. *J. Cell Biol.*, **52**, 1–14.

CLARK, A. W., MAURO, A., LONGENECKER, H. E. and HURLBUT, W. P. (1970) Effects of black widow spider venom on the frog neuromuscular junction. Effects on the fine structure of the frog neuromuscular junction. *Nature, Lond.*, **225**, 703–705.

CLARKE, E. and O'MALLEY, C. D. (1968) *The Human Brain and Spinal Cord*, Berkeley and Los Angeles: University of California.

CLAUDE, A. (1946) Fractionation of mammalian liver cells by differential centrifugation. I. Problems, methods, and preparation of extract. *J. Exp. Med.*, **84**, 51–59.

CLEMENTI, F., CECCARELLI, B., CERATI, E., DEMONTE, M. L., FELICI, M., MOTTA, M. and PECILE, A. (1970) Subcellular localization of neurotransmitters and releasing factors in the rat median eminence. *J. Endocr.*, **48**, 205–213.

CLEMENTI, F., MANTEGAZZA, P. and BOTTURI, M. (1966a) Pharmacologic and morphologic study on the nature of the dense-core granules present in the presynaptic endings of sympathetic ganglia. *Intern. J. Neuropharmacol.*, **5**, 281–285.

CLEMENTI, F., WHITTAKER, V. P. and SHERIDAN, M. N. (1966b) The yield of synaptosomes from the cerebral cortex of guinea pigs estimated by a polystyrene bead 'tagging' procedure. *Z. Zellforsch.*, **72**, 126–138.

COAKLEY, W. T. (1974) Comparison of conditions of tissue fragmentation. *Brain Res.*, **70**, 281–284.

COHEN, H. A. and McGOVERN, S. A. (1973) Identity of 'dumbbell' profiles in synaptosomal fractions from rat brain. *J. Neurobiol.*, **4**, 583–587.

COLBURN, R. W., GOODWIN, F. K., MURPHY, D. L., BUNNEY, W. E. and DAVIS, J. M. (1968) Quantitative studies of noradrenaline uptake by synaptosomes. *Biochem. Pharmac.*, **17**, 957–964.

COLLIER, B. (1969) The preferential release of newly synthesized transmitter by a sympathetic ganglion. *J. Physiol., Lond.*, **205**, 341–352.

COLLIER, B. and MACINTOSH, F. C. (1969) The source of choline for acetylcholine synthesis in a sympathetic ganglion. *Can. J. Physiol. Pharmacol.*, **47**, 127–135.

COLLIER, B., POON, P. and SALEHMOGHADDAM, S. (1972) The formation of choline and of acetylcholine by brain *in vitro*. *J. Neurochem.*, **19**, 51–60.

COLONNIER, M. (1964) Experimental degeneration in the cerebral cortex. *J. Anat., Lond.*, **98**, 47–53.

COLONNIER, M. (1968) Synaptic patterns on different cell types in the different laminae of the cat visual cortex. An electron microscope study. *Brain Res.*, **9**, 268–287.

COLONNIER, M. and GUILLERY, R. W. (1964) Synaptic organization in the lateral geniculate nucleus of the monkey. *Z. Zellforsch.*, **62**, 333–355.

COOKE, C. T., NOLAN, T. M., DYSON, S. E. and JONES, D. G. (1974) Pentobarbital-induced configurational changes at the synapse. *Brain Res.*, **76**, 330–335.

COSTIN, A., COTMAN, V., HAFEMANN, D. R. and HERSCHMANN, H. R. (1972) Effect of antibrain synaptosomal fraction serum and complement on evoked potentials and impedance. *Experientia,* **28**, 411–412.

COTMAN, C. W. (1968) Doctoral dissertation, Department of Chemistry, Indiana University, Bloomington, Indiana.

COTMAN, C. W. (1972) Principles for the optimization of centrifugation conditions for fractionation of brain tissue. In *Research Methods in Neurochemistry*, **1**, ed. Marks N. and Rodnight, R. Pp. 45–93. New York: Plenum Press.

COTMAN, C., BROWN, D. H., HARRELL, B. W., and ANDERSON, N. G. (1970) Analytical differential centrifugation: an analysis of the sedimentation properties of synaptosomes, mitochondria and lysosomes from rat brain homogenates. *Arch. Biochem. Biophys.*, **136**, 436–447.

COTMAN, C. W. and FLANSBURG, D. A. (1970) An analytical micro-method for electron microscopic study of the composition and sedimentation properties of subcellular fractions. *Brain Res.*, **22**, 152–156.

COTMAN, C., HERSCHMAN, H. and TAYLOR, D. (1971a) Subcellular fractionation of cultured glial cells. *J. Neurobiol.*, **2**, 169–180.

COTMAN, C. W., LEVY, W., BANKER, G. and TAYLOR, D. (1971b) An ultrastructural and chemical analysis of the effect of triton X-100 on synaptic plasma membranes. *Biochim. Biophys. Acta.*, **249**, 406–418.

COTMAN, C., MAHLER, H. R. and ANDERSON, N. G. (1968a) Isolation of a membrane fraction enriched in nerve-end membranes from rat brain by zonal centrifugation. *Biochim. Biophys. Acta*, **163**, 272–275.

COTMAN, C. W., MAHLER, H. R. and HUGLI, T. E. (1968b) Isolation and characterization of insoluble proteins of the synaptic plasma membrane. *Arch. Biochem. Biophys.*, **126**, 821–837.

COTMAN, C. W. and MATTHEWS, D. A. (1971) Synaptic plasma membranes from rat brain synaptosomes: isolation and partial characterization. *Biochim. Biophys. Acta*, **249**, 380–394.

COTMAN, C. W. and TAYLOR, D. A. (1971) Autoradiographic analysis of protein synthesis in synaptosomal fractions. *Brain Res.*, **29**, 366–372.

COTMAN, C. W. and TAYLOR, D. (1972) Isolation and structural studies on synaptic complexes from rat brain. *J. Cell Biol.*, **55**, 696–711.

COTMAN, C., TAYLOR, D. and LYNCH, G. (1973) Ultrastructural changes in synapses in the dentate gyrus of the rat during development. *Brain Res.*, **63**, 205–213.

COTTRELL, G. A. (1966) Separation and properties of subcellular particles associated with 5-hydroxytryptamine, with acetylcholine and with an unidentified cardio-excitatory substance from *Mercenaria* nervous tissue. *Comp. Biochem. Physiol.*, **17**, 891–907.

COUTEAUX, R. (1961) Principaux critères morphologiques et cytochimiques utilisables aujourd' hui pour definir les divers types de synapses. *Act. Neurophysiol.*, **3**, 145–173.

COYLE, J. T. and SNYDER, S. H. (1969) Catecholamine uptake by synaptosomes in homogenates of rat brain: stereospecificity in different areas. *J. Pharmacol. Exp. Ther.*, **170**, 221–231.

CRAGG, B. G. (1968) Are there structural alterations in synapses related to functioning? *Proc. Roy. Soc. Lond. B*, **171**, 319–323.

CRAGG, B. G. (1969a) Structural changes in naive retinal synapses detectable within minutes of first exposure to daylight. *Brain Res.*, **15**, 79–96.

CRAGG, B. G. (1969b) The effects of vision and dark-rearing on the size and density of synapses in the lateral geniculate nucleus measured by electron microscopy. *Brain Res.*, **13**, 53–67.

CRAGG, B. G. (1970) Synapses and membranous bodies in experimental hypothyroidism. *Brain Res.*, **18**, 297–307.

CRAGG, B. G. (1971) Plasticity of synapses. In *Structure and Function of Nervous Tissue*, ed. Bourne, G. H. Vol. 4. Pp. 1–60. Academic Press, New York.

CRAGG, B. G. (1972a) The development of cortical synapses during starvation in the rat. *Brain*, **95**, 143–150.

CRAGG, B. G. (1972b) The development of synapses in cat visual cortex. *Invest. Ophthalmol.*, **11**, 377–385.

CRAIN, B., COTMAN, C., TAYLOR, D. and LYNCH, G. (1973) A quantitative electron microscope study of synaptogenesis in the dentate gyrus of the rat. *Brain Res.*, **63**, 195–204.

CRAIN, S. M. and BORNSTEIN, M. B. (1964) Bioelectric activity of neonatal mouse cerebral cortex during growth and differentiation in tissue culture. *Exptl. Neurol.*, **10**, 425–450.

CREMER, J. E., JOHNSTON, P. V., ROOTS, B. I. and TREVOR, A. J. (1968) Heterogeneity of brain fractions containing neuronal and glial cells. *J. Neurochem.*, **15**, 1361–1370.

SILLIK, B. and JOÓ, F. (1967) Effect of hemicholinium on the number of synaptic vesicles. *Nature, Lond.*, **213**, 508–509.

CSILLIK, B., KNYIHÁR, E., LÁSZLÓ, I. and BONCZ, I. (1974) Electron histochemical evidence for the role of thiamine pyrophosphatase in synaptic transmission, *Brain Res.*, **70**, 179–183.

CUÉNOD, M., SANDRI, C. and AKERT, K. (1970) Enlarged synaptic vesicles as an early sign of secondary degeneration in the optic nerve terminals of the pigeon. *J. Cell Sci.*, **6**, 605–613.

CUÉNOD, M. and SCHÖNBACH, J. (1971) Synaptic proteins and axonal flow in the pigeon visual pathway. *J. Neurochem.*, **18**, 809–816.

CURRAN, R. C., CLARK, A. E. and LOVELL, D. (1965) Acid mucopolysaccharides in electron microscopy. The use of the colloidal iron method *J. Anat., Lond.*, **99**, 427–434.

CURTIS, D. R. and DE GROAT, W. C. (1968) Tetanus toxin and spinal inhibition. *Brain Res.* **10**, 208–212.

CURTIS, D. R., FELIX, D., GAME, C. J. A. and McCULLOCH, R. M. (1973) Tetanus toxin and the synaptic release of GABA. *Brain Res.*, **51**, 358–362.

CURTIS, D. R. and JOHNSTON, G. A. R. (1970) Amino acid transmitters. In *Handbook of Neurochemistry*, ed. Lajtha, A. Vol. 4, pp. 115–134. New York: Plenum Press.

211

CUZNER, M. L. and DAVISON, A. N. (1968) The lipid composition of rat brain myelin and subcellular fractions during development. *Biochem. J.*, **106**, 29–34.

DALE, H. H. (1914) The action of certain esters and ethers of choline, and their relation to muscarine. *J. Pharmacol. Exp. Ther.*, **6**, 147–190.

DALE, H. H. (1935) Pharmacology and nerve endings. *Proc. Roy. Soc. Med.*, **28**, 319–332.

DALE, H. H., FELDBERG, W. and VOGT, M. (1936) Release of acetylcholine at voluntary motor nerve endings. *J. Physiol., Lond.*, **86**, 353–380.

DAVIS, G. and BLOOM, F. E. (1970) Proteins of synaptic junctional complexes. *J. Cell Biol.*, **47**, 46a.

DAVIS, G. A. and BLOOM, F. E. (1973) Isolation of synaptic junctional complexes from rat brain. *Brain Res.*, **62**, 135–154.

DAVIS, R. and KOELLE, G. B. (1967) Electron microscopic localization of acetylcholinesterase and nonspecific cholinesterase at the neuromuscular junction by the gold–thiocholine and gold–thiolacetic acid methods. *J. Cell. Biol.*, **34**, 157–171.

DAY, E. D., MCMILLAN, P. N., MICKEY, D. D. and APPEL, S. H. (1971) Zonal centrifuge profiles of rat brain homogenates: instability in sucrose, stability in iso-osmotic Ficoll–sucrose, *Analyt. Biochem.*, **39**, 29–45.

DE BELLEROCHE, J. S. and BRADFORD, H. F. (1972a) Metabolism of beds of mammalian cortical synaptosomes: response to depolarising influences. *J. Neurochem.*, **19**, 585–602.

DE BELLEROCHE, J. and BRADFORD, H. F. (1972b) The stimulus-induced release of acetylcholine from synaptosome beds and its calcium dependence. *J. Neurochem.*, **19**, 1817–1819.

DE BELLEROCHE, J. S. and BRADFORD, H. F. (1973a) Amino acids in synaptic vesicles from mammalian cerebral cortex: a reappraisal. *J. Neurochem.*, **21**, 441–451.

DE BELLEROCHE, J. S. and BRADFORD, H. F. (1973b) The synaptosome: an isolated, working, neuronal compartment. In *Progress in Neurobiology*, ed. Kerkut, G. A. and Phillis, J. W. Vol. **1**, pp. 275–298. Oxford: Pergamon.

DE BELLEROCHE, J. S., BRADFORD, H. F. and JONES, D. G. (1975) Amino acid release from nerve-endings isolated from sheep basal ganglia. Unpublished.

DE DUVE, C. (1963a) The lysosome concept. In *Lysosomes, CIBA Foundation Symposium*, ed. De Reuck, A. V. S. and Cameron, M.P. Pp. 1–35. London: Churchill.

DE DUVE, C. (1963b) The scope and limitations of cell fractionation. *Biochem. Soc. Symp.* 1–7.

DE DUVE, C., BERTHET, J., BERTHET, L. and APPELMANS, F., (1951) Permeability of mitochondria. *Nature, Lond.*, **167**, 389–390.

DEKIRMENJIAN, H. and BRUNNGRABER, E. G. (1969) Distribution of proteinbound *N*-acetylneuraminic acid in subcellular particulate fractions prepared from whole rat brain. *Biochim. Biophys. Acta*, **177**, 1–10.

DEKIRMENJIAN, H., BRUNNGRABER, E. G., LEMKEY-JOHNSTON, N. and LARRAMENDI, L. M. H. (1969) Distribution of gangliosides, glycoprotein-NANA and acetylcholinesterase in axonal and synaptosomal fractions of cat cerebellum. *Exp. Brain. Res.*, **8**, 97–104.

DEL CASTILLO, J. and KATZ, B. (1954) Quantal components of the end-plate potential. *J. Physiol., Lond.*, **124**, 560–573.

DEL CASTILLO, J. and KATZ, B. (1955) Local activity at a depolarized nerve-muscle junction. *J. Physiol., Lond.*, **128**, 396–411.

DEL CASTILLO, J. and KATZ, B. (1956) Biophysical aspects of neuromuscular transmission. *Progr. Biophys.*, **6**, 121–170.

DEL CASTILLO, J. and KATZ, B. (1957) La base 'quantale' de la transmission neuromusculaire. In: *Microphysiologie Comparée des Eléments Excitables*. Coll. Internat. C.N.R.S. Paris, No. 67, pp. 245–258.

DEL CERRO, M. P. and SNIDER, R. S. (1972) Axo-somatic and axo-dendritic synapses in the cerebellum of the newborn rat. *Brain Res.*, **43**, 581–586.

DEL CERRO, M.P., SNIDER, R. S. and OSTER, M. L. (1969) Subcellular fractions of adult and developing rat cerebellum. *Exp. Brain Res.*, **8**, 311–320.

DE LORENZO, A. J. D. (1961) Electron microscopy of the cerebral cortex. I. The ultrastructure and histochemistry of synaptic junctions. *Bull. Johns Hopkins Hosp.*, **108**, 258–279.

DEMPSEY, G. P., BULLIVANT, S. and WATKINS, W. B. (1973) Ultrastructure of the rat posterior pituitary gland and evidence of hormone release by exocytosis as revealed by freeze-fracturing. *Z. Zellforsch.*, **143**, 465–484.

DENNISON, M. E. (1971) Electron stereoscopy as a means of classifying synaptic vesicles. *J. Cell Sci.*, **8**, 525–539.

DE POTTER, W. P., SMITH, A. D. and DE SCHAEPDRYVER, A. F. (1970) Subcellular fractionation of splenic nerve: ATP, chromagranin A and dopamine β-hydroxylase in noradrenergic vesicles. *Tissue and Cell*, **2**, 529–546.

DERMER, G. B. (1973) Specificity of phosphotungstic acid used as a section stain to visualize surface coats of cells. *J. Ultrastruct. Res.*, **45**, 183–191.

DE ROBERTIS, E. (1956) Submicroscopic changes of the synapse after nerve section in the acoustic ganglion of the guinea pig. An electron microscope study. *J. biophys. biochem. Cytol.*, **2**, 503–512.

DE ROBERTIS, E. (1958) Submicroscopic morphology and function of the synapse. *Exp. Cell Res.*, Suppl. **5**, 347–369.

DE ROBERTIS, E. (1959) Submicroscopic morphology of the synapse. *Int. Rev. Cytol.*, **8**, 61–96.

DE ROBERTIS, E. (1964) *Histophysiology of Synapses and Neurosecretion.* Oxford: Pergamon.

DE ROBERTIS, E. (1967) Ultrastructure and cytochemistry of the synaptic region. *Science*, **156**, 907–914.

DE ROBERTIS, E. (1968) Isolation of inhibitory nerve endings from brain. In *Structure and Function of Inhibitory Neuronal Mechanisms*, ed. Von Euler, C., Skoglund, S. and Soderberg, U. Pp. 511–522. Oxford: Pergamon.

DE ROBERTIS, E. (1971) Molecular biology of synaptic receptors. *Science*, **171**, 963–971.

DE ROBERTIS, E., ALBERICI, M., RODRIGUEZ DE LORES ARNAIZ, G. and AZCURRA, J. M. (1966a) Isolation of different types of synaptic membranes from the brain cortex. *Life Sci.*, **5**, 577–582.

DE ROBERTIS, E., AZCURRA, J. M. and FISZER, S. (1967a) Ultrastructure and cholinergic binding capacity of junctional complexes isolated from rat brain. *Brain Res.*, **5**, 45–56.

DE ROBERTIS, E. D. P. and BENNETT, H. S. (1954) Submicroscopic vesicular component in the synapse. *Fed. Proc.*, **13**, 35.

DE ROBERTIS, E. D. P. and BENNETT, H. S. (1955) Some features of the submicroscopic morphology of synapses in frog and earthworm. *J. biophys. biochem. Cytol.*, **1**, 47–58.

DE ROBERTIS, E. and FRANCHI, C. M. (1956) Electron microscope observations on synaptic vesicles in synapses of the retinal rods and cones. *J. biophys. biochem. Cytol.*, **2**, 307–318.

DE ROBERTIS, E., LAPETINA, E., SAAVEDRA, J. P. and SOTO, E. F. (1966) In vivo and in vitro action of antisera against isolated nerve endings of brain cortex. *Life Sci.*, **5**, 1979–1989.

DE ROBERTIS, E., LAPETINA, E. G. and WALD, F. (1968) The effect of antiserum against nerve-ending membranes from cat cerebral cortex on the ultrastructure of isolated nerve endings and mollusc neurons. *Exptl. Neurol.*, **21**, 322–335.

DE ROBERTIS, E., PELLEGRINO DE IRALDI, A., RODRIGUEZ, G. and GOMEZ, C. J. (1961a) On the isolation of nerve endings and synaptic vesicles. *J. biophys. biochem. Cytol.*, **9**, 229–235.

DE ROBERTIS, E., PELLEGRINO DE IRALDI, A., RODRIGUEZ DE LORES ARNAIZ, G.

and SALGANICOFF, L. (1961b) Electron microscope observations on nerve endings isolated from rat brain. *Anat. Rec.,* **139**, 220.

DE ROBERTIS, E., PELLEGRINO DE IRALDI, A., RODRIGUEZ DE LORES ARNAIZ, G. and SALGANICOFF, L. (1962a) Cholinergic and non-cholinergic nerve endings in rat brain I. *J. Neurochem.,* **9**, 23–35.

DE ROBERTIS, E., PELLEGRINO DE IRALDI, A., RODRIGUEZ DE LORES ARNAIZ, G. and ZIEHER, L. M. (1965) Synaptic vesicles from the rat hypothalmus, isolation and norepinephrine content. *Life Sci.,* **4**, 193–201.

DE ROBERTIS, E., RODRIGUEZ DE LORES ARNAIZ, G., ALBERICI, M., BUTCHER, R. W. and SUTHERLAND, E. W. (1967b) Subcellular distribution of adenyl cyclase and cyclic phosphodiesterase in rat brain cortex. *J. Biol. Chem.,* **242**, 3487–3493.

DE ROBERTIS, E., RODRIGUEZ DE LORES ARNAIZ, G. and PELLEGRINO DE IRALDI, A. (1962b) Isolation of synaptic vesicles from nerve endings of the rat brain. *Nature, Lond.,* **194**, 794–795.

DE ROBERTIS, E., RODRIGUEZ DE LORES ARNAIZ, G., SALGANICOFF, L., PELLEGRINO DE IRALDI, A., and ZIEHER, L. M. (1963) Isolation of synaptic vesicles and structural organization of the acetylcholine system within brain nerve endings. *J. Neurochem.,* **10**, 225–235.

DE ROBERTIS, E., RODRIGUEZ DE LORES ARNAIZ, G. and SELLINGER, O. Z. (1966b) Nerve endings isolated from rats convulsed by methionine sulphoximine. *Nature, Lond.,* **212**, 537–538.

DE ROBERTIS, E., SELLINGER, O. Z., RODRIGUEZ DE LORES ARNAIZ, G., ALBERICI, M. and ZIEHER, L. M. (1967c) Nerve endings in methionine sulphoximine convulsant rats, a neurochemical and ultrastructural study. *J. Neurochem.,* **14**, 81–89.

DESCARRIES, L. and DROZ, B. (1970) Intraneuronal distribution of exogenous norepine-phrine in the central nervous system of the rat. *J. Cell Biol.,* **44**, 385–399.

DESCARRIES, L. and HAVRANKOVA, J. (1970) Catécholamines endogènes marquées dans le systeme nerveux central. Etude radioautographique après L–3, 4-dihydroxyphenylalanine tritée (DOPA–^{3}H). *C. R. Acad. Sci. Paris,* **271**, 2392–2395.

DE VRIES, G. H., NORTON, W. T. and RAINE, C. S. (1972) Axons: isolation from mammalian central nervous system. *Science,* **172**, 1370–1372.

DIAMOND, I. and KENNEDY, E. P. (1969) Carrier-mediated transport of choline into synaptic nerve endings. *J. Biol. Chem.,* **244**, 3258–3263.

DI GIAMBERARDINO, L., BENNETT, G., KOENIG, H. L. and DROZ, B. (1973) Axonal migration of protein and glycoprotein to nerve endings. III. Cell fraction analysis of chicken ciliary ganglion after intracerebral injection of labelled precursors of proteins and glyco-proteins. *Brain Res.,* **60**, 147–159.

DILLY, P. N., GRAY, E. G. and YOUNG, J. Z. (1963) Electron microscopy of optic nerves and optic lobes of *Octopus* and *Eledone*. *Proc. Roy. Soc. Lond. B,* **158**, 446–456.

DIXON, W. E. (1906) Vagus inhibition. *Brit. Med. J.,* **2**, 1807.

DOBBING, J. (1968) Effects of experimental undernutrition on development of the nervous system. In *Malnutrition, Learning and Behaviour*, ed. Scrimshaw, N. S. and Gordon, J. E. Pp. 181–202. Boston: M.I.T. Press.

DOBBING, J. (1972) Vulnerable periods of brain development. In *Lipids, Malnutrition and the Developing Brain*. Ciba Foundation Symposium. Pp. 9–29. Amsterdam: Elsevier.

DOBBING, J. and SANDS, J. (1970) Growth and development of the brain and spinal cord of the guinea pig. *Brain Res.,* **17**, 115–123.

DODGE, F. A. and RAHAMIMOFF, R. (1967) Cooperative action of calcium ions in trans-mitter release at the neuromuscular junction. *J. Physiol., Lond.,* **193**, 419–432.

DOGGENWEILER, C. F. and FRENK, S. (1965) Staining properties of lanthanum on cell membranes. *Proc. Natl. Acad. Sci., U.S.A.,* **53**, 425–430.

DOLIVO, M. and ROUILLER, Ch. (1969) Changes in ultrastructure and synaptic transmission in the sympathetic ganglion during various metabolic conditions. *Prog. Brain Res.*, **31**, 111–123.

DORAN, G. A. and JONES, D. G. (1971) Synaptic ultrastructure in a marsupial, *Setonix brachyurus*. *Experientia*, **27**, 1198–1199.

DOUGLAS, W. W. and NAGASAWA, J. (1971) Membrane vesiculation at sites of exocytosis in the neurohypophysis, adenohypophysis and adrenal medulla; a devise for membrane conservation. *J. Physiol., Lond.*, **218**, 94P–95P.

DOUGLAS, W. W., NAGASAWA, J. and SCHULTZ, R. A. (1971a) Coated microvesicles in neurosecretory terminals of posterior pituitary glands shed their coats to become smooth 'synaptic' vesicles. *Nature, Lond.*, **232**, 340–341.

DOUGLAS, W. W., NAGASAWA, J. and SCHULTZ, R. (1971b) Electron microscopic studies on the mechanism of secretion of posterior pituitary hormones and significance of micro-vesicles ('synaptic vesicles'): evidence of secretion by exocytosis and formation of micro-vesicles as a by-product of this process. *Mem. Soc. Endocr.*, **19**, 353–378.

DOUNCE, A. L. (1943) Enzyme studies on isolated cell nuclei of rat liver. *J. Biol. Chem.*, **147**, 685–698.

DOWDALL, M. J. and SIMON, E. J. (1973) Comparative studies on synaptosomes: uptake of [N–Me–^{3}H] choline by synaptosomes from squid optic lobes. *J. Neurochem.*, **21**, 969–982.

DOWDALL, M. J. and WHITTAKER, V. P. (1973) Comparative studies in synaptosome formation: the preparation of synaptosomes from the head ganglion of the squid, *Loligo pealii*. *J. Neurochem.*, **20**, 921–935.

DOWDALL, M. J. and ZIMMERMAN, H. (1974) Evidence for heterogeneous pools of acetyl-choline in isolated cholinergic synaptic vesicles. *Brain Res.*, **71**, 160–166.

DROCHMANS, P. (1963) Techniques for the isolation of particulate glycogen and its examina-tion in the electron microscope. *Biochem. Soc. Symp.*, **23**, 127–137.

DROZ, B. (1967) Synthèse et transfert des protéines cellulaires dans les neurones ganglion-naires. Étude radioautographique quantitative en microscopie électronique. *J. Microscopie*, **6**, 201–228.

DROZ, B. (1969) Metabolic information derived from radioautography. *Handbook of Neuro-chemistry*, ed. Lajtha, A. Vol. **2**, pp. 505–523. New York: Plenum.

DROZ, B. and BARONDES, S. H. (1969) Nerve endings: rapid appearance of labeled protein shown by electron microscope radioautography. *Science*, **165**, 1131–1133.

DROZ, B. and DI GIAMBERARDINO, L. (1973) Critical analysis of the rates of axonal migration estimated from radioautographs. *Brain Res.*, **60**, 122–127.

DROZ, B. and KOENIG, H. L. (1969) The turnover of proteins in axons and nerve endings. In *Cellular Dynamics of the Neuron*, ed. Barondes, S. H. Pp. 35–50. New York: Academic Press.

DROZ, B. and KOENIG, H. L. (1971) Dynamic condition of protein in axons and axon terminals. *Acta Neuropath., Berl., Suppl.* **5**, 109–118.

DROZ, B., KOENIG, H. L. and DI GIAMBERARDINO, L. (1973) Axonal migration of protein and glycoprotein to nerve endings. I. Radio-autographic analysis of the renewal of protein in nerve endings of chicken ciliary ganglion after intracerebral injection of [^{3}H] lysine *Brain Res.*, **60**, 93–127.

DUNANT, Y., GAUTRON, J., ISRAËL, M., LESBATS, B. and MANARANCHE, R. (1971) Acetylcholine turnover investigated at a subcellular level in the electric organ of *Torpedo*. *Experientia*, **27**, 4–5.

DUNANT, Y., GAUTRON, J., ISRAËL, M., LESBATS, B. and MANARANCHE, R. (1972) Les compartiments d'acetylcholine de l'organe electrique de la torpille et leurs modifications par la stimulation. *J. Neurochem.*, **19**, 1987–2002.

EAYRS, J. T. and GOODHEAD, B. (1959) Postnatal development of the cerebral cortex of the rat. *J. Anat., Lond.*, **93**, 385–402.

ECCLES, J. C. (1964) *The Physiology of Synapses.* Berlin: Springer-Verlag.

ECCLES, J. C., ITO, M. and SZENTAGOTHAI, J. (1967) *The Cerebellum as a Neuronal Machine.* Berlin: Springer-Verlag.

EDWARDSON, J., BENNETT, G. and BRADFORD, H. F. (1972) The release of amino acids and neurosecretory substances following electrical and potassium stimulation from nerve endings (synaptosomes) of the hypothalamus. *Nature, Lond.*, **240**, 554–556.

EHINGER, B. (1970) Autoradiographic identification of rabbit retinal neurons that take up GABA. *Experientia*, **26**, 1063.

EHINGER, B. and FALCK, B. (1971) Autoradiography of some suspected neurotransmitter substances: GABA, glycine, glutamic acid, histamine, dopamine and L-DOPA. *Brain Res.*, **33**, 157–172.

EICHBERG, J., WHITTAKER, V. P. and DAWSON, R. M. C. (1964) The distribution of lipids in subcellular particles of guinea-pig brain. *Biochem. J.*, **92**, 91–100.

EIDE, E., FEDINA, L., JANSEN, J., LUNDBERG, A. and VYKLICKÝ, L. (1967) Unitary excitatory postsynaptic potentials in Clarke's column neurones. *Nature, Lond.*, **215**, 1176–1177.

ELFVIN, L. G. (1963) The ultrastructure of the superior cervical sympathetic ganglion of the cat. II. The structure of the preganglionic end fibers and the synapses as studied by serial sections. *J. Ultrastruct. Res.*, **8**, 441–476.

ELLIOTT, K. A. C. and VAN GELDER, N. M. (1958) Occlusion and metabolism of γ-aminobutyric acid by brain tissue. *J. Neurochem.*, **3**, 28–40.

ELLIOTT, T. R. (1904) On the action of adrenalin. *J. Physiol., Lond.*, **31**, xx–xxi.

ELIMQVIST, D. and QUASTEL, D. M. J. (1965) Presynaptic action of hemicholinium at the neuromuscular junction. *J. Physiol., Lond.*, **177**, 463–482.

ESCUETA, A. V. and APPEL, S. N. (1969) Biochemical studies of synapses *in vitro*. II. Potassium transport. *Biochemistry*, **8**, 725–733.

EVANS, E. M. (1966) On the ultrastructure of the synaptic region of visual receptors in certain vertebrates. *Z. Zellforsch.*, **71**, 499–516.

FAHN, S., RODMAN, J. S. and CÔTÉ, L. J. (1969) Association of tyrosine hydroxylase with synaptic vesicles in bovine caudate nucleus. *J. Neurochem.*, **16**, 1293–1300.

FARROW, J. T. and O'BRIEN, R. D. (1971) Metabolites of (^{3}H) acetate bound to synaptic vesicles isolated from rat cerebral cortex. *J. Neurochem.*, **18**, 963–973.

FATT, P. and KATZ, B. (1950) Some observations on biological noise. *Nature, Lond.*, **166**, 597–598.

FATT, P. and KATZ, B. (1952) Spontaneous subthreshold activity at motor nerve endings. *J. Physiol., Lond.*, **117**, 109–128.

FAWCETT, D. W. (1965) Surface specialization of absorbing cells. *J. Histochem. Cytochem.*, **13**, 75–91.

FEHÉR, O., JOÓ, F. and HALÁSZ, N. (1972) Effect of stimulation on the number of synaptic vesicles in nerve fibres and terminals of the cerebral cortex in the cat. *Brain. Res.*, **47**, 37–48.

FEIT, H. and BARONDES, S. H. (1970) Colchicine – binding activity in particulate fractions of mouse brain. *J. Neurochem.*, **17**, 1355–1364.

FELDBERG, W. (1945) Present views on the mode of action of acetylcholine in the central nervous system. *Physiol. Rev.*, **25**, 596–642.

FELDBERG, W. and GADDUM, J. H. (1934) The chemical transmitter at synapses in a sympathetic ganglion. *J. Physiol., Lond.*, **81**, 305–319.

FELDBERG, W. and VARTIANEN, A. (1934) Further observations on the physiology and pharmacology of a sympathetic ganglion. *J. Physiol., Lond.*, **83**, 103–128.

FERNANDEZ–MORÁN, H. (1957) Electron microscopy of nervous tissue. In *Metabolism of the Nervous System*, ed. Richter, D. Pp. 1–34. London: Pergamon.

FESTOFF, B. W., APPEL, S. H. and DAY, E. (1971) Incorporation of [^{14}C] glucosamine into synaptosomes *in vitro*. *J. Neurochem.*, **18**, 1871–1886.

FEWSTER, M. E., SCHEIBEL, A. B. and MEAD, J. F. (1967) The preparation of isolated glial cells from rat and bovine white matter. *Brain Res.*, **6**, 401–408.

FIFKOVÁ, E. (1972) Effect of visual deprivation and light on synapses of the inner plexiform layer. *Exptl. Neurol.*, **35**, 458–469.

FINE, R. E. and BRAY, D. (1971) Actin in growing nerve cells. *Nature, Lond.*, **234**, 115–118.

FISZER, S. and DE ROBERTIS, E. (1967) Action of Triton X-100 on ultrastructure and membrane-bound enzymes of isolated nerve endings from rat brain. *Brain Res.*, **5**, 31–44.

FISZER, S. and DE ROBERTIS, E. (1969) Subcellular distribution and chemical nature of the receptor for 5–hydroxytryptamine in the central nervous system. *J. Neurochem.*, **16**, 1201–1209.

FLANGAS, A. L. and BOWMAN, R. E. (1968) Neuronal perikarya of rat brain isolated by zonal centrifugation. *Science*, **161**, 1025–1027.

FLEXNER, L. B., GAMBETTI, P., FLEXNER, J. B. and ROBERTS, R. B. (1971) Studies on memory: distribution of peptidyl-puromycin in subcellular fractions of mouse brain. *Proc. Natl. Acad. Sci. U.S.A.*, **68**, 26–28.

FLORENDO, N. T., BARRNETT, R. J. and GREENGARD, P. (1971) Cyclic 3′, 5′–nucleotide phosphodiesterase: cytochemical localization in cerebral cortex. *Science*, **173**, 745–747.

FLOREY, E. (1963) Acetylcholine in invertebrate nervous systems. *Can. J. Biochem. Physiol.*, **41**, 2619–2626.

FLOREY, E. and WINESDORFER, J. (1968) Cholinergic nerve endings in *Octopus* brain. *J. Neurochem.*, **15**, 169–177.

FOLKOW, B. and HAGGENDAHL, J. (1970) Some aspects of the quantal release of the adrenergic transmitter. In *Bayer Symposium II*, ed. Schumann, H. J. and Kroneberg, G. Pp. 91–97. New York: Springer-Verlag.

FONNUM, F. (1967) The 'compartmentation' of choline acetyltransferase within the synaptosome. *Biochem. J.*, **103**, 262–270.

FONNUM, F. (1968) The distribution of glutamate decarboxylase and aspartate transaminase in subcellular fractions of rat and guinea-pig brain. *Biochem. J.*, **106**, 401–412.

FONNUM, F., STORM-MATHISEN, J. and WALBERG, F. (1970) Glutamate decarboxylase in inhibitory neurons. A study of the enzyme in Purkinje cell axons and boutons in the cat. *Brain Res.*, **20**, 259–275.

FOREL, A–H (1887) Einige hirnanatomische Betrachtungen und Ergebnisse. *Arch. Psychiat. NervKrankh.*, **18**, 162–198.

FOX, C. A. and BARNARD, J. W. (1957) A quantitative study of the Purkinje cell dendritic branchlets and their relationship to afferent fibres. *J. Anat., Lond.*, **91**, 299–313.

FOX, C. A., HILLMAN, D. E., SIEGESMUND, K. A. and DUTTA, C. R. (1967) The primate cerebellar cortex—a Golgi and electron microscopic study. *Prog. Brain Res.*, **25**, 174–225.

FRAENKEL-CONRAT, H. and OLCOTT, H. S. (1945) Esterification of proteins with alcohols of low molecular weight. *J. Biol. Chem.*, **161**, 259–268.

FRIEND, D. S. and FARQUHAR, M. G. (1967) Functions of coated vesicles during protein absorption in the rat vas deferens. *J. Cell Biol.*, **35**, 357–376.

FROESCH, D. and MARTIN, R. (1972) Heterogeneity of synaptic vesicles in the squid giant fibre system. *Brain Res.*, **43**, 573–579.

FRONTALI, N. and PIERANTONI, R. (1973) Autoradiographic localization of ^{3}H–GABA in the cockroach brain. *Comp. Biochem. Physiol.*, **44**, 1369–1372.

217

FRONTALI, N. and TOSCHI, G. (1958) Subcellular fractions from the electric tissue of *Torpedo*—morphological aspect and cholinesterase content. *Exp. Cell Res.*, **15**, 446–450.

FRYE, L. D. and EDIDIN, M. (1970) The rapid intermixing of cell surface antigens after formation of mouse-human heterokaryons. *J. Cell Sci.*, **7**, 319–335.

FUKAMI, Y. (1969) Two types of synaptic bulb in snake and frog spinal cord, the effect of fixation. *Brain Res.*, **14**, 137–145.

FURSHPAN, E. J. and POTTER, D. D. (1957) Mechanism of nerve-impulse transmission at a crayfish synapse. *Nature, Lond.*, **180**, 342–343.

FURSHPAN, E. J. and POTTER, D. D. (1959) Transmission at the giant synapses of the crayfish. *J. Physiol., Lond.*, **145**, 289–325.

FURUKAWA, T. and FURSHPAN, E. J. (1963) Two inhibitory mechanisms in the Mauthner neurons of goldfish. *J. Neurophysiol.*, **26**, 140–176.

FUXE, K., GROBECKER, H., HÖKFELT, T. and JONSSON, G. (1967) Identification of dopamine, noradrenaline and 5-hydroxytryptamine varicosities in a fraction containing nerve ending particles. *Brain Res.*, **6**, 475–480.

FUXE, K., HÖKFELT, T., RITZEN, M. and UNGERSTEDT U. (1968) Studies on uptake of intraventricularly administered tritiated noradrenaline and 5-hydroxytryptamine with combined fluorescence histochemical and autoradiographic techniques. *Histochemie*, **16**, 186–194.

GADDUM, J. H. (1965) An improved microbath. *Brit. J. Pharmacol.*, **23**, 613–619.

GAMBETTI, P., AUTILIO-GAMBETTI, L., GONATAS, N. K., SHAFER, B. and STIEBER, A. (1972) Synapses and malnutrition. Morphological and biochemical study of synaptosomal fractions from rat cerebral cortex. *Brain Res.*, **47**, 477–484.

GAREY, R., HARPER, J., BEST, J. B. and GOODMAN, A. B. (1972) Preparative resolution and identification of synaptic components of rat neocortex. *J. Neurobiol.*, **3**, 163–195.

GEFFEN, L. B. and LIVETT, B. G. (1971) Synaptic vesicles in sympathetic neurons. *Physiol. Rev.*, **51**, 98–157.

GEFFEN, L. B., LIVETT, B. G. and RUSH, R. A. (1969) Immunological localization of chromogranins in sheep sympathetic neurones, and their release by nerve impulses. *J. Physiol., Lond.*, **204**, 58P–59P.

GEISON, R. L., FLANGAS, A. L. and KORNGUTH, S. E. (1972) Ganglioside content of membrane fractions from developing pig cerebellar and cerebral cortex separated in a CsC1–sucrose gradient by zonal centrifugation. *Brain Res.*, **43**, 303–308.

GERLACH, J. VON (1872) Über die Structur der grauern Substanz des menschlichen Grosshirus. Vorläufige Mittheilung. *Zbl. med. Wiss.*, **10**, 273–275.

GERMAIN, M. and PROULX, P. (1965) Adenosinetriphosphatase activity in synaptic vesicles of rat brain. *Biochem. Pharmacol.*, **14**, 1815–1819.

GERSCHENFELD, H. M., TRAMEZZANI, J. H. and DE ROBERTIS, E. (1960) Ultrastructure and function in neurohypophysis of the toad. *Endocrinology*, **66**, 741–762.

GERWIRTZ, G. P. and KOPIN, I. J. (1970) Release of dopamine-β-hydroxylase with norepinephrine during cat splenic nerve stimulation. *Nature, Lond.*, **227**, 406–407.

GFELLER, E., KUHAR, M. J. and SNYDER, S. H. (1971) Neurotransmitter-specific synaptosomes in rat corpus striatum: morphological variations. *Proc. Natl. Acad. Sci. U.S.A.*, **68**, 155–159.

GIACOBINI, E., HÖKFELT, T., KERPEL-FRONIUS, S., KOSLOW, S. H., MITCHARD, M. and NORÉ, B. (1971) A micro-scale procedure for the preparation of subcellular fractions from individual autonomic ganglia. *J. Neurochem.*, **18**, 223–231.

GLEES, P. and SHEPPARD, B. L. (1964) Electron microscopical studies of the synapse in the developing chick spinal cord. *Z. Zellforsch.*, **62**, 356–362.

GLEZER, I. I. (1970) Morphogenesis of synapses in neocortex of the albino rat. *Neurosci. Transl.*, **11**, 51–58.

GLOBUS, A., LUX, H. D. and SCHUBERT, P. (1968) Somadendritic spread of intracellularly injected tritiated glycine in cat spinal motoneurons. *Brain Res.*, **11**, 440–445.

GOBEL, S. (1968) Electron microscopical studies of the cerebellar molecular layer. *J. Ultrastruct. Res.*, **21**, 430–458.

GOLDSTEIN, M. A. (1969) Anionic binding of ruthenium red in fish extraocular muscle. *Z. Zellforsch.*, **102**, 459–465.

GOLGI, C. (1883) Recherches sur l'histologie des centres nerveux. *Archs. ital. Biol.*, **3**, 285–317.

GONATAS, N. K., AUTILIO–GAMBETTI, L., GAMBETTI, P. and SHAFER, B. (1971) Morphological and biochemical changes in rat synaptosome fractions during neonatal development. *J. Cell Biol.*, **51**, 484–498.

GRAFSTEIN, B. (1969) Axonal transport: communication between soma and synapse. *Advanc. Biochem. Psychopharmacol.*, **1**, 11–25.

GRAFSTEIN, B. (1971) Transneuronal transfer of radioactivity in the central nervous system. *Science*, **172**, 177–179.

GRAHAM, L. T. (1972) Intraretinal distribution of GABA content and glutamic acid decarboxylase activity. *Brain Res.*, **36**, 476–479.

GRAY, E. G. (1959a) Axosomatic and axodendritic synapses of the cerebral cortex: an electron microscopic study. *J. Anat., Lond.*, **93**, 420–433.

GRAY, E. G. (1959b) Electron microscopy of synaptic contacts on dendritic spines of the cerebral cortex. *Nature, Lond.*, **183**, 1592–1593.

GRAY, E. G. (1961) The granule cells, mossy synapses and Purkinje spine synapses of the cerebellum: light and electron microscope observations. *J. Anat., Lond.*, **95**, 345–356.

GRAY, E. G. (1962) Electron microscopy of synaptic organelles of the central nervous system. In *IV International Congress of Neuropathology*, ed. Jacob, H. Vol. **2**, pp. 57–61. Stuttgart: Thieme.

GRAY, E. G. (1963) Electron microscopy of presynaptic organelles of the spinal cord. *J. Anat., Lond.*, **97**, 101–106.

GRAY, E. G. (1964) Tissue of the central nervous system. In *Electron Microscopic Anatomy*, Kurtz, S. M. ed. Pp. 369–417. New York: Academic Press.

GRAY, E. G. (1966) Problems of interpreting the fine structure of vertebrate and invertebrate synapses. *Int. Rev. Gen. exp. Zool.*, **2**, 139–170.

GRAY, E. G. (1969a) Electron microscopy of excitatory and inhibitory synapses: a brief review. *Prog. Brain Res.*, **31**, 141–155.

GRAY, E. G. (1969b) Round and flat synaptic vesicles in the fish central nervous system. In *Cellular Dynamics of the Neuron*, ed. Barondes, S. H. Pp. 211–227. New York: Academic Press.

GRAY, E. G. (1970a) The fine structure of nerve. *Comp. Biochem. Physiol.*, **36**, 419–448.

GRAY, E. G. (1970b) The fine structure of the vertical lobe of *Octopus* brain. *Trans. Roy. Soc. Lond. B*, **258**, 379–394.

GRAY, E. G. (1970c) The question of relationship between Golgi vesicles and synaptic vesicles in *Octopus* neurons. *J. Cell Sci.*, **7**, 189–201.

GRAY, E. G. (1971) The fine structural characterization of different types of synapse. *Prog. Brain Res.*, **34**, 149–160.

GRAY, E. G. (1972) Are the coats of coated vesicles artefacts? *J. Neurocytol.*, **1**, 363–382.

GRAY, E. G. (1973) The cytonet, plain and coated vesicles, reticulosomes, multivesicular bodies and nuclear pores. *Brain Res.*, **62**, 329–336.

GRAY, E. G. and GUILLERY, R. W. (1963) A note on the dendritic spine apparatus. *J. Anat., Lond.*, **97**, 389–392.

GRAY, E. G. and GUILLERY, R. W. (1966) Synaptic morphology in the normal and degenerating nervous system. *Int. Rev. Cytol.*, **19**, 111–182.

GRAY, E. G. and HAMLYN, L. H. (1962) Electron microscopy of experimental degeneration in the avian optic tectum. *J. Anat., Lond.*, **96**, 309–316.

GRAY, E. G. and PEASE, H. (1971) On understanding the organization of the retinal receptor synapses. *Brain Res.*, **35**, 1–15.

GRAY, E. G. and WHITTAKER, V. P. (1960) The isolation of synaptic vesicles from the central nervous system. *J. Physiol. Lond.*, **153**, 35P–37P.

GRAY, E. G. and WHITTAKER, V. P. (1962) The isolation of nerve endings from brain: an electron microscopic study of cell fragments derived by homogenization and centrifugation. *J. Anat., Lond.*, **96**, 79–87.

GRAY, E. G. and WILLIS, R. A. (1968) Problems of electron stereoscopy of biological tissue. *J. Cell Sci.*, **3**, 309–326.

GRAY, E. G. and WILLIS, R. A. (1970) On synaptic vesicles, complex vesicles and dense projections. *Brain Res.*, **24**, 149–168.

GRAY, E. G. and YOUNG, J. Z. (1964) Electron microscopy of synaptic structure in *Octopus* brain. *J. Cell Biol.*, **21**, 87–103.

GREEN, A. I., SNYDER, S. H. and IVERSEN, L. L. (1969) Separation of catecholamine-storing synaptosomes in different regions of rat brain. *J. Pharmacol. Exp. Ther.*, **168**, 264–271.

GREEN, J. D. and VAN BREEMEN, V. L. (1955) Electron microscopy of the pituitary and observations on neurosecretion. *Am. J. Anat.*, **97**, 177–227.

GREENE, L. J., HIRS, C. H. W. and PALADE, G. E. (1963) On the protein composition of bovine pancreatic zymogen granules. *J. Biol. Chem.*, **238**, 2054–2070.

GREENGARD, P., McAFEE, D. A. and KEBABIAN, J. W. (1972) On the mechanism of action of cyclic AMP and its role in synaptic transmission. In *Physiology and Pharmacology of Cyclic AMP*, Advances in Cyclic Nucleotide Research, ed. Greengard, P. and Robison, G. A. Vol. **1** pp. 337–355. New York: Raven Press.

GRIFFITH, D. L. and BONDAREFF, W. (1973) Localization of thiamine pyrophosphatase in synaptic vesicles. *Amer. J. Anat.*, **136**, 549–556.

GRILLO, M. A. (1966) Electron microscopy of sympathetic tissues. *Pharmacol. Rev.*, **18**, 387–399.

GROVE, W. E., BONDAREFF, W. and VEIS, A. (1973) A sampling technique for quantitative electron microscopy of subcellular fractions. *J. Neurochem.*, **21**, 703–704.

GRYNZSPAN–WINOGRAD, O. (1971) Morphological aspects of exocytosis in the adrenal medulla. *Trans. Roy. Soc. Lond. B.*, **261**, 291–292.

GÜLDNER, F–H. and WOLFF, J. R. (1973) Neurono-glial. synaptoid contacts in the median eminence of the rat: ultrastructure, staining properties and distribution of tanycytes. *Brain Res.*, **61**, 217–234.

GURD, J. W., JONES, L. R., MAHLER, H. R. and MOORE, W. J. (1974) Isolation and partial characterization of rat brain synaptic plasma membranes. *J. Neurochem.*, **22**, 281–290.

GUTH, P. S. (1969) Acetylcholine binding by isolated synaptic vesicles *in vitro. Nature, Lond.*, **224**, 384–385.

HAGA, T. (1971) Synthesis and release of [^{14}C]-acetylcholine in synaptosomes. *J. Neurochem.*, **18**, 781–798.

HAGADORN, I. R., BERN, H. A. and NISHIOKA, R. S. (1963) The fine structure of the supraesophageal ganglion of the rhynchobdellid leech, *Theromyzon rude*, with special reference to neurosecretion. *Z. Zellforsch.*, **58**, 714–758.

HAGEN, P., BARNETT, R. J. and LEE, F. L. (1959) Biochemical and electron microscopic study of particles isolated from mastocytoma cells. *J. Pharmacol.*, **126**, 91–108.

HAGIWARA, S. and MORITA, H. (1962) Electrotonic transmission between two nerve cells in leech ganglion. *J. Neurophysiol.*, **25**, 721–731.

HAJÓS, F., TAPIA, R., WILKIN, G., JOHNSON, A. L. and BALÁZS, R. (1974) Subcellular fractionation of rat cerebellum: an electron microscopic and biochemical investigation. I. Preservation of large fragments of the cerebellar glomeruli. *Brain Res.*, **70**, 261–279.

HALE, C. W. (1946) Histochemical demonstration of acid polysaccharides in animal tissues. *Nature, Lond.*, **157**, 802.

HAMBERGER, A., BLOMSTRAND, C. and LEHNINGER, A. L. (1970) Comparative studies on mitochondria isolated from neuron-enriched and glia-enriched fractions of rabbit and beef brain. *J. Cell Biol.*, **45**, 221–234.

HAMLYN, L. H. (1961) Electron microscopy of mossy fibre endings in Ammon's Horn. *Nature, Lond.*, **190**, 645–646.

HAMLYN, L. H. (1962) The fine structure of the mossy fibre endings in the hippocampus of the rabbit. *J. Anat., Lond.*, **96**, 112–120.

HAMLYN, L. H. (1963) An electron microscope study of pyramidial neurons in the Ammon's Horn of the rabbit. *J. Anat., Lond.*, **97**, 189–201.

HAMMERSTADT, J. P., MURRAY, J. E. and CUTLER, R. W. P. (1971) Efflux of amino acid neurotransmitters from rat spinal cord slices. II. Factors influencing the electrically induced efflux of [^{14}C]-glycine and ^{3}H–GABA. *Brain Res.*, **35**, 357–367.

HÁMORI, J. and DYACHKOVA, L. N. (1964) Electron microscope studies on developmental differentiation of ciliary ganglion synapses in the chick. *Acta. biol. Acad. Sci. hung.*, **15**, 213–230.

HANNIG, K. (1967) Preparative electrophoresis. In *Electrophoresis*, ed. Bier, M. Pp. 423–471. New York: Academic Press.

HANZON, V. and TOSCHI, G. (1959) Electron microscopy on microsomal fractions from rat brain. *Expt. Cell Res.*, **16**, 256–271.

HEBB, C. O., LING, G. M., MCGEER, E. G., MCGEER, P. L. and PERKINS, D. (1964). Effect of locally applied hemicholinium on the acetylcholine content of the caudate nucleus. *Nature, Lond.*, **204**, 1309–1311.

HEBB, C. O. and SMALLMAN, B. N. (1956) Intracellular distribution of choline acetylase. *J. Physiol., Lond.*, **134**, 385–392.

HEBB, C. O. and WHITTAKER, V. P. (1958) Intracellular distributions of acetylcholine and choline acetylase. *J. Physiol. Lond.*, **142**, 187–196.

HEILBRONN, E. (1972) Action of phospholipase A on synaptic vesicles. A model for transmitter release? *Prog. Brain. Res.*, **36**, 29–40.

HEILBRONN, E., HAUSE, S. and LUNDGREN, G. (1971) Chemical identification of acetylcholine in squid-head ganglion. *Brain Res.*, **33**, 431–437.

HENDLER, R. W. (1971) Biological membrane ultrastructure. *Physiol. Rev.*, **51**, 66–97.

HENDRICKSON, A. E. (1972) Electron microscopic distribution of axoplasmic transport. *J. Comp. Neurol.*, **144**, 381–397.

HENN, F. A. and HAMBERGER, A. (1971) Glial cell function: uptake of transmitter substances. *Proc. Nat. Acad. Sci. U.S.A.*, **68**, 2686–2690.

HENN, F. A., HANSSON, H.–A. and HAMBERGER, A. (1972) Preparation of plasma membrane from isolated neurons. *J. Cell Biol.*, **53**, 654–661.

HERSCHMANN, H. R., COTMAN, C. W. and MATTHEWS, D. A. (1972) Serological specificities of brain subcellular organelles. I. Antisera to synaptosomal fractions. *J. Immunol.*, **108**, 1362–1369.

HERTZ, L. (1969) The biochemistry of brain tissue. In *The Biological Basis of Medicine*, Bittar, E. E. and Bittar, N. eds. Vol. **5**, pp. 1–37. London: Academic Press.

HEUSER, J. E. and REESE, T. S. (1973) Evidence for recycling of synaptic vesicle membrane during transmitter release at the frog neuromuscular junction. *J. Cell Biol.*, **57**, 315–344.

HIRANO, A. and DEMBITZER, H. M. (1973) Cerebellar alterations in the weaver mouse. *J. Cell Biol.*, **56**, 478–486.

HIRATA, Y. (1966) Occurrence of cylindrical synaptic vesicles in the central nervous system perfused with buffered formalin. *Arch. Histol. Japan (Okayama)*, **26**, 269–279.

HIRIPI, L., SÁLANKI, J., ZS-NAGY, I. and MUSKÓ, I. (1973) Subcellular distribution of biogenic monoamines in the central nervous system of *Anodonta cygnea* L. as revealed by density gradient centrifugation. *J. Neurochem.*, **21**, 791–797.

HIS, W. (1887) Zur Geschichte des menschlichen Rückenmarkes und der Nervenwurzelen. *Abh. K. säch. Ges. Wiss.*, **13**, 477–514.

HODGE, A. T. and SCHMITT, F. O. (1960) The charge profile of the tropocollagen macromolecule and the packing arrangement in native-type collagen fibrils. *Proc. Natl. Acad. Sci., U.S.A.*, **46**, 186–197.

HOFFER, B. J., BLOOM, F. E., SIGGINS, G. R. and WOODWARD, D. J. (1972) The development of synapses in the rat cerebellar cortex. In *Sleep and the Maturing Nervous System*, Clemente, C. D., Purpura, D. P. and Meyer, F. E. eds. Pp. 33–48. New York: Academic Press.

HOFMANN, W. W., STRUPPLER, A., WEINDL, A. and VELHO, F. (1973) Neuromuscular transmission with colchicine-treated nerves. *Brain Res.*, **49**, 208–213.

HOGEBOOM, G. H., SCHNEIDER, W. C. and PALADE, G. E. (1948) Cytochemical studies of mammalian tissue. I. Isolation of intact mitochondria from rat liver; some biochemical properties of mitochondria and submicroscopic particulate material. *J. Biol. Chem.*, **172**, 619–635.

HÖKFELT, T. (1965) *In vitro* studies on central and peripheral monoamine neurons at the ultrastructural level. *Z. Zellforsch.*, **91**, 1–74.

HÖKFELT, T. (1966) The effect of reserpine on the intraneuronal vesicles of the rat vas deferens. *Experientia*, **22**, 56.

HÖKFELT, T. (1967a) On the ultrastructural localization of noradrenaline in the central nervous system of the rat. *Z. Zellforsch.*, **79**, 110–117.

HÖKFELT, T. (1967b) Ultrastructural studies on adrenergic nerve terminals in the albino rat iris after pharmacological and experimental treatment. *Acta Physiol. Scand.*, **69**, 125–126.

HÖKFELT, T. (1968) *In vitro* studies on central and peripheral monoamine neurons at the ultrastructural level. *Z. Zellforsch.*, **91**, 1–74.

HÖKFELT, T. (1969) Distribution of noradrenaline storing particles in peripheral adrenergic neurons as revealed by electron microscopy. *Acta physiol. Scand.*, **76**, 427–440.

HÖKFELT, T., JONSSON, G. and LIDBRINK, P. (1970) Electron microscopic identification of monoamine nerve ending particles in rat brain homogenates. *Brain Res.*, **22**, 147–151.

HÖKFELT, T. and LJUNGDAHL, A. (1970) Cellular localization of labelled gamma-aminobutyric acid (^{3}H–GABA) in rat cerebellar cortex: an autoradiographic study', *Brain Res.*, **22**, 391–396.

HÖKFELT, T. and LJUNGDAHL, A. (1971a) Light and electron microscopic autoradiography on spinal cord slices after incubation with labeled glycine. *Brain Res.*, **32**, 189–194.

HÖKFELT, T. and LJUNGDAHL, A. (1971b) Uptake of ^{3}H-noradrenaline and γ–^{3}H–aminobutyric acid in isolated tissues of rat: an autoradiographic and fluorescence microscopic study. *Prog. Brain Res.*, **34**, 87–102.

HÖKFELT, T. and LJUNGDAHL, A. (1972) Autoradiographic identification of cerebral and cerebellar cortical neurons accumulating labeled gamma-aminobutyric acid (^{3}H–GABA). *Exp. Brain Res.*, **14**, 354–362.

HOLMES, R. L. (1964) Comparative observations on inclusions in nerve fibres of the mammalian neurohypophysis. *Z. Zellforsch.*, **64**, 474–492.

HOLMES, R. L. and KNOWLES, F. G. W. (1960) 'Synaptic vesicles' in the neurohypophysis. *Nature, Lond.*, **185**, 710–711.

HOLST, M.C. (1974) Personal communication.

HOLTZMAN, E., FREEMAN, A. R. and KASHNER, L. A. (1971) Stimulation-dependent alterations in peroxidase uptake at lobster neuromuscular junctions. *Science*, **173**, 733–736.

HOLTZMAN, E., NOVIKOFF, A. B. and VILLAVERDE, H. (1967) Lysosomes and GERL in normal and chromatolytic neurons of the rat ganglion nodosum. *J. Cell Biol.*, **33**, 419–435.

HOPKIN, J. M. and NEAL, M. J. (1970) The release of ^{14}C-glycine from electrically stimulated rat spinal cord slices. *Br. J. Pharmac.*, **40**, 136P–138P.

HORNE, R. W. (1965) Negative staining methods. In *Techniques for Electron Microscopy*, ed. Kay, D. H. Pp. 328–355. Oxford: Blackwell.

HORNE, R. W. and WHITTAKER, V. P. (1962) The use of the negative staining method for the electron-microscopic study of subcellular particles from animal tissues. *Z. Zellforsch.*, **58**, 1–16.

HOSIE, R. J. A. (1965) The localization of adenosine triphosphatases in morphologically characterized subcellular fractions of guinea-pig brain. *Biochem. J.*, **96**, 404–412.

HUBBARD, J. I. (1970) Mechanism of transmitter release. *Progr. Biophys. Mol. Biol.*, **21**, 33–124.

HUBBARD, J. I. (1971) Mechanism of transmitter release from nerve terminals. *Ann. N.Y. Acad. Sci.*, **183**, 131–146.

HUBBARD, J. I. and KWANBUNBUMPEN, S. (1968) Evidence for the vesicle hypothesis. *J. Physiol., Lond.*, **194**, 407–420.

HUGHES, D. E., WIMPENNY, J. W. T. and LLOYD, D. (1971) The disintegration of micro-organisms. In *Methods in Microbiology*, ed. Norris, J. R. and Ribbons, D. W. Vol. 5B. Pp. 1–54. New York: Academic Press.

HUXLEY, H. E. and ZUBAY, G. (1961) Preferential staining of nucleic acid-containing structures for electron microscopy. *J. biophys. biochem., Cytol.*, **11**, 273–296.

HYDÉN, H. (1959) Quantitative assay of compounds in isolated, fresh nerve cells and glial cells from control and stimulated animals. *Nature, Lond.*, **184**, 433–435.

INOUYE, A., KATAOKA, K. and SHINAGAWA, Y. (1963) Intracellular distribution of brain noradrenalin and De Robertis' non-cholinergic nerve endings. *Biochim. Biophys. Acta*, **71**, 491–493.

IQBAL, Z. and TALWAR, G. P. (1971) Acetylcholinesterase in developing chick embryo brain. *J. Neurochem.*, **18**, 1261–1267.

ISHII, T. and FRIEDE, R. L. (1967) Distribution of a catecholamine-binding mechanism in rat brain. *Histochemie*, **9**, 126–135.

ISHII, T. and FRIEDE, R. L. (1968) Tissue binding of tritiated norepinephrine in pigmented nuclei of human brain. *Amer. J. Anat.*, **122**, 139–144.

ISRAËL, M. (1970) Localisation de l'acétylcholine des synapses myoneurales et nerf-électro-plaque. *Arch. Anat. Miscrosc.*, **59**, 67–98.

ISRAËL, M. and GAUTRON, J. (1969) Cellular and subcellular localization of acetylcholine in electric organs. In *Cellular Dynamics of the Neuron*, ed. Barondes, S. H. Pp. 137–152. New York: Academic Press.

ISRAËL, M., GAUTRON, J. and LESBATS, B. (1968) Isolement des vésicules synaptiques de l'organe electrique de la Torpille et localisation de l'acétylcholine à leur niveau. *C. R. Acad. Sci.*, **266**, 273–275.

ISRAËL, M., GAUTRON, J. and LESBATS, B. (1970) Fractionnement de l'organe electrique de la Torpille: localisation subcellulaire de l'acétylcholine. *J. Neurochem.*, **17**, 1441–1450.

ISRAËL, M. and WHITTAKER, V. P. (1965) The isolation of mossy fibre endings from the granular layer of the cerebellar cortex. *Experientia*, **21**, 325–326.

IVERSEN, L. L. (1967) *The Uptake and Storage of Noradrenaline in Sympathetic Nerves*. London: Cambridge University Press.

IVERSEN, L. L. and BLOOM, F. E. (1972) Studies of the uptake of ^{3}H–GABA and

[³H]glycine in slices and homogenates of rat brain and spinal cord by electron microscopic autoradiography. *Brain Res.*, **41**, 131–143.

IVERSEN, L. L. and JOHNSTON, G. A. R. (1971) GABA uptake in rat central nervous system: comparison of uptake in slices and homogenates and the effects of some inhibitors. *J. Neurochem.*, **18**, 1939–1950.

IVERSEN, L. L., MITCHELL, J. F. and SRINIVASAN, V. (1971) The release of γ-aminobutyric acid during inhibition in the cat visual cortex. *J. Physiol., Lond.*, **212**, 519–534.

IVERSEN, L. L. and NEAL, M. J. (1968) The uptake of ³H–GABA by slices of rat cerebral cortex. *J. Neurochem.*, **15**, 1141–1149.

IVERSEN, L. L. and SCHON, F. E. (1973) The use of autoradiographic techniques for the identification and mapping of transmitter-specific neurones in CNS. In *New Concepts in Neurotransmitter Regulation*, ed. Mandell, A. J. Pp. 153–193. New York: Plenum Press.

IVERSEN, L. L. and SNYDER, S. H., (1968) Synaptosomes: different populations storing catecholamines and gamma-aminobutyric acid in homogenates of rat brain. *Nature, Lond.*, **220**, 796–798.

JABONERO, V. (1964) Ueber die Brauchbarkeit der Osmiumtetroxyd Zinkjodid–Methode Zur Analyse der vegetativen Peripherie. *Acta Neuroveg. (Wien)*, **26**, 184–210.

JACOB, S. T. and BHARGAVA, P. M. (1962) A new method for the preparation of liver cell suspensions. *Exp. Cell Res.*, **27**, 453–467.

JAMIESON, J. D. and PALADE, G. E. (1971) Synthesis, intracellular transport, and discharge of secretory proteins in stimulated pancreatic exocrine cells. *J. Cell Biol.*, **50**, 135–158.

JANKOVIĆ, B. D., RAKIĆ, L. J. and SESTOVIĆ, M. (1969) Changes in electrical activity of the cockroach *Blatta orientalis* L. brain induced by anti-lobster brain antibody. *Experientia*, **25**, 1049–1050.

JÄRLFORS, U. and SMITH, D. S. (1969) Association between synaptic vesicles and neuro-tubules. *Nature, Lond.*, **224**, 710–711.

JAROSCH, E. and PRECHT, W. (1972) Effects of antibodies directed toward membrane fragments of synaptosomes on cerebellar field potentials. *Brain Res.*, **42**, 225–229.

JASPER, H. H. and KOYAMA, I. (1969) Rate of release of amino acids from the cerebral cortex in the cat as affected by brainstem and thalamic stimulation. *Can. J. Physiol. Pharmac.* **47**, 889–905.

JOHNSON, D. G., THOA, N. B., WEINSHILBOUM, R., AXELROD, J. and KOPIN, I. J. (1971) Enhanced release of dopamine–β–hydroxylase from sympathetic nerves by calcium and phenoxybenzamine and its reversal by prostaglandins, *Proc. Nat. Acad. Sci. U.S.A.*, **68**, 2227–2230.

JOHNSON, G. A., BOUKMA, S. J., LAHTI, R. A. and MATHEWS, J. (1973) Cyclic AMP and phosphodiesterase in synaptic vesicles from mouse brain. *J. Neurochem.*, **20**, 1387–1392.

JOHNSON, J. L. (1972) Glutamic acid as a synaptic transmitter in the nervous system, a review. *Brain Res.*, **37**, 1–19.

JOHNSON, M. K., and WHITTAKER, V. P. (1963) Lactate dehydrogenase as a cytoplasmic marker in brain. *Biochem. J.*, **88**, 404–409.

JOHNSON, R. and ARMSTRONG-JAMES, M. (1970) Morphology of superficial postnatal cerebral cortex with special reference to synapses. *Z. Zellforsch.*, **110**, 540–558.

JOHNSTON, G. A. R. and IVERSEN, L. L. (1971) Glycine uptake in rat central nervous system slices and homogenates: evidence for different uptake systems in spinal cord and cerebral cortex. *J. Neurochem.*, **18**, 1951–1961.

JOHNSTON, P. V. and ROOTS, B. I. (1965) The neurone surface. *Nature, Lond.*, **205**, 778–780.

JOHNSTON, P. V. and ROOTS, B. I. (1970) Neuronal and glial perikarya preparations: an appraisal of present methods. *Int. Rev. Cytol.*, **29**, 265–281.

JOHNSTON, P. V. and ROOTS, B. I. (1972) *Nerve Membranes.* Oxford: Pergamon.

JONES, D. G. (1967) An electron-microscope study of subcellular fractions of *Octopus* brain. *J. Cell Sci.,* **2**, 573–586.

JONES, D. G. (1968) The fine structure of the synaptic membrane adhesions on octopus synaptosomes. *Z. Zellforsch.,* **88**, 457–469.

JONES D. G. (1969) The morphology of the contact region of vertebrate synaptosomes. *Z. Zellforsch.,* **95**, 263–279.

JONES, D. G. (1970a) A further contribution to the study of the contact region of *Octopus* synaptosomes. *Z. Zellforsch.,* **103**, 48–60.

JONES, D. G. (1970b) A study of the presynaptic network of *Octopus* synaptosomes. *Brain Res.,* **20**, 145–158.

JONES, D. G. (1970c) The isolation of synaptic vesicles from octopus brain. *Brain Res.,* **17**, 181–193.

JONES, D. G. (1971) The negative staining of *Octopus* synaptosomes. *Brain Res.,* **29**, 378–382.

JONES, D. G. (1972) On the ultrastructure of the synapse: the synaptosome as a morphological tool! In *The Structure and Function of Nervous Tissue,* ed. Bourne, G. H. Vol. 6, pp. 81–129. New York: Academic Press.

JONES, D. G. (1973a) Some factors affecting the PTA staining of synaptic junctions; a preliminary comparison of PTA stained junctions in various regions of the CNS. *Z. Zellforsch.,* **143**, 301–312.

JONES, D. G. (1973b) Subunits and unit membranes. *J. Anat., Lond.,* **114**, 162.

JONES, D. G. (1973c) Synaptogenesis in guinea-pig cerebral cortex: dense projections as a criterion of maturity. *IRCS Medical Science,* (73–7) 5–5–3.

JONES, D. G. (1973d) The integrity of synaptosomes: a morphological approach. *Abstracts of Fourth International Neurochemistry Meeting, Tokyo,* 155–156.

JONES, D. G. (1974) Unpublished observations.

JONES, D. G. and BRADFORD, H. F. (1971a) Observations on the morphology of mammalian synaptosomes following their incubation and electrical stimulation. *Brain Res.,* **28**, 491–499.

JONES, D. G. and BRADFORD, H. F. (1971b) The relationship between complex vesicles, dense-cored vesicles and dense projections in cortical synaptosomes. *Tissue and Cell,* **3**, 177–190.

JONES, D. G., and BREARLEY, R. F. (1972a) Further studies on synaptic junctions I. Ultrastructural features in intact rat cerebral cortex. *Z. Zellforsch.,* **125**, 415–431.

JONES, D. G. and BREARLEY, R. F. (1972b) Further studies on synaptic junctions. II. A comparison of synaptic ultrastructure in fractionated and intact cerebral cortex. *Z. Zellforsch.,* **125**, 432–447.

JONES, D. G. and BREARLEY, R. F. (1973) An analysis of some aspects of synaptosomal ultrastructure using serial sections. *Z. Zellforsch.,* **140**, 481–496.

JONES, D. G., BREARLEY, R. F. and DORAN, G. A. (1972) The organization of dense projections in synapses of the brain of a marsupial. *Setonix brachyurus. Anat. Rec.,* **174**, 39–46.

JONES, D. G., DITTMER, M. M. and READING, L. C. (1974) Synaptogenesis in guinea-pig cerebral cortex: a glutaraldehyde–PTA study. *Brain Res.,* **70**, 245–259.

JONES, D. G., and REVELL, E. (1970a) The postnatal development of the synapse: a morphological approach utilizing synaptosomes. I. General features. *Z. Zellforsch.,* **111**, 179–194.

JONES, D. G. and REVELL, E. (1970b) The postnatal development of the synapse: a morphological approach utilizing synaptosomes. II. Paramembranous densities. *Z. Zellforsch.,* **111**, 195–208.

JONES, E. G. and POWELL, T. P. S. (1970) An electron microscopic study of terminal degeneration in the neocortex of the cat. *Trans. Roy. Soc. Lond. B.,* **257**, 29–43.

JONES, E. G. and ROCKEL, A. J. (1973) Observations on complex vesicles, neurofilamentous hyperplasia and increased electron density during terminal degeneration in the inferior colliculus. *J. Comp. Neurol.*, **147**, 93–118.

JONES, S. F. and KWANBUNBUMPEN, S. (1970) The effects of nerve stimulation and hemicholinium on synaptic vesicles at the mammalian neuromuscular junction. *J. Physiol., Lond.*, **207**, 31–50.

JUORIO, A. V. (1970) The distribution of catecholamines in the nervous system of an Octopoda mollusc. *Brit. J. Pharmacol.*, **39**, 240–242.

JUORIO, A. V. (1971) Catecholamines and 5-hydroxytryptamine in nervous tissue of cephalopods. *J. Physiol., Lond.*, **216**, 213–226.

KADOTA, K. and KADOTA, T. (1973a) A nucleoside diphosphate phosphohydrolase present in a coated-vesicle fraction from synaptosomes of guniea-pig whole brain. *Brain Res.*, **56**, 371–376.

KADOTA, K. and KADOTA, T. (1973b) Isolation of coated vesicles, plain synaptic vesicles and fine particles from synaptosomes of guinea-pig whole brain. *J. Electron Miscrosc.*, **22**, 91–98.

KADOTA, K. and KADOTA, T. (1973c) Isolation of coated vesicles, plain synaptic vesicles, and flocculent material from a crude synaptosome fraction of guinea-pig whole brain. *J. Cell Biol.*, **58**, 135–151.

KADOTA, K., KAMIYA, H. and KUMEGAWA, M. (1970) Localization of acetylcholine in a smooth synaptic vesicle fraction of synaptic vesicle preparation from guinea-pig brain. *Abstracts of 47th General Meeting of the Physiological Society of Japan, Tokyo*, 406.

KADOTA, K. and KANASEKI, T. (1969) Isolation of a synaptic vesicle fraction from guinea-pig brain with the use of DEAE–Sephadex column chromatography and some of its properties. *J. Biochem., Tokyo*, **65**, 839–842.

KAMIYA, H., KADOTA, K. and KADOTA, T. (1972) Localization of acetylcholine and choline in plain synaptic vesicles and coated vesicles isolated from guinea-pig whole brain. *Abstracts of General Meeting of the Japanese Pharmacological Society, Sendai, Japan*, 86.

KANASEKI, K. (1973) A morphological study of the synaptic and coated vesicles isolated from the nerve endings of vertebrate brain. *Abstracts of Fourth International Neurochemistry Meeting, Tokyo*, 165.

KANASEKI, T. and KADOTA, K. (1969) The 'vesicle in a basket'. A morphological study of the coated vesicle isolated from the nerve endings of the guinea-pig brain, with special reference to the mechanism of membrane movements. *J. Cell Biol.*, **42**, 202–220.

KARLIN, A. (1965) The association of acetylcholinesterase and membrane in subcellular fractions of the electric tissue of *Electrophorus*. *J. Cell Biol.*, **25**, 159–169.

KARLSSON, J. O. and SJÖSTRAND, J. (1971) Synthesis, migration and turnover of protein in retinal ganglion cells. *J. Neurochem.*, **18**, 749–767.

KARLSSON, U. (1966) Three-dimensional study of neurons in the lateral geniculate nucleus of the rat. II. Environment of perikarya and proximal parts of their branches. *J. Ultrastruct. Res.*, **16**, 482–504.

KARLSSON, U. (1967) Observations on the postnatal development of neuronal structures in the lateral geniculate nucleus of the rat by electron microscopy. *J. Ultrastruct. Res.*, **17**, 158–175.

KARNOVSKY, M. J. (1964) The localization of cholinesterase activity in rat cardiac muscle by electron miscrosopy. *J. Cell. Biol.*, **23**, 217–232.

KÁSA, P. (1971) Ultrastructural localization of choline acetyltransferase and acetylcholinesterase in central and peripheral nervous tissue. *Prog. Brain Res.*, **34**, 337–344.

KÁSA, P., MANN, S. P. and HEBB, C. (1970a) Localization of choline acetyltransferase. *Nature, Lond.*, **226**, 812–814.

KÁSA, P., MANN, S. P. and HEBB, C. (1970b) Ultrastructural localization in spinal neurones. *Nature, Lond.*, **226**, 814–816.

KÁSA, P., MANN, S. P., KARCSU, S., TÓTH, L. and JORDAN, S. (1973) Transport of choline acetyltransferase and acetylcholinesterase in the rat sciatic nerve: a biochemical and electron histochemical study. *J. Neurochem.*, **21**, 431–436.

KÁSA, P. and MORRIS, D. (1972) Inhibition of choline acetyltransferase and its histochemical localization. *J. Neurochem.*, **19**, 1299–1304.

KATAOKA, K. (1962) Subcellular distribution of 5-hydroxytryptamine in the rabbit brain. *Jap. J. Physiol.*, **12**, 623–638.

KATAOKA, K. and DE ROBERTIS, E. (1967) Histamine in isolated small nerve endings and synaptic vesicles of rat brain cortex. *J. Pharmacol. Exp. Ther.*, **156**, 114–125.

KATZ, B. (1962) The transmission of impulses from nerve to muscle, and the subcellular unit of synaptic action. *Proc. Roy. Soc., Lond., B.*, **155**, 455–477.

KATZ, B. (1966) *Nerve, Muscle, and Synapse.* New York: McGraw-Hill.

KATZ, B. (1969) *The Release of Neural Transmitter Substances.* Liverpool: Liverpool University Press.

KATZ, B. (1971) Quantal mechanism of neural transmitter release. *Science*, **173**, 123–126.

KATZ, B. and MILEDI, R. (1963) A study of spontaneous miniature potentials in spinal motoneurones. *J. Physiol., Lond.*, **168**, 389–422.

KATZ, B. and MILEDI, R. (1965) The measurement of synaptic delay, and the time course of acetylcholine release at the neuromuscular junction. *Proc. Roy. Soc. Lond. B*, **161**, 483–495.

KATZ, N. L. (1972) The effects on frog neuromuscular transmission of agents which act upon microtubules and microfilaments. *Europ. J. Pharmacol.*, **191**, 88–93.

KAWANA, E., AKERT, K. and SANDRI, C. (1969) Zinc iodide–osmium tetroxide impregnation of nerve terminals in the spinal cord. *Brain Res.*, **16**, 325–331.

KEEN, P. and WHITE, T. D. (1970) Light scattering technique for study of the permeability of rat brain synaptosomes *in vitro. J. Neurochem.*, **17**, 565–571.

KELLY, P., LUTTGES, M., JOHNSON, T. and GROVE, W. (1974) Maturation-dependent alterations in (^{3}H) GABA compartmentalization in neural tissue *in vivo. Brain Res.*, **68**, 267–280.

KERKUT, G. A., SEDDEN, C. E. and WALKER, R. J. (1967) Uptake of dopa and 5-hydroxytryptophan by monoamine-forming neurones in the brain of *Helix aspersa. Comp. Biochem. Physiol.*, **23**, 159–162.

KIRKPATRICK, J. B. (1969) Microtubules in brain homogenates. *Science*, **163**, 187–188.

KLEIN, R. L. and THURESON-KLEIN, Å. (1971) An electron microscopic study of noradrenaline storage vesicles isolated from bovine nerve trunk. *J. Ultrastruct. Res.*, **34**, 473–491.

KNOWLES, F. and BERN, H. A. (1966) The function of neurosecretion in endocrine regulation. *Nature, Lond.*, **210**, 271–272.

KNYIHÁR, E., LÁSZLÓ, I. and CSILLIK, B. (1973) Thiamine pyrophosphatase activity in neurotubuli and synaptic vesicles. *Neurobiology*, **3**, 327–334.

KOCH, R. B. (1969) Fractionation of olfactory tissue homogenates. Isolation of a concentrated plasma membrane fraction. *J. Neurochem.*, **16**, 145–157.

KOELLE, G. B. and FOROGLOU-KERAMEOS, C. (1965) Electron microscopic localization of cholinesterases in a sympathetic ganglion by a gold-thiolacetic acid method. *Life Sci.*, **4**, 417–424.

KOENIG, H. (1967) Quelques particularités ultrastructurales des zones synaptiques dans le ganglion ciliaire du poulet. *Bull. Ass. Anat., Orsay*, **138**, 711–719.

KOENIG, H. L. and DROZ, B. (1971) Transports axonaux de protéines aux terminaisons nerveuses du ganglion ciliaire du poulet, après injection intraventriculaire cérébrale de leucine – ^{3}H. *C. R. Acad. Sci., Paris*, **272**, 2812–2815.

KOPIN, I. J. (1968) False adrenergic transmitters. *Ann. Rev. Pharmacol.*, **8**, 377–394.

227

KOPIN, I. J., BREESE, G. R., KRAUSS, K. R. and WEISE, V. K. (1968) Selective release of newly synthesized norepinephrine from the cat spleen during sympathetic nerve stimulation. *J. Pharmacol. Exp. Ther.*, **161**, 271–278.

KORNELIUSSEN, H. (1972) Ultrastructure of normal and stimulated motor endplates. With comments on the origin and fate of synaptic vesicles. *Z. Zellforsch.*, **130**, 28–57.

KORNGUTH, S. E., ANDERSON, J. W. and SCOTT, G. (1969) Isolation of synaptic complexes in a caesium chloride density gradient: electron microscopic and immunohistochemical studies. *J. Neurochem.*, **16**, 1017–1024.

KORNGUTH, S. E., ANDERSON, J. W., SCOTT, G. and KUBINSKI, H. (1967) Fractionation of subcellular elements from rat central nervous tissue in a cesium chloride gradient. *Exp. Cell Res.*, **45**, 656–670.

KORNGUTH, S. E., FLANGAS, A. L., SIEGEL, F. L., GEISON, R. L., O'BRIEN, J. F., LAMAR, C. and SCOTT, G. (1971) Chemical and metabolic characteristics of synaptic complexes from brain isolated by zonal centrifugation in a cesium chloride gradient. *J. Biol. Chem.*, **246**, 1177–1184.

KORNGUTH, S. E., FLANGAS, A. L., GEISON, R. L. and SCOTT, G. (1972) Morphology, isopycnic density and lipid content of synaptic complexes isolated from developing cerebellums and different brain regions. *Brain Res.* **37**. 53–68.

KORR, I. M., WILKINSON, P. N. and CHORNOCK, F. W. (1967) Axonal delivery of neuroplasmic components to muscle cells. *Science*, **155**, 342–345.

KRNJEVIĆ, K. (1970) Glutamate and γ-aminobutyric acid in brain. *Nature, Lond.*, **228**, 119–124.

KRNJEVIĆ, K. and MITCHELL, J. F. (1961) The release of acetylcholine in the isolated rat diaphragm. *J. Physiol., Lond.*, **155**, 246–262.

KUENZLE, C. C., PELLONI, R. R. and KISTLER, G. S. (1972) Zonal centrifugation of neuronal perikarya and isolation of neuronal membranes rich in acetylcholinesterase. *J. Neurochem.*, **19**, 2333–2339.

KUHAR, M. J. and AGHAJANIAN, G. K. (1973) Selective accumulation of ^{3}H-serotonin by nerve terminals of raphé neurons: an autoradiographic study. *Nature, New Biol.*, **241**, 187–189.

KUHAR, M. J., GREEN, A. I., SNYDER, S. H. and GFELLER, E. (1970) Separation of synaptosomes storing catecholamines and gamma-aminobutyric acid in rat corpus striatum. *Brain Res.*, **21**, 405–417.

KUHAR, M. J., SHASKAN, E. G. and SNYDER, S. H. (1971) The subcellular distribution of endogenous and exogenous serotonin in brain tissue: comparison of synaptosomes storing serotonin, norepinephrine and γ-aminobutyric acid. *J. Neurochem.*, **18**, 333–343.

KUNO, M. (1964) Quantal components of excitatory synaptic potentials in spinal motoneurones. *J. Physiol., Lond.*, **175**, 81–99.

KUNO, M. (1971) Quantum aspects of central and ganglionic synaptic transmission in vertebrates. *Physiol. Rev.*, **51**, 647–678.

KURIYAMA, K., ROBERTS, E. and KAKEFUDA, T. (1968a) Association of the γ-aminobutyric acid system with a synaptic vesicle fraction from mouse brain. *Brain Res.*, **8**, 132–152.

KURIYAMA, K., ROBERTS, E. and VOS, J. (1968b) Some characteristics of binding of γ-aminobutyric acid and acetylcholine to a synaptic vesicle fraction from mouse brain. *Brain Res.*, **9**, 231–252.

KURIYAMA, K., SISKEN, B., ITO, J., SIMONSEN, D. G., HABER, B. and ROBERTS, E. (1968c) The γ-aminobutyric acid system in the developing chick embryo cerebellum. *Brain Res.*, **11**, 412–430.

KURIYAMA, K., WEINSTEIN, H. and ROBERTS, E. (1969) Uptake of GABA by mitochondria and synaptosomal fractions from mouse brain. *Brain Res.*, **16**, 479–492.

KUROKAWA, M., SAKAMOTO, T. and KATO, M. (1965a) A rapid isolation of nerve-ending particles from brain. *Biochim. Biophys. Acta*, **94**, 307–309.

KUROKAWA, M., SAKAMOTO, T. and KATO, M. (1965b) Distribution of sodium-plus-potassium-stimulated adenosine-triphosphate activity in isolated nerve ending particles. *Biochem. J.*, **97**, 833–844.

LABELLA, F. S., BEAULIEU, G. and REIFFENSTEIN, R. J. (1962) Evidence for the existence of separate vasopressin and oxytocin-containing granules in the neurohypophysis. *Nature, Lond.*, **193**, 173–174.

LABELLA, F. S., REIFFENSTEIN, R. J. and BEAULIEU, G. (1963) Subcellular fractionation of bovine posterior pituitary glands by centrifugation. *Arch. Biochem. Biophys.*, **100**, 399–408.

LABELLA, F. S. and SANWAL, M. (1965) Isolation of nerve endings from the posterior pituitary gland. Electron microscopy of fractions obtained by centrifugation. *J. Cell Biol.*, **25**, 179–193.

LAGERCRANTZ, H. and PERTOFT, H. (1972) Separation of catecholamine storing synaptosomes in colloidal silica density gradients. *J. Neurochem.*, **19**, 811–823.

LAM, D. M. K. and STEINMAN, L. (1971) The uptake of γ-^{3}H-aminobutyric acid in the goldfish retina. *Proc. Nat. Acad. Sci., U.S.A.*, **68**, 2777–2781.

LAPETINA, E. G., SOTO, E. F. and DE ROBERTIS, E. (1968) Lipids and proteolipids in isolated subcellular membranes of rat brain cortex. *J. Neurochem.*, **15**, 437–445.

LARRAMENDI, L. M. H. (1969) Analysis of synaptogenesis in the cerebellum of the mouse. In *Neurobiology of Cerebellar Evolution and Development*, ed. Llinás, R. Pp. 803–843. Chicago: Amer. Med. Ass.

LARRAMENDI, L. M. H., FICKENSCHER, L. and LEMKEY-JOHNSTON, N. (1967) Synaptic vesicles of inhibitory and excitatory terminals in the cerebellum. *Science*, **156**, 967–969.

LARRAMENDI, L. M. H. and VICTOR, T. (1967) Synapses on the Purkinje cell spines in the mouse. An electronmicroscopic study. *Brain Res.*, **5**, 15–30.

LAVERTY, R., MICHAELSON, I. A., SHARMAN, D. G. and WHITTAKER, V. P. (1963) The subcellular localization of dopamine and acetylcholine in the dog caudate nucleus. *Br. J. Pharmac.*, **21**, 482–490.

LAWLER, H. C. (1964) The preparation of a soluble acetylcholinesterase from brain. *Biochim. Biophys. Acta*, **81**, 280–288.

LEDUC, E. H. and BERNHARD, W. (1961) Ultrastructural cytochemistry: enzyme and acid hydrolysis of nucleic acids and protein. *J. biophys. biochem. Cytol.*, **10**, 437–455.

LEHNINGER, A. L. (1968) The neuronal membrane. *Proc. Nat. Acad. Sci., U.S.A.*, **60**, 1055–1101.

LEHRER, G. M. and ORNSTEIN, L. (1959) A diazo coupling method for the electron microscopic localization of cholinesterase. *J. biophys. biochem. Cytol.*, **6**, 399–406.

LEMKEY-JOHNSTON, N. and DEKIRMENJIAN, H. (1970) The identification of fractions enriched in nonmyelinated axons from rat whole brain. *Exp. Brain Res.*, **11**, 392–410.

LEMKEY-JOHNSTON, N. and LARRAMENDI, L. M. H. (1968) The separation and identification of fractions of nonmyelinated axons from the cerebellum of the cat. *Exp. Brain Res.*, **5**, 326–340.

LEMKEY-JOHNSTON, N. and LARRAMENDI, L. M. H. (1970) Identification of axons in fractions from caudate nucleus. *J. Cell Biol.*, **47**, 119–120.

LEMKEY-JOHNSTON, N. and LARRAMENDI, L. M. H. (1973) Identification of unmyelinated axons in fractions from caudate-putamen in the rat. *Exp. Brain Res.*, **17**, 124–132.

LENN, N. J. (1967) Localization of uptake of tritiated norepinephrine by rat brain *in vivo* and *in vitro* using electron microscopic autoradiography. *Am. J. Anat.*, **120**, 377–390.

LENN, N. J. and REESE, T. S. (1966) The fine structure of nerve endings in the nucleus of the trapezoid body and the ventral cochlear nucleus. *Am. J. Anat.*, **118**, 375–390.

LENTZ, T. L. (1972) Distribution of leucine-^{3}H during axoplasmic transport within regenerating neurons as determined by electron-microscope radioautography. *J. Cell Biol.*, **52**, 719–732.

LEVI, R. and MAYNERT, E. W. (1964) The subcellular localization of brain stem norepinephrine and 5-hydroxytryptamine in stressed rats. *Biochem. Pharmacol.*, **13**, 615–621.

LEWIS, P. R. and SHUTE, C. C. D. (1966) The distribution of cholinesterase in cholinergic neurons demonstrated with the electron microscope. *J. Cell Sci.*, **1**, 381–390.

LILEY, A. W. (1956) The effects of presynaptic polarization on the spontaneous activity at the mammalian neuromuscular junction. *J. Physiol., Lond.*, **134**, 427–443.

LIM, R. and HSU, L.-W. (1971) Studies on brain specific membrane proteins. *Biochim. Biophys. Acta.*, **249**, 569–582.

LING, C. M. and ABDEL-LATIF, A. A. (1968) Studies on sodium transport in rat brain nerve ending particles. *J. Neurochem.*, **15**, 721–729.

LIVETT, B. G., ROSTAS, J. A. P., JEFFREY, P. L. and AUSTIN, L. (1974) Antigenicity of isolated synaptosomal membranes. *Exptl. Neurol.*, **43**, 330–338.

LJUNGDAHL, A., HÖKFELT, T., JONSSON, G. and SACHS, C. (1971) Autoradiographic demonstration of uptake and accumulation of ^{3}H-6-hydroxydopamine in adrenergic nerves. *Experientia*, **27**, 297–299.

LOE, P. R. and FLOREY, E. (1966) The distribution of acetylcholne and cholinesterase in the nervous system and in innervated organs of *Octopus dofleini*. *Comp. Biochem. Physiol.*, **17**, 509–522.

LOEWI, O. (1921) Über humorale Übertragbarkeit der Herznervenwirkung. *Pflugers Arch. ges. Physiol.*, **189**, 239–242.

LOGAN, W. J. and SNYDER, S. H. (1971) Unique high affinity uptake systems for glycine, glutamic acid and aspartate in central nervous tissue of the rat. *Nature, Lond.*, **234**, 297–299.

LOGAN, W. J. and SNYDER, S. H. (1972) High affinity uptake systems for glycine, glutamic and aspartic acids in synaptosomes of rat central nervous tissues. *Brain Res.*, **42**, 413–431.

LONGENECKER, H. E., HURLBUT, W. P., MAURO, A. and CLARK, A. W. (1970) Effects of black widow spider venom on the frog neuromuscular junction. Effects on end-plate potential, miniature end-plate potential, and nerve terminal spike. *Nature, Lond.*, **225**, 701–703.

LUFT, J. H. (1965) The fine structure of hyaline cartilage matrix following ruthenium red fixative and staining. *J. Cell Biol.*, **27**, 61A.

LUFT, J. H. (1966) Fine structure of capillary and endocapillary layer as revealed by ruthenium red. *Fed. Proc.*, **25**, 1773–1783.

LUFT, J. H. (1971a) Ruthenium red and violet. I. Chemistry, purification, methods of use for electron microscopy and mechanism of action. *Anat. Rec.*, **171**, 347–368.

LUFT, J. H. (1971b) Ruthenium red and violet. II. Fine structural localization in animal tissues. *Anat. Rec.*, **171**, 369–416.

LUND, R. D. (1969) Synaptic patterns of the superficial layers of the superior colliculus of the rat. *J. Comp. Neurol.*, **135**, 179–208.

LUND, R. D. and LUND, J. S. (1972) Development of synaptic patterns in the superior colliculus of the rat. *Brain Res.*, **42**, 1–20.

LUND, R. D. and WESTRUM, L. E. (1966) Synaptic vesicle differences after primary formalin fixation. *J. Physiol., Lond.*, **185**, 7P–9P.

LUST, W. D. and ROBINSON, J. D. (1968) ATP dependent calcium accumulation by isolated nerve ending particles from brain. *Fed. Proc.*, **25**, 752.

LUST, W. D. and ROBINSON, J. D. (1970a) Calcium accumulation by isolated nerve endings from brain. I. Site of energy dependent accumulation. *J. Neurobiol.*, **1**, 303–316.

LUST, W. D. and ROBINSON, J. D. (1970b) Calcium accumulation by isolated nerve endings from brain. II. Factors influencing calcium accumulation. *J. Neurobiol.*, **1**, 317–328.

McBride, W. J. and Cohen, H. (1972) Cytochemical localization of acetylcholinesterase on isolated synaptosomes. *Brain Res.*, **41**, 489–493.

McBride, W. J., Mahler, H. R., Moore, W. J. and White, F. P. (1970) Isolation and characterization of membranes from rat cerebral cortex. *J. Neurobiol.*, **2**, 73–92.

McCaman, R. E., Rodriguez de Lores Arnaiz, G. and De Robertis, E. (1965) Species differences in subcellular distribution of choline acetylase in the C.N.S. *J. Neurochem.*, **12**, 927–935.

McGovern, S., Maguire, M. E., Gurd, R. S., Mahler, H. R. and Moore, W. J. (1973) Separation of adrenergic and cholinergic synaptosomes from immature rat brain. *FEBS letters*, **31**, 193–198.

McIlwain, H. (1955) *Biochemistry and the Central Nervous System*. London: Churchill.

McIlwain, H. and Bachelard, H. S. (1971) *Biochemistry and the Central Nervous System*, 4th edition. Edinburgh: Churchill Livingstone.

McIlwain, H. and Joanny, P. (1963) Characteristics required in electrical pulses of rectangular time-voltage relationships for metabolic change and ion movements in mammalian cerebral tissues. *J. Neurochem.*, **10**, 313–323.

MacIntosh, F. C. (1959) Formation, storage and release of acetylcholine at nerve endings. *Canad. J. Biochem.*, **37**, 343–356.

Mahaley, M. S., Day, E. D., Anderson, N., Wilfong, R. F. and Brater, C. (1968) Zonal centrifugation of adult, fetal, and malignant brain tissue. *Cancer Res.*, **28**, 1783–1789.

Mahler, H. R. and Cotman, C. W. (1970) Insoluble-proteins of the synaptic plasma membrane. In *Protein Metabolism of the Nervous System*, ed. Lajtha, A. Pp. 151–184. New York: Plenum Press.

Mahler, H. R., McBride, W. and Moore, W. J. (1970) Isolation and characterisation of membranes from rat cerebral cortex. In *Drugs and Cholinergic Mechanisms in the CNS*, ed. Heibronn, E. and Winter, A. Pp. 225–244. Res. Inst. of Natl. Def., Stockholm. Stockholm: Almqvist and Wiksell.

Maillet, M. (1962) La technique de Champy à l'osmium ioduré de potassium et la modification de Maillet à l'osmium-ioduré de zinc. *Trab. Inst. Cajal Invest. biol.*, **54**, 1–36.

Malinský, J. (1972) An introductory report on the development of synapses in human spinal cord. *Acta Universitatis Palackianae Olomucensis*, **6**, 25–43.

Malmfors, T. (1969) Histochemical studies on the effect of nerve impulses on exogenous catecholamines taken up into the adrenergic nerves of reserpine-pretreated animals. *Pharmacology*, **2**, 193–208.

Mangan, J. L. and Whittaker, V. P. (1966) The distribution of free amino acids in subcellular fractions of guinea-pig brain. *Biochem. J.*, **98**, 128–137.

Marchbanks, R. M. (1967) The osmotically sensitive potassium and sodium compartments of synaptosomes. *Biochem. J.*, **104**, 148–157.

Marchbanks, R. M. (1968a) Exchangeability of radioactive acetylcholine with the bound acetylcholine of synaptosomes and synaptic vesicles. *Biochem. J.*, **106**, 87–95.

Marchbanks, R. M. (1968b) The uptake of (^{14}C)choline into synaptosomes *in vitro*. *Biochem. J.*, **110**, 533–541.

Marchbanks, R. (1969) The conversion of ^{14}C-choline to ^{14}C-acetylcholine in synaptosomes *in vitro*. *Biochem. Pharmacol.*, **18**, 1763–1766.

Marchbanks, R. M., and Israël, M. (1971) Aspects of acetylcholine metabolism in the electric organ of *Torpedo marmorata*. *J. Neurochem.*, **18**, 439–448.

Marchbanks, R. M. and Israël, M. (1972) The heterogeneity of bound acetylcholine and synaptic vesicles. *Biochem. J.*, **129**, 1049–1061.

Marchbanks, R. M. and Whittaker, V. P. (1969) The biochemistry of synaptosomes. In *The Biological Basis of Medicine*, ed. Bittar, E. E. Vol. 5, pp. 39–76. New York: Academic Press.

231

MARRINOZZI, V. (1968) Phosphotungstic acid (PTA) as a stain for polysaccharides and glycoproteins in electron microscopy. *Proc. Fourth Europ. Reg. Conf. Electron Microscopy, Rome,* pp. 55–56.

MARTIN, A. R. (1955) A further study of the statistical composition of the end plate potential. *J. Physiol., Lond.,* **130,** 114–122.

MARTIN, A. R. (1966) Quantal nature of synaptic transmission. *Physiol. Rev.,* **46,** 51–66.

MARTIN, D. L. and Smith, A. A. (1972) Ions and the transport of GABA by synaptosomes. *J. Neurochem.,* **19,** 841–855.

MARTIN, R. (1968) Fine structure of the neurosecretory system of the vena cava in *Octopus. Brain Res.,* **8,** 201–205.

MARTIN, R., BARLOW, J. and MIRALTO, A. (1969) Application of the zinc iodide–osmium tetroxide impregnation of synaptic vesicles in cephalopod nerves. *Brain Res.,* **15,** 1–16.

MASUOKA, D. (1965) Monoamines in isolated nerve-ending particles. *Biochem. Pharmacol.,* **14,** 1688–1689.

MASUROVSKY, E. B., BENITEZ, H. H. and MURRAY, M. R. (1971) Synaptic development in long-term organized cultures of murine hypothalamus. *J. Comp. Neurol.,* **143,** 263–278.

MATHEWS, J. and BUTHALA, D. A. (1970) Centrifugal sedimentation of virus particles for electron microscopic counting. *J. Virol.,* **5,** 598–603.

MATHEWS, M. B. (1964) Structural factors in cation binding to anionic polysaccharides of connective tissues. *Arch. Biochem., Biophys.,* **104,** 394–404.

MATSUSAKA, T. (1971) The fine structure of the inner limiting membrane of the rat retina as revealed by ruthenium red staining. *J. Ultrastruct. Res.,* **36,** 312–317.

MATUS, A. I. (1970) Ultrastructure of the superior cervical ganglion fixed with zinc iodide and osmium tetroxide. *Brain Res.,* **17,** 195–203.

MATUS, A. I., and DENNISON, M. E. (1971) Autoradiographic localization of tritiated glycine at 'flat vesicle' synapses in spinal cord. *Brain Res.,* **32,** 195–197.

MATUS, A. I. and DENNISON, M. E. (1972) An autoradiographic study of uptake of exogenous glycine by vertebrate spinal cord slices *in vitro. J. Neurocytol.,* **1,** 27–34.

MELLER, K., BREIPOHL, W. and GLEES, P. (1968) The cytology of the developing molecular layer of mouse motor cortex. An electron microscopical and a Golgi impregnation study. *Z. Zellforsch.,* **86,** 171–183.

MELLER, K., BREIPOHL, W. and GLEES, P. (1969) Ontogeny of the mouse motor cortex. The polymorph layer or layer VI. A Golgi and electronmicroscopical study. *Z. Zellforsch.,* **99,** 443–458.

MESZLER, R. M., PAPPAS, G. D., and BENNETT, M. V. L. (1972) Morphological demonstration of electrotonic coupling of neurons by way of presynaptic fibers. *Brain Res.,* **36,** 412–415.

METZGER, H. P., CUÉNOD, M., GRYNBAUM, A. and WAELSCH, H. (1967) The use of tritium oxide as a biosynthetic precursor of macromolecules in brain and liver. *J. Neurochem.,* **14,** 99–104.

MEYER, W. J. (1969) Phosphotungstic acid section staining of synaptic junctions of rat brain. *J. Cell Biol.,* **43,** 92a.

MEYER, W. J. (1970) Distribution of phosphotungstic acid-stained carbohydrate moieties in the brain. Dissertation. Los Angeles: University of California.

MICHAELSON, I. A. and DOWE, G. H. C. (1963) The subcellular distribution of histamine in brain tissue. *Biochem. Pharmacol.,* **12,** 949–956.

MICHAELSON, I. A. and WHITTAKER, V. P. (1962) The distribution of hydroxytryptamine in brain fractions. *Biochem. Pharmacol.,* **11,** 505–506.

MICHAELSON, I. A. and WHITTAKER, V. P. (1963) The subcellular localization of 5-hydroxytryptamine in guinea-pig brain. *Biochem. Pharmacol.,* **12,** 203–211.

MICHAELSON, I. A., WHITTAKER, V. P., LAVERTY, R. and SHARMAN, D. F. (1963)

Localization of acetylcholine, 5-hydroxytryptamine and noradrenaline within subcellular particles derived from guinea-pig subcortical brain tissue. *Biochem. Pharmacol.*, **12**, 1450–1453.

MICKEY, D. D., MCMILLAN, P. N., APPEL, S. H. and DAY, E. D. (1971) Specificity and cross-reactivity of antisynaptosome antibodies as determined by sequential absorption analysis. *J. Immunol.*, **107**, 1599–1610.

MIHAILOVIĆ, L. and JANKOVIĆ, B. D. (1961) Effects of intravenously injected anti-*N. caudatus* antibody on the electrical activity of the cat brain. *Nature, Lond.*, **192**, 665–666.

MILHAILOVIĆ, L. and JANOKOVIĆ, B. D. (1965) Effects of anticerebral antibodies on electrical activity and behavior. *Neurosci. Res. Program Bull.*, **3**, 8–17.

MIHAILOVIĆ, L., JANKOVIĆ, B. D., BELESLIN, B., MILOŜEVIĆ, D. and CUPIC, D. (1965) Effects on antilobster nerve antibody on membrane potentials of the giant axon of *Palinurus vulgaris*. *Nature, Lond.*, **206**, 904–905.

MILEDI, R. (1966) Miniature synaptic potentials in squid nerve cells. *Nature, Lond.*, **212**, 1240–1242.

MILEDI, R. (1967) Spontaneous synaptic potentials and quantal release of transmitter in the stellate ganglion of the squid. *J. Physiol. Lond.*, **192**, 379–406.

MILEDI, R. and SLATER, C. R. (1970), On the degeneration of rat neuromuscular junctions after nerve section. *J. Physiol., Lond.*, **207**, 507–528.

MILHAUD, M. and PAPPAS, G. D. (1966a) Postsynaptic bodies in the habenula and interpeduncular nuclei of the cat. *J. Cell Biol.*, **30**, 437–441.

MILHAUD, M. and PAPPAS, G. D. (1966b) The fine structure of neurons and synapses of the habenula of the cat with special reference to subjunctional bodies. *Brain Res.*, **3**, 158–173.

MIZUNO, N. and NAKAMURA, Y. (1974) An electron microscope study of terminal degeneration of the fasciculus retroflexus Meynerti within the interpeduncular nucleus of the rabbit. *Brain Res.*, **65**, 165–169.

MODEL, P. G., BORNSTEIN, M. B., CRAIN, S. M. and PAPPAS, G. D. (1971) An electron microscopic study of the development of synapses in cultured fetal mouse cerebrum continuously exposed to xylocaine. *J. Cell Biol.*, **49**, 362–371.

MOLENAAR, P. C., NICKOLSON, V. J. and POLAK, R. L. (1971) Preferential release of newly synthesized acetylcholine from rat cerebral cortex *in vitro*. *J. Physiol. Lond.*, **213**, 64P–65P.

MOLENAAR, P. C., NICKOLSON, V. J. and POLAK, R. L. (1973a) Preferential release of newly synthesized ^{3}H-acetylcholine from rat cerebral cortex slices *in vitro*. *Br. J. Pharmac.*, **47**, 97–108.

MOLENAAR, P. C. and POLAK, R. L. (1973) Newly formed acetylcholine in synaptic vesicles in brain tissue. *Brain Res.*, **62**, 537–542.

MOLENAAR, P. C., POLAK, R. L., and NICKOLSON, V. K. (1973b) Subcellular localization of newly-formed [^{3}H]acetylcholine in rat cerebral cortex *in vitro*. *J. Neurochem.*, **21**, 667–678.

MØLLGAARD, K., DIAMOND, M. C., BENNETT, E. L., ROSENZWEIG, M. R. and LINDNER, B. (1971) Quantitative synaptic changes with differential experience in rat brain. *Int. J. Neurosci.*, **2**, 113–128.

MOLLIVER, M. E. and VAN DER LOOS, H. (1970) The ontogenesis of cortical circuitry: the spatial distribution of synapses in somesthetic cortex of newborn dog. *Ergebnisse der Anatomie*, **42**, 1–53.

MONNERON, A. and BERNHARD, W. (1966) Action de certaines enzymes sur des tissus inclus en epon. *J. Microscopie*, **5**, 697–714.

MOOR, H. (1966) Use of freeze-etching in the study of biological ultrastructure. *Int. Rev. Exp. Pathol.*, **5**, 179–216.

MOOR, H. and MÜHLETHALER, K. (1963) Fine structure in frozen-etched yeast cells. *J. Cell Biol.*, **17**, 609–628.

MOOR, H., PFENNINGER, K. and AKERT, K. (1969) Synaptic vesicles in electron micrographs of freeze-etched nerve terminals. *Science*, **164**, 1405–1407.

MORGAN, I. G., REITH, M., MARINARI, U., BRECKENRIDGE, W. C. and GOMBOS, G. (1972) The isolation and characterization of synaptosomal plasma membranes. In *Glycolipids, Glycoproteins and Mucopolysaccharides of the Nervous System*, ed. Zambotti, V., Tettamanti, G. and Arrigoni, M. Pp. 209–228. New York: Plenum Press.

MORGAN, I. G., WOLFE, L. S., MANDEL, P. and GOMBOS, G. (1971) Isolation of plasma membranes from rat brain. *Biochim. Biophys. Acta*, **241**, 737–751.

MORI, S., MAEDA, T. and SHIMIZU, N. (1964) Electron-microscopic histochemistry of cholinesterases in the rat brain. *Histochemie*, **4**, 65–72.

MORRIS, J. H., HUDSON, A. R., and WEDDELL, G. (1972a) A study of degeneration and regeneration in the divided rat sciatic nerve based on electron microscopy. I. The traumatic degeneration of myelin in the proximal stump of the divided nerve. *Z. Zellforsch.*, **124**, 76–102.

MORRIS, J. H., HUDSON, A. R. and WEDDELL, G. (1972b) A study of degeneration and regeneration in the divided rat sciatic nerve based on electron microscopy. II. The development of the 'regenerating unit'. *Z. Zellforsch.*, **124**, 103–130.

MORRIS, J. H., HUDSON, A. R. and WEDDELL, G. (1972c) A study of degeneration and regeneration in the divided rat sciatic nerve based on electron microscopy. III. Changes in the axons of the proximal stump. *Z. Zellforsch.*, **124**, 131–164.

MORRIS, J. H., HUDSON, A. R. and WEDDELL, G. (1972d) A study of degeneration and regeneration in the divided rat sciatic nerve based on electron microscopy. IV. Changes in fascicular microtopography, perineurium and endoneurial fibroblasts. *Z. Zellforsch.* **124**, 165–203.

MORRIS, S. J. (1973) Removal of residual amounts of acetylcholinesterase and membrane contamination from synaptic vesicles isolated from the electric organ of *Torpedo. J. Neurochem.*, **21**, 713–715.

MOWRY, R. W. (1958) Improved procedure for the staining of acidic polysaccharides by Müller's colloidal (hydrous) ferric oxide and its combination with the Feulgen and the periodic acid-Schiff reactions. *Lab. Invest.*, **7**, 566–576.

MOWRY, R. (1963) The special value of methods that color both acidic and vicinal hydroxyl groups in the histochemical study of mucins. *Ann. N.Y. Acad. Sci.*, **106**, 402–407.

MUGNAINI, E. (1970) The relation between cytogenesis and the formation of different types of synaptic contact. *Brain Res.*, **17**, 169–179.

MUGNAINI, E. and FORSTRØNEN, P. F. (1967) Ultrastructural studies on the cerebellar histogenesis. I. Differentiation of granule cells and development of *glomeruli* in the chick embryo. *Z. Zellforsch.*, **77**, 115–143.

MUGNAINI, E. and WALBERG, F. (1967) An experimental electron microscopic study on the mode of termination of cerebellar corticovestibular fibres in the cat lateral vestibular nucleus (Dieter's nucleus). *Exp. Brain Res.*, **4**, 212–236.

MUGNAINI, E., WALBERG, F. and BRODAL, A. (1967a) Mode of termination of primary vestibular fibres in the lateral vestibular nucleus. An experimental electron microscopical study in the cat. *Exp. Brain Res.*, **4**, 187–211.

MUGNAINI, E., WALBERG, F. and HAUGLIE-HANSSEN, E. (1967b) Observations on the fine structure of the lateral vestibular nucleus (Deiters' Nucleus) in the cat. *Exp. Brain Res.*, **4**, 146–186.

MULDER, A. H., GEUZE, J. J. and DE WIED, D. (1970) Studies on the subcellular localization of corticotrophin releasing factor (CRF) and vasopressin in the median eminence of rat. *Endocrinology*, **87**, 61–79.

MUNN, E. A. (1968). On the structure of mitochondria and the value of ammonium molybdate as a negative stain for osmotically sensitive structures. *J. Ultrastruct. Res.*, **25**, 362–380.

MUSCATELLO, U., and HORNE, R. W. (1968) Effect of the tonicity of some negative-staining solutions on the elementary structure of membrane-bounded systems. *J. Ultrastruct. Res.*, **25**, 73–83.

NACHMANSOHN, D. (1971) Chemical events in conducting and synaptic membranes during electrical activity. *Proc. Nat. Acad. Sci. U.S.A.*, **68**, 3170–3174.

NAGASAWA, J. and DOUGLAS, W. W. (1972) Thorium dioxide uptake into adrenal medullary cells and the problem of recapture of granule membrane following exocytosis. *Brain Res.*, **37**, 141–145.

NAGASAWA, J., DOUGLAS, W. W. and SCHULTZ, R. A. (1970) Ultrastructural evidence of secretion by exocytosis and of 'synaptic vesicle' formation in posterior pituitary glands. *Nature, Lond.*, **227**, 407–409.

NAGASAWA, J., DOUGLAS, W. W. and SCHULTZ, R. A. (1971) Micropinocytotic origin of coated and smooth microvesicles ('synaptic vesicles') in neurosecretory terminals of posterior pituitary glands demonstrated by incorporation of horse-radish peroxidase. *Nature, Lond.*, **232**, 341–342.

NATHANIEL, E. J. H. and NATHANIEL, D. R. (1966) The ultrastructural features of the synapses in the posterior horn of the spinal cord in the rat. *J. Ultrastruct. Res.*, **14**, 540–555.

NEAL, M. J. (1971) The uptake of ^{14}C-glycine by slices of mammalian spinal cord. *J. Physiol., Lond.*, **215**, 103–118.

NEAL, M. J. and IVERSEN, L. L. (1969) Subcellular distribution of endogenous and ^{3}H-GABA in rat cortex. *J. Neurochem.*, **16**, 1245–1252.

NEAL, M. J. and IVERSEN, L. L. (1972) Autoradiographic localization of ^{3}H-GABA in rat retina. *Nature, New Biol.*, **235**, 217–218.

NEAL, M. J. and PICKLES, H. (1969) Uptake of ^{14}C-glycine by rat spinal cord. *Nature, Lond.*, **223**, 679–680.

NICHOLSON, J. L. and ALTMAN, J. (1972a) Synaptogenesis in the rat cerebellum: effects of early hypo- and hyperthyroidism. *Science*, **176**, 530–532.

NICHOLSON, J. L. and ALTMAN, J. (1972b) The effects of early hypo- and hyperthyroidism on the development of rat cerebellar cortex. I. Cell proliferation and differentiation. *Brain Res.*, **44**, 13–23.

NICHOLSON, J. L. and ALTMAN, J. (1972c) The effects of early hypo- and hyperthyroidism on the development of the rat cerebellar cortex. II. Synaptogenesis in the molecular layer. *Brain Res.*, **44**, 25–36.

NICKEL, E. and GRIESHABER, E. (1969) Elektronenmikroskopische Darstellung der Muskelkapillaren im Gefrierätzbild. *Z. Zellforsch.*, **95**, 445–461.

NICKEL, E. and POTTER, L. T. (1970) Synaptic vesicles in freeze-etched electric tissue of *Torpedo*. *Brain Res.*, **23**, 95–100.

NICKEL, E., VOGEL, A. and WASER, P. G. (1967) Coated vesicles in der Ungebung der Neuro-muskulären Synapsen. *Z. Zellforsch.*, **78**, 261–266.

NIEBAUER, G., KRAWCZYK, W. S., KIDD, R. L. and WILGRAM, G. F. (1969) Osmium zinc iodide reactive sites in the epidermal Langerhans cell. *J. Cell Biol.*, **43**, 80–89.

NILSSON, S. E. G. and CRESCITELLI, F. (1969) Changes in ultrastructure and electroretinogram of bullfrog retina during development. *J. Ultrastruct. Res.*, **27**, 45–62.

NILSSON, S. E. G., and CRESCITELLI, F. (1970) A correlation of ultrastructure and function in the developing retina of the frog tadpole. *J. Ultrastruct. Res.*, **30**, 87–102.

NISHI, S. and KOKETSU, K. (1960) Electrical properties and activities of single sympathetic neurons in frogs. *J. Cell. Comp. Physiol.*, **55**, 15–30.

NOBACK, C. R. and PURPURA, D. P. (1961) Postnatal ontogenesis of neurons in cat neo-cortex. *J. Comp. Neurol.*, **117**, 291–307.

NOLAN, T. M. (1974) Personal communication.

NOLAN, T. M. and JONES, D. G. (1973a) Equidensitometric analysis of synaptic ultrastruc-ture. *J. Anat., Lond.*, **116**, 469.

NOLAN, T. M. and JONES, D. G. (1973b) Morphometry of synaptic ultrastructure using equidensitometry. *Am. J. Anat.*, **138**, 527–532.

NOLAN, T. M. and JONES, D. G. (1974) Equidensitometric analytical techniques applied to the study of synaptic ultrastructure. *J. Neurocytol.*, **3**, 327–340.

NORTON, W. T. and PODUSLO, S. E. (1970) Neuronal soma and whole neuroglia of rat brain: a new isolation technique. *Science*, **167**, 1144–1146.

NYMAN, M. and WHITTAKER, V. P. (1963) The distribution of adenosine triphosphate in subcellular fractions of brain tissue. *Biochem. J.*, **87**, 248–255.

OBERJAT, T. and HOWARD, B. D. (1973) Age dependent changes in synaptosome buoyant density. *Nature New Biol.*, **244**, 248–250.

OCHI, J. (1967) Electron microscopic study of the olfactory bulb of the rat during develop-ment. *Z. Zellforsch.*, **76**, 339–349.

OCHS, S. (1972) Fast transport of materials in mammalian nerve fibers. *Science*, **176**, 252–260.

OGAWA, K., HIRANO, H., SAITO, T. and AGO, Y. (1970) Ultracytochemistry of intracellular membranes. I. Findings obtained by an *in situ* phosphotungstic acid staining. Ultracyto-chemistry *sine* osmium tetroxide. *Arch. histol. jap.*, **31**, 209–222.

OHLENBUSCH, H. H., OLIVERA, B. M., TUAN, D. and DAVIDSON, N. (1967) Selective dissociation of histones from calf thymus nucleoprotein. *J. Mol. Biol.*, **25**, 299–315.

OKAMOTO, M., LONGENECKER, H. E., RIKER, W. F. and SONG, S. K. (1971) Distribution of mammalian motor nerve terminals by black widow spider venom. *Science*, **172**, 733–736.

OPPENHEIM, R. W. and FOELIX, R. F. (1972) Synaptogenesis in the chick embryo spinal cord. *Nature, New Biol.*, **235**, 126–128.

ORD, M. G., and THOMPSON, R. H. S. (1951) The preparation of soluble cholinesterases from mammalian heart and brain. *Biochem., J.*, **49**, 191–199.

ORKAND, P. M. and KRAVITZ, E. A. (1971) Localization of the sites of γ-aminobutyric acid (GABA) uptake in lobster nerve-muscle preparations. *J. Cell Biol.*, **49**, 75–89.

OSBORNE, R. H. and BRADFORD, R. F. (1973) Tetanus toxin inhibits amino acid release from nerve endings *in vitro*. *Nature, Lond.*, **244**, 157–158.

OSBORNE, R. H., BRADFORD, H. F. and JONES, D. G. (1973) Patterns of amino acid release from nerve-endings isolated from spinal cord and medulla. *J. Neurochem.*, **21**, 407–419.

PALADE, G. E. (1951) Intracellular distribution of acid phosphatase in rat liver cells. *Arch. Biochem.*, **30**, 144–158.

PALADE, G. E. (1954) Electron microscope observations of interneuronal and neuromuscular synapses. *Anat. Rec.*, **118**, 335–336.

PALADE, G. E. and SIEKEVITZ, P. (1956a) Liver microsomes. An integrated morphological and biochemical study. *J. biophys. biochem. Cytol.*, **2**, 171–200.

PALADE, G. E. and SIEKEVITZ, P. (1956b) Pancreatic microsomes. An integrated morpho-logical and biochemical study. *J. biophys. biochem. Cytol.*, **2**, 671–690.

PALAY, S. L. (1954) Electron microscope study of the cytoplasm of neurons. *Anat. Rec.*, **118**, 336.

PALAY, S. L. (1956) Synapses in the central nervous system. *J. biophys. biochem. Cytol.*, **2**, suppl. 193–202.

PALAY, S. L. (1957) The fine structure of the neurohypophysis. In *Prog. Neurobiology*, **2**, 31–49.

PALAY, S. (1963) Alveolate vesicles in Purkinje cells of rat's cerebellum. *J. Cell Biol.*, **19**, 89A–90A.

PALAY, S. L. (1967) Principles of cellular organisation in the nervous system. In *The Neuro-*

sciences, ed. Quarton, G. C., Melnechuk, T. and Schmitt, F. O. Pp. 24–31. New York: Rockefeller University Press.

PALAY, S. L., SOTELO, C., PETERS, A. and ORKAND, P. M. (1968) The axon hillock and the initial segment. *J. Cell Biol.*, **38**, 193–201.

PANNESE, E., LUCIANO, L., IURATO, S. and REALE, E. (1971) Cholinesterase activity in spinal ganglia neuroblasts: a histochemical study at the electron microscope. *J. Ultrastruct. Res.*, **36**, 46–67.

PAPPAS, G. D. (1966) Electron microscopy of neuronal junctions involved in transmission in the central nervous system. In *Nerve as a Tissue*, ed. Rodahl, K. and Issekutz, B. Pp. 49–87. New York: Harper and Row.

PAPPAS, G. D., ASADA, Y. and BENNETT, M. V. L. (1971) Morphological correlates of increased coupling resistance at an electrotonic synapse. *J. Cell Biol.*, **49**, 173–188.

PAPPAS, G. D. and BENNETT, M. V. L. (1966) Specialized junctions involved in electrical transmission between neurons. *Ann. N.Y. Acad. Sci.*, **137**, 495–508.

PAPPAS, G. D. and PURPURA, D. P. (1961) Fine structure of dendrites in the superficial neocortical neuropil. *Expl. Neurol.*, **4**, 507–530.

PAPPAS, G. D. and PURPURA, D. P. (1964) Electron microscopy of immature human and feline neocortex. *Prog. Brain Res..*, **4**, 176–186.

PAPPAS, G. D. and WAXMAN, S. G. (1972) Synaptic fine structure – morphological correlates of chemical and electronic transmission. In *Structure and Function of Synapses*, ed. Pappas, G. D. and Purpura, D. P. Pp. 1–43. New York: Raven Press.

PÁRDUCZ, A. and FEHÉR, O. (1970) Fine structural alterations of presynaptic endings in the superior cervical ganglion of the cat after exhausting preganglionic stimulation. *Experientia*, **26**, 629–630.

PÁRDUCZ, A., FEHÉR, O. and JOÓ, F. (1971a) Effects of stimulation and hemicholinium (HC-3) on the fine structure of nerve endings in the superior cervical ganglion of the cat. *Brain Res.*, **34**, 61–72.

PÁRDUCZ, A., HALÁSZ, N. and JOÓ, F. (1971b) Lack of correlation between the zinc iodide–osmium positivity of cholinergic terminals and the cholinergic transmission in the sympathetic ganglia of the cat. *J. Neurochem.*, **18**, 97–100.

PARSONS, D. F., WILLIAMS, G. R. and CHANCE, B. (1966) Characteristics of isolated and purified preparations of the outer and inner membranes of mitochondria. *Ann. N.Y. Acad. Sci.*, **137**, 643–666.

PEASE, D. C. (1966) Polysaccharides associated with the exterior surface of epithelial cells: kidney, intestine, brain. *J. Ultrastruct. Res.*, **15**, 555–588.

PEASE, D. C. (1970) Phosphotungstic acid as a specific electron stain for complex carbohydrates. *J. Histochem. Cytochem.*, **18**, 455–458.

PELLEGRINO DE IRALDI, A. and DE ROBERTIS, E. (1963) Action of reserpine, iproniazid and pyrogallol on nerve endings in the pineal gland. *Int. J. Neuropharmacol.*, **2**, 231–239.

PELLEGRINO DE IRALDI, A., DUGGAN, H. F. and DE ROBERTIS, E. (1963) Adrenergic synaptic vesicles in the anterior hypothalamus of the rat. *Anat. Rec.*, **145**, 521–531.

PELLEGRINO DE IRALDI, A. and GUEUDET, R. (1968) Action of reserpine on the osmium tetroxide–zinc iodide reactive site of synaptic vesicles in the pineal nerves of the rat. *Z. Zellforsch.*, **91**, 178–185.

PELLEGRINO DE IRALDI, A. and GUEUDET, R. (1969) Osmium tetroxide–zinc iodide reactive sites in the photoreceptor cells of the retina of the rat. *Z. Zellforsch.*, **101**, 203–211.

PELLEGRINO DE IRALDI, A. and SUBURO, A. M. (1970) Electron staining of synaptic vesicles using the Champy–Maillet technique. *J. Microscopy*, **91**, 99–103.

PELLEGRINO DE IRALDI, A. and SUBURO, A. M. (1972) Effect of tyramine on the compartments of the granulated vesicles in rat pineal nerve endings. *Eur. J. Pharmacol.*, **19**, 251–259.

PERRI, V., SACCHI, O., RAVIOLA, E. and RAVIOLA, G. (1972) Evaluation of the number and distribution of synaptic vesicles at cholinergic nerve-endings after sustained stimulation. *Brain Res.*, **39**, 526–529.

PETERS, A., PALAY, S. L. and WEBSTER, H. DE F. (1970) *The Fine Structure of the Nervous System – The Cells and Their Processes.* New York: Harper and Row.

PETERS, A., PROSKAUER, C. C. and KAISERMAN-ABRAMOF, I. R. (1968) The small pyramidal neuron of the rat cerebral cortex. The axon hillock and initial segment. *J. Cell Biol.*, **39**, 604–619.

PETERS, R. A. (1963) *Biochemical Lesions and Lethal Synthesis.* Oxford: Pergamon Press.

PETRUSHKA, E. and GIUDITTA, A. (1959) Electron microscopy of two subcellular fractions isolated from cerebral cortex homogenate. *J. biophys. biochem. Cytol.*, **6**, 129–132.

PFENNINGER, K. H. (1971a) The cytochemistry of synaptic densities. I. An analysis of the bismuth iodide impregnation method. *J. Ultrastruct. Res.*, **34**, 103–122.

PFENNINGER, K. H. (1971b) The cytochemistry of synaptic densities. II. Proteinaceous components and mechanism of synaptic connectivity. *J. Ultrastruct. Res.*, **35**, 451–475.

PFENNINGER, K. (1972) Synaptic morphology and cytochemistry. *Prog. Histochem. Cytochem.*, **5**, 1–83.

PFENNINGER, K., AKERT, K., MOOR, H. and SANDRI, C. (1971) Freeze-fracturing of presynaptic membranes in the central nervous system. *Trans. Roy. Soc. Lond. B.*, **261**, 387.

PFENNINGER, K., AKERT, K., MOOR, H. and SANDRI, C. (1972) The fine structure of freeze-fractured presynaptic membranes. *J. Neurocytol.*, **1**, 129–149.

PFENNINGER, K., AKERT, K. and SANDRI, C. (1970) Structural organization of the synaptic cleft: polyionic binding between pre- and postsynaptic membranes. In *Seventh Int. Congress of Electron Microscopy, Grenoble*, pp. 715–716.

PFENNINGER, K., SANDRI, C., AKERT, K. and EUGSTER, C. H. (1969) Contribution to the problem of structural organization of the presynaptic area. *Brain Res.*, **12**, 10–18.

PHILLIS, J. W. (1970) *The Pharmacology of Synapses.* Oxford: Pergamon.

PILCHER, C. W. T. and JONES, D. G. (1970) The distribution of 5′-nucleotidase in subcellular fractions of mouse cerebellum. *Brain Res.*, **24**, 143–147.

PIRAS, M. M., SZIJAN, I. and GÓMEZ, C. J. (1970) Enzymatic and ultrastructural changes in subcellular fractions from developing rat brain. *Acta Physiol. Latinoam.*, **20**, 252–264.

PLATTNER, H. (1970) A study on the interpretation of freeze-etched animal tissues and cell organelles. *Mikroskopie*, **26**, 233–250.

PODUSLO, S. E. and NORTON, W. T. (1972) The bulk separation of neuroglia and perikarya. In *Research Methods in Neurochemistry*, ed. Marks, N. and Rodnight, R. **1**, pp. 19–32. New York: Plenum Press.

POISNER, A. M. (1973) Mechanisms of exocytosis. *Life Sci.*, **13**, cxxxi–cxxxiv.

POTTER, L. T. (1968) Uptake of choline by nerve endings isolated from rat cerebral cortex. In *The Interaction of Drugs and Subcellular Components in Animal Cells*, ed. Campbell, P. N. Pp. 293–304. London: Churchill.

POTTER, L. T. (1970) Synthesis, storage and release of [^{14}C] acetylcholine in isolated rat diaphragm muscles. *J. Physiol., Lond.*, **206**, 145–166.

POTTER, L. T. and AXELROD, J. (1963a) Subcellular localization of catecholamines in tissues of the rat. *J. Pharmacol. Expt. Therap.*, **142**, 291–298.

POTTER, L. T. and AXELROD, J. (1963b) Properties of norepinephrine storage particles of the rat heart. *J. Pharmacol. Expt. Therap.*, **142**, 299–305.

POTTS, W. T. W. (1954) The inorganic composition of the blood of *Mytilus edulis* and *Anodonta cygnea. J. exp. Biol.*, **31**, 376–385.

PRICE, J. L. and POWELL, T. P. S. (1970) Synaptology of the granule cells of the olfactory bulb. *J. Cell Sci.*, **7**, 125–155.

PURPURA, D. P. (1973) Analysis of morphophysiological developmental processes. In *Biological and Environmental Determinants of Early Development*, ed., Nurnberger, J. I. Pp. 79–112. Baltimore: Williams and Wilkins.

PURPURA, D. P., SHOFER, R. J., HOUSEPIAN, E. M. and NOBACK, C. R. (1964) Comparative ontogenesis of structure-function relations in cerebral and cerebellar cortex. *Prog. Brain Res.*, **4**, 187–221.

PUSZKIN, S. and BERL, S. (1972) Actomyosin-like protein from brain. Separation and characterization of the actin-like component. *Biochim. Biophys. Acta.*, **256**, 695–709.

PUSZKIN, S., BERL, S., PUSZKIN, E. and CLARKE, D. D. (1968) Actomyosin-like protein isolated from mammalian brain. *Science*, **161**, 170–171.

PUSZKIN, S., NICKLAS, W. J. and BERL, S. (1972) Actomyosin-like protein in brain subcellular distribution. *J. Neurochem.*, **19**, 1319–1333.

PYSH, J. J. (1969) The development of the extracellular space in neonatal rat inferior colliculus: an electron microscopic study. *Amer. J. Anat.*, **124**, 411–430.

PYSH, J. J. (1970) Mitochondrial changes in rat inferior colliculus during postnatal development: an electron microscopic study. *Brain Res.*, **18**, 325–342.

PYSH, J. J. and WILEY, R. G. (1972) Morphologic alterations of synapses in electrically stimulated superior cervical ganglia of the cat. *Science*, **176**, 191–193.

PYSH, J. J. and WILEY, R. G. (1974) Synaptic vesicle depletion and recovery in cat sympathetic ganglia electrically stimulated *in vivo*. Evidence for transmitter secretion by exocytosis. *J. Cell Biol.*, **60**, 365–374.

QUASTEL, J. H. (1969) Carbohydrate metabolism. In *The Structure and Function of Nervous Tissue*, ed. Bourne, G. H. Vol. 3, pp. 80–107. New York: Academic Press.

QUILLIAM, J. P. and TAMARIND, D. L. (1973) Local vesicle populations in rat superior cervical ganglia and the vesicle hypothesis. *J. Neurocytol.*, **2**, 59–75.

QUINTARELLI, G., CIFONELLI, J. A. and ZITO, R. (1971a) On phosphotungstic acid staining. II. *J. Histochem., Cytochem.*, **19**, 648–653.

QUINTARELLI, G., ZITO, R. and CIFONELLI, J. A. (1971b) On phosphotungstic acid staining. I. *J. Histochem. Cytochem.*, **19**, 641–647.

RABIÉ, A. and LEGRAND, J. (1973) Effects of thyroid hormone and undernourishment on the amount of synaptosomal fraction in the cerebellum of the young rat. *Brain Res.*, **61**, 267–278.

RAINE, C. S., PODUSLO, S. E., and NORTON, W. T. (1971) The ultrastructure of purified preparations of neurons and glial cells. *Brain Res.*, **27**, 11–24.

RAITERI, M. and BERTOLLINI, A. (1974) Specificity and cross-reactivity of antisynaptosome antibodies. *Brain Res.*, **65**, 297–302.

RAITERI, M., BERTOLLINI, A. and LA BELLA, R. (1972) Synaptosome antisera affect permeability of synaptosomal membranes in vitro. *Nature, New Biol.*, **238**, 242–243.

RALSTON, H. J. (1965) The organization of the substantia gelatinosa Rolandi in the cat lumbosacral spinal cord. *Z. Zellforsch.*, **67**, 1–23.

RALSTON, H. J. (1968) The fine structure of neurons in the dorsal horn of the cat spinal cord. *J. Comp. Neurol.*, **132**, 275–301.

RAMBOURG, A. (1967) Détection des glycoprotéines en microscopie électronique: coloration de la surface cellulaire et l'appareil de Golgi par un mélange acide chromique phosphotungstique. *C.R. Acad., Paris*, **265**, 1426–1428.

RAMBOURG, A. (1971) Morphological and histochemical aspects of glycoproteins at the surface of animal cells. *Int. Rev. Cytol.*, **31**, 57–114.

RAMBOURG, A., HERNANDEZ, W. and LEBLOND, C. P. (1969) Detection of complex carbohydrates in the Golgi apparatus of rat cells. *J. Cell Biol.*, **40**, 395–414.

RAMBOURG, A. and LEBLOND, C. P. (1967) Electron microscope observations on the carbohydrate-rich cell coat present at the surface of cells in the rat. *J. Cell Biol.*, **32**, 27–53.

RAMÓN Y CAJAL, S. (1888) Estructura de los centros nerviosos de los aves. *Rev. trimest. Histol. norm. patol.*, **1**, 305–315.

RAMÓN Y CAJAL, S. (1911) *Histologie du Système Nerveux de l'Homme et des Vertébrés.* Vol. II. Paris: Maloine.

RAMÓN Y CAJAL, S. (1933) Neuronismo o reticularismo? Las pruebas objectivas de la unidad anatómica, de la celulas nerviosas. *Archos. Neurobiol.*, **13**, 217–291, 579–646.

RASSIN, D. K. (1972) Amino acids as putative transmitters: failure to bind to synaptic vesicles of guinea pig cerebral cortex. *J. Neurochem.*, **19**, 139–148.

REICHETT, K. L. and FONNUM, F. (1969) Subcellular localization of *N*-acetylaspartyl glutamate, *N*-acetyl glutamate and glutathione in brain. *J. Neurochem.*, **16**, 1409–1416.

REVEL, J. P. (1964) A stain for the ultrastructural localization of acid mucopolysaccharides. *J. Microscopie*, **3**, 535–544.

RICHARDSON, K. C. (1966) Electron microscopic identification of autonomic nerve endings. *Nature, Lond.*, **210**, 756.

RICHTER, J. A. and MARCHBANKS, R. M. (1971a) Synthesis of radioactive acetylcholine from [^{3}H]choline and its release from cerebral cortex slices *in vitro. J. Neurochem.*, **18**, 691–703.

RICHTER, J. A. and MARCHBANKS, R. M. (1971b) Isolation of [^{3}H]acetylcholine pools by subcellular fractionation of cerebral cortex slices incubated with [^{3}H]choline. *J. Neurochem.*, **18**, 705–712.

ROBERTS, P. J. and MITCHELL, J. F. (1972) The release of amino acids from the hemisected spinal cord during stimulation. *J. Neurochem.*, **19**, 2473–2481.

ROBERTSON, J. D. (1956) The ultrastructure of a reptilian myoneural junction. *J. biophys. biochem. Cytol.*, **2**, 381–394.

ROBERTSON, J. D. (1959) The ultrastructure of cell membranes and their derivatives. *Biochem. Soc. Symposia*, **16**, 1–43.

ROBERTSON, J. D. (1966) Granulo-fibrillar and globular substructure in unit membranes. *Ann. N.Y. Acad. Sci.*, **137**, 421–440.

ROBERTSON, J. D. BODENHEIMER, T. S. and STAGE, D. E. (1963) The ultrastructure of Mauthner cell synapses and nodes in goldfish brains. *J. Cell Biol.*, **19**, 159–199.

RODNIGHT, R., WELLER, M. and GOLDFARB, P. S. G. (1969) Large scale preparation of a crude membrane fraction from ox brain. *J. Neurochem.*, **16**, 1591–1597.

RODRIGUEZ DE LOREZ ARNAIZ, G. (1964) Subcellular localization of cholinesterase in brain. *J. Histochem. Cytochem.*, **12**, 696–699.

RODRIGUEZ DE LORES ARNAIZ, G., ALBERICI, M., and DE ROBERTIS, E. (1967) Ultrastructural and enzymic studies of cholinergic and non-cholinergic synaptic membranes isolated from brain cortex. *J. Neurochem.*, **14**, 215–225.

RODRIGUEZ DE LORES ARNAIZ, G., ALBERICI DE CANAL, M. and DE ROBERTIS, E. (1971) Turnover of proteins in subcellular fractions of rat cerebral cortex. *Brain Res.*, **31**, 179–184.

RODRIGUEZ DE LORES ARNAIZ, G., ZIEHER, L. M. and DE ROBERTIS, E. (1970) Neurochemical and structural studies on the mechanism of action of hemicholinium-3, in central cholinergic synapses. *J. Neurochem.*, **17**, 221–229.

ROGERS, S. C. (1968) Fine structure of smooth muscle and neuromuscular junctions in the optic tentacles of *Helix aspersa* and *Limax flavus. Z. Zellforsch.*, **89**, 80–94.

ROOTS, B. I. and JOHNSTON, P. V. (1964) Neurons of ox brain nuclei: their isolation and appearance by light and electron microscopy. *J. Ultrastruct. Res.*, **10**, 350–361.

ROOTS, B. I. and JOHNSTON, P. V. (1965) Isolated rabbit neurones: electron microscopical observations. *Nature, Lond.*, **207**, 315–316.

ROSE, S. P. R. (1965) Preparation of enriched fractions from cerebral cortex containing isolated, metabolically active neuronal cells. *Nature, Lond.*, **206**, 621–622.

ROSE, S. P. R. (1967) Preparation of enriched fractions from cerebral cortex containing isolated, metabolically active neuronal and glial cells. *Biochem. J.*, **102**, 33–43.

ROSE, S. P. R. (1968) Glucose and amino acid metabolism in isolated neuronal and glial cell fractions *in vitro*. *J. Neurochem.*, **15**, 1415–1429.

ROSE, S. P. R. (1969) Neurons and glia: separation techniques and biochemical interrelationships. In *Handbook of Neurochemistry*, ed. Lajtha, A. Vol. 2, pp. 183–193. New York: Plenum Press.

ROSE, S. P. R. and SINHA, A. K. (1969) Some properties of isolated neuronal cell fractions. *J. Neurochem.*, **16**, 1319–1328.

ROSENBLUTH, J. (1962) Subsurface cisterns and their relationship to the neuronal plasma membrane. *J. Cell Biol.*, **13**, 405–421.

ROSENBLUTH, J. (1973) Postjunctional membrane specialization at cholinergic myoneural junctions in the leech. *J. Comp. Neurol.*, **151**, 399–406.

ROSENBLUTH, J. and WISSIG, S. L. (1964) The distribution of exogenous ferritin in toad spinal ganglia and the mechanism of its uptake by neurons. *J. Cell Biol.*, **23**, 307–325.

ROSS, L. L., ANDREOLI, V. M. and MARCHBANKS, R. M. (1971) A morphological and biochemical study of subcellular fractions of the guinea pig spinal cord. *Brain Res.*, **25**, 103–119.

ROSTAS, J. A. P. and JEFFREY, P. L. (1973) Histochemical localization of axosynaptic antigens. *Proc. Aust. Physiol. Pharmacol. Soc.*, **4**, 169.

ROTH, T. F. and PORTER, K. R. (1962) Specialized sites on the cell surface for protein uptake. In *Electron Microscopy: Fifth Int. Congress for Electron Microscopy*, ed. Breese, S. S. Vol. 2, p. LL4. New York: Academic Press.

ROTH, T. F. and PORTER, K. R. (1963) Membrane differentiation for protein uptake. *Fedn. Proc. Fedn. Am. Socs. exp. Biol.*, **22**, 178.

ROTH, T. F. and PORTER, K. R. (1964) Yolk protein uptake in the oocyte of the mosquito *Aedes aegypti* L. *J. Cell Biol.*, **20**, 313–332.

RYALL, R. W. (1964) The subcellular distributions of acetylcholine, substance P, 5-hydroxytryptamine, γ-aminobutyric acid and glutamic acid in brain homogenates. *J. Neurochem.*, **11**, 131–145.

RYAN, K. J., KALANT, H. and THOMAS, E. L. (1971) Free-flow electrophoretic separation and electrical surface properties of subcellular particles from guinea-pig brain. *J. Cell Biol.*, **49**, 235–246.

SACHS, H. (1961) Studies in the intracellular distribution of vasopressin. *J. Neurochem.*, **10**, 289–297.

SAELENS, J. K. and POTTER, L. T. (1966) Subcellular localization of choline acetyltransferase in rat brain cortex. *Fed. Proc.*, **25**, 451.

SALGANICOFF, L. and DE ROBERTIS, E. (1963) Subcellular distribution of glutamic decarboxylase and gamma-aminobutyric alphaketoglutamic transaminase. *Life Sci.*, **2**, 85–91.

SALGANICOFF, L. and DE ROBERTIS, E. (1965) Subcellular distribution of the enzymes of the glutamic acid, glutamine and γ-aminobutyric acid cycles in rat brain. *J. Neurochem.*, **12**, 287–309.

SANDRI, C., AKERT, K., LIVINGSTON, R. B. and MOOR, H. (1972) Particle aggregations at specialized sites in freeze-etched postsynaptic membranes. *Brain Res.*, **41**, 1–16.

SATAKE, M. and ABE, S. (1966) Preparation and chacterization of nerve cell perikaryon from rat cerebral cortex. *J. Biochem. (Tokyo)*, **59**, 72–75.

SATAKE, M., HASEGAWA, S-I., ABE, S. and TANAKE, R. (1968) Preparation and characterization of nerve cell perikaryon from pig brain stem. *Brain Res.*, **11**, 246–250.

SATTIN, A. (1966) The synthesis and storage of acetylcholine in the striatum. *J. Neurochem.*, **13**, 515–524.

SCHADÉ, J. P. and BAXTER, C. (1960) Changes during growth in the volume and surface area of the cortical neurons in the rabbit. *Exptl. Neurol.*, **2**, 158–178.

SCHARRER, E. and BROWN, S. (1961) Neurosecretion. XII. The formation of neurosecretory granules in the earthworm, *Lumbricus terrestris* L. *Z. Zellforsch.*, **54**, 530–540.

SCHEIBEL, M. E., and SCHEIBEL, A. B. (1964) Some structural and functional substrates of development in young cats. *Prog. Brain Res.*, **9**, 6–25.

SCHEIBEL, M. E. and SCHEIBEL, A. B. (1968) On the nature of dendritic spines – reports of a workshop. *Communications in Behavioral Biology, Part A*, **1**, 231–265.

SCHMIDT, S. Y. and LOLLEY, R. N. (1973) Cyclic-nucleotide phosphodiesterase. An early defect in inherited retinal degeneration of C3H mice. *J. Cell Biol.*, **57**, 117–123.

SCHMITT, F. O. (1969) Brain cell membranes and their microenvironment. *Neurosci. Res. Program Bull.*, **7**, 281–300.

SCHMITT, F. O. and SAMSON, F. E. (1969) Brain cell microenvironment. *Neurosci. Res. Program Bull.*, **7**, 277–417.

SCHNEIDER, W. C. (1946) Intracellular distribution of enzymes. I. The distribution of succinic dehydrogenase, cytochrome oxidase, adenosinetriphosphatase, and phosphorus compounds in normal rat tissues. *J. Biol. Chem.*, **165**, 585–593.

SCHNEIDER, W. C. and HOGEBOOM, G. H. (1951) Cytochemical studies of mammalian tissues: The isolation of cell components by differential centrifugation: A review. *Cancer Res.*, **11**, 1–22.

SCHON, F. and IVERSEN, L. L. (1972) Selective accumulation of ^{3}H-GABA by stellate cells in rat cerebellar cortex *in vivo*. *Brain Res.*, **42**, 503–507.

SCHÖNBACH, J., SCHÖNBACH, C. and CUÉNOD, M. (1971) Rapid phase of axoplasmic flow and synaptic proteins: an electron microscopical autoradiographic study. *J. Comp. Neurol.*, **141**, 485–498.

SCHUBERTH, J., SPARF, B., and SUNDWALL, A. (1969) A technique for the study of acetylcholine turnover in mouse brain *in vivo*. *J. Neurochem.*, **16**, 695–700.

SCHULTZ, R. L. and KARLSSON, U. (1966) Spine apparatus occurrence during different fixation procedures. *J. Ultrastruct. Res.*, **14**, 268–276.

SCHWARTZ, I. R. (1972) Axonal endings in the cat medial superior olive: coated vesicles and intercellular substance. *Brain Res.*, **46**, 187–202.

SCHWARTZ, I. R., PAPPAS, G. D. and PURPURA, D. P. (1968) Fine structure of neurons and synapses in the feline hippocampus during postnatal ontogenesis. *Exptl. Neurol.*, **22**, 394–407.

SCOTT, J. E. and GLICK, D. (1971) The invalidity of 'phosphotungstic acid as a specific electron stain for complex carbohydrates'. *J. Histochem. Cytochem.*, **19**, 63–64.

SELLINGER, O. Z. and BORENS, R. N. (1969) Zonal density gradient electrophoresis of intracellular membranes of brain cortex. *Biochim. Biophys. Acta*, **173**, 176–184.

SELLINGER, O. Z., LODIN, Z. and AZCURRA, J. M. (1972) A comparison of enzyme patterns in the granular and molecular layers of the rabbit cerebellar cortex. *Brain Res.*, **42**, 159–175.

SEMINARIO, L. M., HREN, N. and GOMEZ, C. J. (1964) Lipid distribution in subcellular fractions of the rat brain. *J. Neurochem.*, **11**, 197–207.

SHAPIRA, R., BINKLEY, F., KIBLER, R. F. and WUNDRAM, I. J. (1970) Preparation of purified myelin of rabbit brain by sedimentation in a continuous sucrose gradient. *Proc, Soc. exp. Biol. (N.Y.)*, **133**, 238–245.

SHAPIRO, S., VUKOVICH, K. and GLOBUS, A. (1973) Effects of neonatal thyroxine and hydrocortisone administration on the development of dendritic spines in the visual cortex of rats. *Exptl. Neurol.*, **40**, 286–296.

SHASKAN, E. A. and SNYDER, S. H. (1970) Kinetics of serotonin uptake into slices from different regions of rat brain. *J. Pharmac. Exp. Ther.*, **175**, 404–418.

242

SHAW, R. K. and HEINE, J. D. (1965) Ninhydrin positive substances present in different areas of normal rat brain. *J. Neurochem.*, **12**, 151–155.

SHELANSKI, M. L., ALBERT, S., DE VRIES, G. H. and NORTON, W. T. (1971) Isolation of filaments from brain. *Science*, **174**, 1242–1245.

SHERIDAN, M. N. (1965) The fine structure of the electric organ of *Torpedo marmorata*. *J. Cell Biol.*, **24**, 129–141.

SHERIDAN, M. N., WHITTAKER, V. P. and ISRAËL, M. (1966) The subcellular fractionation of the electric organ of *Torpedo*. *Z. Zellforsch.*, **74**, 291–307.

SHERIDAN, W. F. and BARRNETT, R. J. (1967) Cytochemical studies of chromosomal ultrastructure. *J. Cell Biol.*, **35**, 125a.

SHERRINGTON, C. S. (1897) The central nervous system. In *A Textbook of Physiology*, ed. Forster, Sir Michael. Vol. 3, 7th edition. London: MacMillan.

SHOLL, D. A. (1956) *The Organization of the Cerebral Cortex*, London: Methuen.

SHUTE, C. C. D. and LEWIS, P. R. (1966) Electron microscopy of cholinergic terminals and acetylcholinesterase-containing neurones in the hippocampal formation of the rat. *Z. Zellforsch.*, **69**, 334–343.

SIAKOTOS, A. N. ROUSER, G. and FLEISCHER, S. (1969) Isolation of highly purified human and bovine brain endothelial cells and nuclei and their phospholipid composition. *Lipids*, **4**, 234–239.

SIEGESMUND, K. A., SANCES, A. and LARSON, S. J. (1969) Effects of electroanesthesia on synaptic ultrastructure. J. *neurol. Sci.*, **9**, 89–96.

SILVERMAN, L. and GLICK, D. (1969) The reactivity and staining of tissue proteins with phosphotungstic acid. *J. Cell Biol.*, **40**, 761–767.

SINGER, S. T. and NICOLSON, G. L. (1972) The fluid mosaic model of the structure of cell membranes. *Science*, **175**, 720–731.

SJÖSTRAND, F. S. (1953) Ultrastructure of retinal rod synapses of guinea-pig eye. *J. Appl. Physics*, **24**, 1422–1423.

SLOPER, J. J. and POWELL, T. P. S. (1973) Observations on the axon initial segment and other structures in the neocortex using conventional staining and ethanolic phosphotungstic acid. *Brain Res.*, **50**, 163–169.

SMITH, A. D. (1971) Secretion of proteins (chromogranin A and dopamine β-hydroxylase) from a sympathetic neuron. *Trans. Roy. Soc. Lond.*, B., **261**, 363–370.

SMITH, D. S. (1971) On the significance of cross-bridges between microtubules and synaptic vesicles. *Trans. Roy. Soc. Lond.* B, **261**, 395–405.

SMITH, D. S. and TREHERNE, J. E. (1965) The electron microscopic localization of cholinesterase activity in the central nervous system of an insect, *Periplaneta americana* L. *J. Cell Biol.*, **26**, 445–465.

SMITH, U. (1970) The origin of small vesicles in neurosecretory axons. *Tissue and Cell*, **2**, 427–433.

SNODGRASS, S. R., HEDLEY-WHITE, E. T. and LORENZO, A. V. (1973) GABA transport by nerve ending fractions of cat brain. *J. Neurochem.*, **20**, 771–782.

SNYDER, S. H. (1970) Putative neurotransmitters in the brain: selective neuronal uptake, subcellular localization, and interactions with centrally acting drugs. *Biological Psychiatry*, **2**, 367–389.

SNYDER, S. H., KUHAR, M. J., GREEN, A. I., COLE, J. T. and SHASKAN, E. G. (1970) Uptake and subcellular localization of neurotransmitters in the brain. *Int. Rev. Neurobiol.*, **13**, 127–158.

SNYDER, S. H., YAMAMURA, H. I., PERT, C. B., LOGAN, W. J. and BENNETT, J. P. (1973) Neuronal uptake of neurotransmitters and their precursors: studies with 'transmitter' amino acids and choline. In *New Concepts in Neurotransmitter Regulation*, ed. Mandell, A. J. Pp. 195–222. New York: Plenum Press.

SOIFER, D., and WHITTAKER, V. P. (1972) Morphology of subcellular fractions derived from the electric organ of *Torpedo. Biochem. J.*, **128**, 845–846.

SOMOGYI, J. (1968) The effect of proteases on the (Na$^+$+K$^+$)-activated adenosine triphosphatase system of rat brain. *Biochim. Biophys. Acta*, **151**, 421–428.

SOSULA, L. and GLOW, P. H. (1971) Increase in number of synapses in the inner plexiform layer of light deprived retinae: quantitative electron microscopy. *J. Comp. Neurol.*, **141**, 427–452.

SOTELO, C. (1968) Permanence of postsynaptic specializations in the frog sympathetic ganglion cells after denervation. *Exp. Brain Res.*, **6**, 294–305.

SOTELO, C. (1969) Ultrastructural aspects of the cerebellar cortex of the frog. In *Neurobiology of Cerebellar Evolution and Development*, ed. Llinas, R. Pp. 327–371. American Medical Association.

SOTELO, C. (1971a) General features of the synaptic organization in the central nervous system. In *Chemistry and Brain Development*, ed. Paoletti, R. and Davison, A. N. Pp. 239–280. New York: Plenum Press.

SOTELO, C. (1971b) The fine structural localization of norepinephrine-^{3}H in the substantia nigra and area postrema of the rat. An autoradiographic study. *J. Ultrastruct. Res.*, **36**, 824–841.

SOTELO, C. and PALAY, S. L. (1970) The fine structure of the lateral vestibular nucleus in the rat. II. Synaptic organization. *Brain Res.*, **18**, 93–115.

SOTELO, C., PRIVAT, A. and DRIAN, M-J. (1972) Localization of (^{3}H) GABA in tissue culture of rat cerebellum using electron microscopy radioautography. *Brain Res.*, **45**, 302–308.

SOTELO, C. and TAXI, J. (1973) On the axonal migration of catecholamines in constricted sciatic nerve of the rat. A radioautographic study. *Z. Zellforsch.*, **138**, 345–370.

SPANNER, S. (1972) Methods of separating the subcellular components of brain tissue. In *Glycolipids, Glycoproteins and Mucopolysaccharides of the Nervous System*, ed. Zambotti, V., Tettamanti, G. and Arrigoni, M. Pp. 195–207. New York: Plenum Press.

SPANNER, S. and ANSELL, G. B. (1970) The use of zonal centrifugation in the preparation of subcellular fractions from brain tissue. *Biochem. J.*, **119**, 45P.

SPANNER, S. and ANSELL, G. B. (1971) Preparation of subcellular fractions from brain tissue. In *Separations with Zonal Rotors*, ed. Reid, E. Pp. V–3, 1–3, 7. Guildford: Wolfon Bioanalytical Centre of the University of Surrey.

SPENCE, M. W. and WOLFE, L. S. (1967) Gangliosides in developing rat brain. Isolation and composition of subcellular membranes enriched in gangliosides. *Can. J. Biochem.*, **45**, 671–688.

SRINIVASAN, V., NEAL, M. J. and MITCHELL, J. F. (1969) The effect of electrical stimulation and high potassium concentrations on the efflux of ^{3}H-γ-aminobutyric acid from brain slices. *J. Neurochem.*, **16**, 1235–1244.

STAHL, W. L. and SWANSON, P. D. (1969) Uptake of calcium by subcellular fractions isolated from ouabain-treated cerebral tissues. *J. Neurochem.*, **16**, 1553–1563.

STEDMAN, E. and STEDMAN, E. (1937) The mechanism of the biological synthesis of acetylcholine. I. The isolation of acetylcholine produced by brain tissue *in vitro. Biochem. J.*, **31**, 817–827.

STEDMAN, E. and STEDMAN, E. (1939) The mechanism of the biological synthesis of acetylcholine. II. *Biochem. J.*, **33**, 811–821.

STEERE, R. L. (1957) Electron microscopy of structural detail in frozen biological specimens. *J. biophys. biochem. Cytol.*, **3**, 45–60.

STELZNER, D. J. (1971) The relationship between synaptic vesicles, Golgi apparatus, and smooth endoplasmic reticulum a developmental study using the zinc iodide–osmium technique. *Z. Zellforsch.*, **120**, 332–345.

STELZNER, D. J., MARTIN, A. H. and SCOTT, G. L. (1973) Early stages of synaptogenesis in the cervical spinal cord of the chick embryo. *Z. Zellforsch.*, **138**, 475–488.

STOECKENIUS, W. (1961) Electron microscopy of DNA molecules 'stained' with heavy metal salts. *J. biophys. biochem. Cytol.*, **11**, 297–310.

STOECKENIUS, W. and ENGELMAN, D. M. (1969) Current models for the structure of biological membranes. *J. Cell Biol.*, **42**, 613–646.

STREIT, P., AKERT, K., SANDRI, C., LIVINGSTON, R. B. and MOOR, H. (1972) Dynamic ultrastructure of presynaptic membranes at nerve terminals in the spinal cord of rats. Anesthetized and unanesthetized preparations compared. *Brain Res.*, **48**, 11–26.

SVENSSON, H. (1960) Zonal density gradient electrophoresis. In *A Laboratory Manual of Analytical Methods of Protein Chemistry*, ed., Alexander, P. and Block, R. J. Pp. 193. London: Pergamon.

SWANSON, P. D., BRADFORD, H. F. and MCILWAIN, H. (1964) Stimulation and solubilization of sodium ion-activated adenosine triphosphatase of cerebral microsomes by surface-active agents, specially polyoxyethylene ethers: actions of phospholipases and neuraminidase. *Biochem. J.*, **92**, 235–247.

SWANSON, P. D., HARVEY, F. H. and STAHL, W. L. (1973) Subcellular fractionation of postmortem brain. *J. Neurochem.*, **20**, 465–475.

SWANSON, P. D. and MCILWAIN, H. (1963) Solubilization and stimulation of the sodium-activated adenosine triphosphatase of cerebral microsomes by surface active agents. *Biochem. J.*, **88**, 68P.

SZENTÁGOTHAI, J. (1962) Anatomical aspects of junctional transformation. In *Information Processing in the Nervous System*, ed., Gerard, R. W. and Duyff, J. W. Pp. 119–136. Intr. Congr. Series no. **49**, Amsterdam: Excerpta Medica.

SZERB, J. C. (1961) The estimation of acetylcholine, using leech muscle in a microbath. *J. Physiol., Lond.*, **158**, 8P–9P.

TAPIA, R., HAJÓS, F., WILKIN, G., JOHNSON, A. L. and BALÁZS, R. (1974) Subcellular fractionation of rat cerebellum: an electron microscopical and biochemical investigation. II. Resolution of morphologically characterized fractions. *Brain Res.*, **70**, 285–299.

TAXI, J. (1961) Étude de l'ultrastructure des zones synaptiques dans les ganglions sympathiques de Grenouille. *C.R. Acad. Sci., Paris*, **252**, 174–176.

TAXI, J. (1965) Contribution à l'étude des connexions des neurones moteurs du système nerveux autonome. *Ann. Sci. nat. Zool.*, **7**, 413–674.

TAXI, J. (1967) Observations on the ultrastructure of the ganglionic neurons and synapses of the frog, *Rana esculenta* L. In *The Neuron*, ed., Hydèn, H. Pp. 221–254. Amsterdam: Elsevier.

TAXI, J. (1969) Morphological and cytochemical studies on the synapses in the autonomic nervous system. *Prog. Brain Res.*, **31**, 5–20.

TENNYSON, V. M. (1970) The fine structure of the developing nervous system. In *Developmental Neurobiology*, ed., Himwich, W. A. Pp. 47–116. Springfield: Thomas.

TENNYSON, V. M. and BRZIN, M. (1970) The appearance of acetylcholinesterase in the dorsal root neuroblast of the rabbit embryo. A study by electron microscope cytochemistry and microgasometric analysis with the magnetic diver. *J. Cell Biol.*, **46**, 64–80.

TERAVAINEN, H. (1969) Histochemical localization of acetylcholinesterase in isolated brain synaptosomes. *Histochemie*, **18**, 191–194.

TISSARI, A. H., SCHÖNHÖFER, P. S., BOGDANSKI, D. F. and BRODIE, B. B. (1969) Mechanism of biogenic amine transport. II. Relationship between Na^+ and the mechanism of ouabain blockade of the accumulation of serotonin and noradrenaline by synaptosomes. *Mol. Pharmacol.*, **5**, 593–604.

TONOSAKI, A. (1965) The fine structure of the retinal plexus in *Octopus vulgaris*. *Z. Zellforsch.*, **67**, 521–532.

TRANZER, J. P. and SNIPES, R. L. (1968) Fine structural localization of noradrenaline in sympathetic nerve terminals: a critical study on the influence of fixation. *Proceedings of the 4th European Regional Conference on Electron Microscopy, Rome*, **2**, 519–520.

TRANZER, J. P. and THOENEN, H. (1967) Significance of 'empty vesicles' in postganglionic sympathetic nerve terminals. *Experientia*, **23**, 123–124.

TRANZER, J. P., THOENEN, H., SNIPES, R. L. and RICHARDS, J. G. (1969) Recent developments on the ultrastructural aspect of adrenergic nerve endings in various experimental conditions. *Prog. Brain Res.*, **31**, 33–46.

TUČEK, S. (1966) On subcellular localization and binding of choline acetyltransferase in the cholinergic nerve endings of the brain. *J. Neurochem.*, **13**, 1317–1327.

TUČEK, S. (1967) Subcellular distribution of acetyl-Co A synthetase, ATP citrate lyase, citrate synthase, choline acetyltransferase, fumarate hydratase and lactate dehydrogenase in mammalian brain tissue. *J. Neurochem.* **14**, 531–545.

TURKANIS, S. A. (1973) Some effects of vinblastine and colchicine on neuromuscular transmission. *Brain Res.*, **54**, 324–329.

UCHIZONO, K. (1965) Characteristics of excitatory and inhibitory synapses in the central nervous system of the cat. *Nature, Lond.*, **207**, 642–643.

UCHIZONO, K. (1967) Inhibitory synapses on the stretch receptor neurone of the crayfish. *Nature, Lond.*, **214**, 833–834.

UCHIZONO, K. (1968) Inhibitory and excitatory synapses in vertebrate and invertebrate animals. In *Structure and Function of Inhibitory Neural Mechanisms*, ed. Von Euler, C., Skoglund, S. and Soderberg, U. Pp. 33–60. Oxford: Pergamon.

ULMAR, G. and WHITTAKER, V. P. (1974a) Immunohistochemical localization and immunoelectrophoresis of cholinergic synaptic vesicle protein constituents from the *Torpedo*. *Brain Res.*, **71**, 155–159.

ULMAR, G. and WHITTAKER, V. P. (1974b) Immunological approach to the characterization of cholinergic vesicular protein. *J. Neurochem.*, **22**, 451–454.

VALDIVIA, O. (1971) Methods of fixation and the morphology of synaptic vesicles. *J. Comp. Neurol.*, **142**, 257–274.

VAN DER KLOOT, W. and KITA, H. (1974) Mechanisms for neurotransmitter release. *Bioscience*, **24**, 13–17.

VAN DER KLOOT, W., KITA, H. and KITA, K. (1974) Excitation-secretion coupling in the release of catecholamines from *in vitro* frog adrenal: effects of K^+, Ca^{2+}, hypertonicity, Na^+ and Ni^{2+}. *Comp. Biochem. Physiol.*, **47A**, 701–711.

VAN DER LOOS, H. (1963) Fine structure of synapses in the cerebral cortex. *Z. Zellforsch.* **60**, 815–825.

VAN DER LOOS, H. (1965) Fine structure of synapses in the cerebral cortex. *Neurosci. Res. Program Bull.*, **3**, 22–24.

VAN GELDER, M. M. (1967) A possible enzyme barrier for γ-aminobutyric acid in the central nervous system. *Prog. Brain Res.*, **29**, 259–268.

VAN HARREVELD, A. V., CROWELL, J. and MALHOTRA, S. K. (1965) A study of extracellular space in central nervous tissue by freeze-substitution. *J. Cell Biol.*, **25**, 117–137.

VAN HARREVELD, A. and KHATTAB, F. I. (1967) Electron microscopy of asphyxiated spinal cords of cats. *J. Neuropath. Exp. Neurol.*, **26**, 521–536.

VAN KEMPEN, G. M. J., VAN DEN BERG, C. J., VAN DER HELM, H. J. and VELDSTRA, H. (1965) Intracellular localization of glutamate decarboxylase, γ-aminobutyrate transaminase and some other enzymes in brain tissue. *J. Neurochem.*, **12**, 581–588.

VÁSQUEZ, C., BARRANTES, F. J., LA TORRE, J. L. and DE ROBERTIS, E. (1970) Electron microscopy of proteolipid macromolecules from cerebral cortex. *J. Mol. Biol.*, **52**, 221–226.

VIVEROS, O. H., ARQUEROS, L. and KIRSHNER, N. (1968) Release of catecholamines and dopamine-β-oxidase from the adrenal medulla. *Life Sci.*, **7**, 609–618.

VOELLER, K., PAPPAS, G. D. and PURPURA, D. P. (1963) Electron microscope study of development of cat superficial neocortex. *Exptl. Neurol.*, 7, 107–130.

VON EULER, U. S. (1971) Adrenergic neurotransmitter functions. *Science*, 173, 202–206.

VON HUNGEN, K., MAHLER, H. R. and MOORE, W. J. (1968) Turnover of protein and RNA in synaptic subcellular fractions from rat brain. *J. Biol. Chem.*, 243, 1415–1423.

VOS, J., KURIYAMA, K. and ROBERTS, E. (1968) Electrophoretic mobilities of brain subcellular particles and binding of γ-aminobutyric acid, acetylcholine, norepinephrine, and 5-hydroxytryptamine. *Brain Res.*, 9, 224–230.

VRENSEN, G. and DE GROOT, D. (1973) Quantitative stereology of synapses: a critical investigation. *Brain Res.*, 58, 25–35.

WALBERG, F. (1965) A special type of synaptic vesicles in boutons in the inferior olive. *J. Ultrastruct. Res.*, 12, 237(B6).

WALBERG, F. (1966) The fine structure of the cuneate nucleus in normal cats and following interruption of afferent fibres. An electron microscopical study with particular reference to findings made in Glees and Nauta sections. *Exp. Brain Res.*, 2, 107–128.

WALD, F., MAZZUCHELLI, A., LAPETINA, E. G. and DE ROBERTIS, E. (1968) The effect of antiserum against nerve-ending membranes from cat cerebral cortex bioelectrical activity of mollusc neurons. *Exptl. Neurol.*, 21, 336–345.

WALDEYER-HARTZ, H. W. G. VON (1891) Über einige neuere Forschungen im Gebiete der Anatomie des Centralnervensystems. *Dt. med. Wschr.*, 17, 1213–1218, 1244–1246, 1267–1269, 1287–1289, 1331–1332, 1352–1356.

WANNAMAKER, B. B., KORNGUTH, S. E., SCOTT, G., DUDLEY, A. W. and KELLY, A. (1973) Isolation and ultrastructure of human synaptic complexes. *J. Neurobiol.*, 4, 541–554.

WASHIZU, Y. (1960) Single spinal motoneurons excitable from two different antidromic pathways. *Jap. J. Physiol.*, 10, 121–131.

WATSON, M. L. (1958) Staining of tissue sections for electron microscopy with heavy metals. *J. biophys. biochem. Cytol.*, 4, 475–478.

WEAKLY, J. N. (1969) Effect of barbiturates on 'quantal' synaptic transmission in spinal motoneurones. *J. Physiol., Lond.*, 204, 63–77.

WEBSTER, H. de F. and AMES, A. (1965) Reversible and irreversible changes in the fine structure of nervous tissue during oxygen and glucose deprivation. *J. Cell Biol.*, 26, 885–909.

WEINSTEIN, H., MALAMED, S. and SACHS, H. (1961) Isolation of vasopressin-containing granules from the neurohypophysis of the dog. *Biochim. Biophys. Acta*, 50, 386–389.

WEINSTEIN, H., ROBERTS, E. and KAKEFUDA, T. (1963) Studies of sub-cellular distribution of γ-aminobutyric acid and glutamic decarboxylase in mouse brain. *Biochem. Pharmacol.*, 12, 503–509.

WEINSTEIN, H., VARON, S., MUHLEMANN, D. R. and ROBERTS, E. (1965) A carrier-mediated transfer mode for the accumulation of ^{14}C-γ-aminobutyric acid by subcellular brain particles. *Biochem. Pharmacol.*, 14, 273–288.

WEISS, B. (1971) Ontogenetic development of adenyl cyclase and phosphodiesterase in rat brain. *J. Neurochem.*, 18, 469–477.

WEISS, B. and COSTA, E. (1968) Regional and subcellular distribution of adenyl cyclase and 3′, 5′-cyclic nucleotide phosphodiesterase in brain and pineal gland. *Biochem. Pharmacol.*, 17, 2107–2116.

WEISS, P. (1947) The problem of specificity in growth and development. *Yale J. Biol. Med.*, 19, 235–278.

WELSCH, F. and DETTBARN, W-D. (1972) The subcellular distribution of acetylcholine, cholinesterases and choline acetyltransferase in optic lobes of the squid *Loligo pealei*. *Brain Res.*, 39, 467–482.

WELSH, J. H. and MOORHEAD, M. (1959) Identification and assay of 5-hydroxytryptamine in molluscan tissues by fluorescence method. *Science*, **129**, 1491–1492.

WERMAN, R., DAVIDOFF, R. A. and APRISON, M. H. (1968) Inhibitory action of glycine on spinal neurons in the cat. *J. Neurophysiol.*, **31**, 81–95.

WEST, M. (1974) Personal communication.

WEST, M. J., COLEMAN, P. D. and WYSS, U. R. (1972) A computerized method of determining the number of synaptic contacts in a volume of cerebral cortex. *J. Microscopy*, **95**, 277–283.

WESTRUM, L. E. (1965) On the origin of synaptic vesicles in the cerebral cortex. *J. Physiol., Lond.*, **179**, 4P–6P.

WESTRUM, L. E. and BLACKSTAD, T. W. (1962) An electron microscopic study of the stratum radiatum of the rat hippocampus (regio superior, CA1) with particular emphasis on synaptology. *J. Comp. Neurol.*, **119**, 281–309.

WESTRUM, L. E. and LUND, R. D. (1966) Formalin perfusion for correlative light- and electron-microscopical studies of the nervous system. *J. Cell Sci.*, **1**, 229–238.

WHITTAKER, V. P. (1959) The isolation and characterization of acetylcholine-containing particles from brain. *Biochem. J.*, **72**, 694–706,

WHITTAKER, V. P. (1965) The application of subcellular fractionation techniques to the study of brain function. *Progr. Biophys. molec. Biol.*, **15**, 39–96.

WHITTAKER, V. P. (1966a) Some properties of synaptic membranes isolated from the central nervous system. *Ann. N.Y. Acad. Sci.*, **137**, 982–998.

WHITTAKER, V. P. (1966b) The binding of acetylcholine by brain particles *in vitro*. *Mechanisms of Release of Biogenic Amines*, ed. Von Euler, U. S., Rosell, S. and Uvnäs, B. Pp. 147–163. New York: Pergamon Press.

WHITTAKER, V. P. (1968a) The morphology of fractions of rat forebrain synaptosomes separated on continuous sucrose density gradients. *Biochem. J.*, **106**, 412–417.

WHITTAKER, V. P. (1968b) The subcellular distribution of amino acids in brain and its relation to a possible transmitter function for these compounds. In *Structure and Function of Inhibitory Neuronal Mechanisms*, ed., Von Euler, C., Skoglund, S. and Soderberg, U. Pp. 487–504. Oxford: Pergamon Press.

WHITTAKER, V. P. (1969a) The nature of the acetylcholine pools in brain tissue. *Prog. Brain Res.*, **31**, 211–222.

WHITTAKER, V. P. (1969b) The subcellular fractionation of nervous tissue. In *The Structure and Function of Nervous Tissue*, ed., Bourne, G. H. Vol. 3, pp. 1–24. New York: Academic Press.

WHITTAKER, V. P. (1969c) The synaptosome. In *Handbook of Neurochemistry*, ed. Lajtha, A. Vol. 2, pp. 327–364. New York: Plenum Press.

WHITTAKER, V. P. (1970) The vesicle hypothesis. In *Excitatory Synaptic Mechanisms*, ed., Andersen, P. and Jansen, J. K. S. Pp. 67–76. Oslo: Universitatsforlaget.

WHITTAKER, V. P. (1971a) Origin and function of synaptic vesicles. *Ann. N.Y. Acad. Sci.*, **183**, 21–32.

WHITTAKER, V. P. (1971b) Subcellular localization of neurotransmitters. *Advances in Cytopharmacology*, **1**, 319–330.

WHITTAKER, V. P. (1972) The use of synaptosomes in the study of synaptic and neural membrane function. In *Structure and Function of Synapses*, ed., Pappas, G. D. and Purpura, D. P. Pp. 87–100. New York: Raven Press.

WHITTAKER, V. P. and DOWE, G. H. C. (1965) The effect of homogenization conditions on subcellular distribution in brain. *Biochem. Pharmacol.*, **14**, 194–196.

WHITTAKER, V. P., ESSMAN, W. B. and DOWE, G. H. C. (1972) The isolation of pure cholinergic synaptic vesicles from the electric organs of elasmobranch fish of the family Torpedinidae. *Biochem. J.*, **128**, 833–845.

WHITTAKER, V. P. and GRAY, E. G. (1962) The synapse: biology and morphology. *Brit. Med. Bull.*, **18**, 223–228.

WHITTAKER, V. P. and GREENGARD, P. (1971) The isolation of synaptosomes from the brain of a teleost fish, *Centriopristes striatus*. *J. Neurochem.*, **18**, 173–176.

WHITTAKER, V. P., DOWDALL, M. J. and BOYNE, A. F. (1972), The storage and release of acetylcholine by cholinergic nerve terminals: recent results with non-mammalian preparations. *Biochem. Soc. Symp.*, **36**, 49–68.

WHITTAKER, V. P., MICHAELSON, I. A. and KIRKLAND, R. J. A. (1964) The separation of synaptic vesicles from nerve-ending particles ('synaptosomes'). *Biochem. J.*, **90**, 293–303.

WHITTAKER, V. P. and SHERIDAN, M. N. (1965) The morphology and acetylcholine content of isolated cerebral cortical synaptic vesicles. *J. Neurochem.*, **12**, 363–372.

WIDLUND, L., KARLSSON, K. A., WINTER, A. and HEILBRONN, E. (1974) Immunochemical studies on cholinergic synaptic vesicles. *J. Neurochem.*, **22**, 455–456.

WILLIAMS, V. and GROSSMAN, R. G. (1970) Ultrastructure of cortical synapses after failure of presynaptic activity in ischemia. *Anat. Rec.*, **166**, 131–142.

WILSON, W. S. and COOPER, J. R. (1972) The preparation of cholinergic synaptosomes from bovine superior cervical ganglia. *J. Neurochem.*, **19**, 2779–2790.

WILSON, W. S., SCHULTZ, R. A. and COOPER, J. R. (1973) Thc isolation of cholinergic synaptic vesicles from bovine superior cervical ganglion and estimation of their acetylcholine content. *J. Neurochem.*, **20**, 659–667.

WOFSEY, A. R., KUHAR, M. J. and SNYDER, S. H. (1971) A unique synaptosomal fraction in brain tissue accumulating glutamic and aspartic acids. *Proc. Natl. Acad. Sci., U.S.A.*, **68**, 1102–1106.

WOLFE, D. E., POTTER, L. T., RICHARDSON, K. C. and AXELROD, J. (1962) Localizing tritiated norepinephrine in sympathetic axons by electron microscopic autoradiography. *Science*, **138**, 440–442.

WOODWARD, D. J., HOFFER, B. J., SIGGINS, G. R. and BLOOM, F. E. (1971) The ontogenetic development of synaptic junctions, synaptic activation and responsiveness to neurotransmitter substances in rat cerebellar Purkinje cells. *Brain Res.*, **34**. 73–97.

WORSFOLD, M., DUNN, R. F. and PETER, J. B. (1969) A simplified technique for preparing isolated subcellular particles for electron microscopy. *J. Lab. clin. Med.*, **74**, 160–165.

YOSHIDA, H., KADOTA, K. and FUJISAWA, H. (1966) ATP dependent binding of calcium to microsomes and nerve endings. *Nature, Lond.*, **212**, 291–292.

YOUNOSZAI, R. (1968) Characterization of a large synaptosome fraction from guinea pig cerebellum. *Anat. Rec.*, **160**, 455.

ZACHS, S. I. and SAITO, A. (1969) Uptake of exogenous horseradish peroxidase (HRP) by coated vesicles in mouse neuromuscular junctions. *J. Histochem., Cytochem.*, **17**, 161–170.

ZIEHER, L. M. and DE ROBERTIS, E. (1963) Subcellular localization of 5-hydroxytryptamine in rat brain. *Biochem. Pharmacol.*, **12**, 596–598.

ZIEHER, L. M. and DE ROBERTIS, E. (1964) Distribución subcelular de noradrenalina y dopamina en el cerebro de rata. *VI Congreso Asociación Latinoamericana de Ciencias Fisológicas*, Viña del Jar, Chile, p. 150.

ZIMMERMANN, H. and WHITTAKER, V. P. (1973) The effect of stimulation on the composition and yield of cholinergic synaptic vesicles. *Abstracts of Fourth International Neurochemistry Meeting, Tokyo*, 321.

ZS-NAGY, I., RÓZSA, K. S., SALÁNKI, J., FÖLDES, I., PERÉNYI, L. and DEMETER, M. (1965) Subcellular localization of 5-hydroxytryptamine in the central nervous system of lamellibranchiates. *J. Neurochem.*, **12**, 245–251.

Index

Page numbers in **boldface** indicate principal reference.